Breathe Again Naturally

and Reclaim Your Life

ASTHMA

BREATHE AGAIN NATURALLY AND RECLAIM YOUR LIFE

MIMI WEISBORD

ST. MARTIN'S GRIFFIN
NEW YORK

Everyone with asthma will react in a different manner and with different sensitivity to any food, herb, or nutrient. Nothing in this book should be used without the advice of a qualified medical practitioner. This book is intended to be informational and is not to be used as a medical manual or as a substitute for medical advice. Neither the publisher nor the author makes warranties for the efficacy or appropriateness of any product or treatment, nor are they liable for any loss or damage to any person from reliance on or other misuse of this book.

Library of Congress Cataloging-in-Publication Data

Weisbord, Mimi.
    Asthma: breathe again naturally and reclaim your life / Mimi
Weisbord.
        p.   cm.
    ISBN 0–312–14544–6
    1. Asthma—Popular works.   I. Title.
RC591.W384   1997
616.2'38—dc21   96–44531

First St. Martin's Griffin edition: June 1997
10 9 8 7 6 5 4 3 2 1

CONTENTS

FOREWORD

BY MARTIN FELDMAN, M.D.

As a complementary physician who has specialized in nutritional and holistic medicine for fifteen years, I have seen that asthma is a very complex disease. The popular notion that asthma patients simply need drugs to regulate their breathing barely hints at the true nature of the "asthmatic state." The reality is, asthma encompasses a host of immune and biochemical breakdowns that manifest themselves in the lungs and respiratory tract.

What physicians diagnose as asthma—that is, a constriction of the muscles in the lungs and irritation of the respiratory lining—ultimately results from a three-pronged attack on the respiratory system. Those three prongs are biochemical, immune, and allergic in nature, and it is the combination of factors that makes the *successful* treatment of asthma so elusive.

Note that I emphasize "successful" treatment. As a complementary doctor, my mandate is to treat the disease state by eliminating its causes, not simply by relieving the symptoms. It is unfortunate, but the orthodox medical community does just the opposite: It focuses primarily on eliminating the symptoms of asthma and gives little thought to the underlying causes.

The hundreds of pulmonary experts and medical doctors who treat asthmatics are mainly committed to drug therapies that prevent the respiratory tract from constricting when an asthmatic attack occurs. This is not to say that drug therapy does not play an important—and sometimes vital—role in the treatment of asthma. The orthodox approach can mean the difference between life and death when a severe asthmatic attack occurs.

However, conventional medicine's focus on the symptoms of asthma leads asthmatic patients to believe that drug therapy is the beginning and end of their treatment options. Nothing could be further from the truth. Once you begin to focus on the causes of the asthmatic state, you will find an array of natural, safe, and effective therapies that focus on correcting the imbalances in body functioning which may trigger or worsen the condition.

Therein lies the value of this book. Through her in-depth look at holistic approaches to the treatment of asthma, Mimi Weisbord opens up a new world for asthma sufferers. She provides the information you need to begin to take control of your own destiny. The book's detailed discussion of non-drug therapies—from vitamins and herbs to Chinese acupressure, exercise, and detoxification—will introduce you to an entirely new way of viewing the disease process that we call asthma. This new point of view—and the crux of the complementary medical model—is to assist the body in healing itself, to rebalance the body systems, and to move them toward their optimal level of functioning.

The greatest strength of this book is that it tells you, the asthmatic patient, what you can do on your own to win the battle against asthma. It is clear that the orthodox medical community is losing this battle with its single-minded focus on suppressing the symptoms of the disease. The number of people who suffer from asthma has continued to climb in recent years, the cases are becoming more severe, and the associated death rate is rising.

With *Asthma: Breathe Again Naturally and Reclaim Your Life* as a guide, you can go beyond orthodox medicine's limited view of asthma and develop a more complete understanding of the asthmatic process. The book includes interviews with medical doctors working at the frontier of the complementary approach to medicine. These doctors are leaders in their fields, and their thinking, diagnostic methods, and treatments are far ahead of the medical mainstream.

These interviews, along with patient narratives, will enable you to educate yourself about the asthmatic condition and its associated problems. Because asthma is not a single, one-diagnosis disease, many patients suffer from subsidiary problems, such as overgrowths of yeast and parasites, hormonal imbalances with the menstrual cycle, multiple food and inhalant allergies, and body toxicity. Better yet, you can repair these imbalances with the safe and effective protocols presented in this book.

Most importantly, the book may serve as a guide and an inspiration to people with asthma.

A COMPLEMENTARY PERSPECTIVE

Before you delve into Ms. Weisbord's book, allow me to add my perspective on the complementary approach to medicine. It was only through a quirk of fate that I became a complementary physician in 1980. Until that time, I practiced medicine as a classically trained neurologist with a biochemically-oriented approach to treatment. I also served as an assistant professor of neurology at Mount Sinai Medical School in New York.

One day a Dr. Benjamin Frank died unexpectedly and I was asked to continue his practice temporarily. Dr. Frank was a leading nutritional physician who used biochemical data to help rebalance the body functioning, rather than suppress its biochemical status with drugs. I had little training in nutrition at the time and, in fact, it was Dr. Frank's nutrition counselor who worked with patients in devising vitamin, mineral, and food recommendations. As I continued the medical part of Dr. Frank's practice, I was pleasantly surprised to see the enormous benefits of these nutritional methods of treatment. I soon became a convert to his nonorthodox approach to medicine.

My move from the orthodox medical community to holistic medicine has given me an unusual vantage point on the value of the complementary approach to treatment. Patients come to my office with a wide variety of health conditions, and I have seen that the orthodox model does not treat many biochemical conditions as effectively as possible because it fails to get to the root causes of the problem.

But in the case of asthma, until the cause of the disease has been eliminated, the asthmatic time bomb continues to tick away in the patient. The orthodox treatment looks to contain the explosion. The complementary approach looks to remove the detonator so that another explosion will not occur.

As you read this book, it will help to have a good understanding of the principles of complementary medicine. A complementary physician's objective is to treat the body as a whole, using all the diagnostic intelligence available to the orthodox community *and* all the natural therapies available to the practitioners of alternative medicine. In short, we "complement" the best of orthodox medicine with the best of holistic health practices.

What does this mean for the person who suffers from asthma, allergies, or another chronic health condition? The most important principle is that a complementary doctor will look at the entire body when treating a given disease. All of the organs, body systems, and biochemical factors are suspect because no one factor accounts for the genesis of a disease. The interdependency of our organs, body systems, and biochemistry ultimately means that any disease process is a multifaceted condition within the body. Moreover, complementary doctors have expanded their treatment models to focus on reducing both internal and external toxicity in the home and work environments.

Complementary medicine demands that the physician cut across many specialty areas, such as pulmonology, internal medicine, infectious-disease analysis, and immunology, in treating the patient and eliminating the disease. This approach requires time, patience, and an understanding of the relationships among body systems. Within the orthodox medical community, many doctors fail to make these connections because they function as specialists. They treat the condition that falls within their field of expertise and leave any other problems—a weak immune system, a hormonal imbalance, or allergies—to the other specialists.

With asthma, in particular, the orthodox community applies a simple formula: Control the symptoms and the asthmatic no longer has difficulty in breathing.

The orthodox approach is effective to a point, but it simply fails to address a larger issue: If you only suppress the symptoms, you allow the imbalances in body functioning to keep producing them. The disease gets a chance to come back day after day because the underlying causes have not been eliminated. The complementary doctor wants to attack those causes and strengthen the body functioning. In the process, he or she will work on relieving the symptoms as well. All of the therapies presented in this book follow that formula.

The point is not that the complementary model will solve every aspect of the asthmatic state. Indeed, this book should not be interpreted as advancing an "us" versus "them" mentality. It is my hope that the book will serve as an inspiration to the many pulmonary experts and medical doctors who want to expand their view of the asthmatic condition. Complementary medicine offers a logical and comprehensive approach to treatment; it makes use of safe, gentle therapies that work in harmony with the body's true functioning. Once the orthodox medical community comes to understand these holistic approaches, there can be a union of the two models.

THE ALLERGY CONNECTION

For just a moment, let's return to the fundamental goal of the complementary model: to identify and treat the causes of a disease. Meeting this goal requires a thorough approach to evaluating patients and probing their medical histories. No stone must be left unturned. The complementary physician is like a medical supersleuth who examines all aspects of body functioning to answer the question that most troubles patients: Why?

For asthma patients, a big piece of that puzzle has been solved by complementary physicians in recent years. In many cases, an allergic reaction is responsible, at least in part, for the asthmatic state. The connection? When a patient is allergic to foods or inhalants, such as dust or chemicals, those allergens set off an allergic response that eventually results in an irritation of the lining and muscles in the lungs.

Complementary doctors are well aware that the allergic process will manifest itself in a variety of "target" organs, be it the digestive tract, the skin, or the nervous system. Therefore, it comes as no surprise that what we call gastritis may result, in part, from an allergic reaction targeted at the digestive tract, or that what we call arthritis may be an allergic reaction targeted at the joints. The same is true of asthma. What we call an asthmatic attack may be an allergic reaction targeted at the lungs.

Most pulmonary specialists do not refer their asthmatic patients to allergists. Even when they do, the classical allergist often restricts his or her diagnosis to the use of IgE Rast testing. This method only identifies the small percentage of allergies caused by dust, molds, pollens, and the like. It does little to isolate allergies to foods, which can be especially problematic if they are "hidden" or "delayed" in nature.

What makes these "hidden" allergies so hard to detect and control is that a negative reaction to a given food may not occur until several days after contact. Moreover, these allergens can be found in both the foods we eat and in the environment. As a result, asthmatic patients must examine both their diet and their home and work environments for possible causes of their attacks.

As you read chapter 7, you will come to appreciate the havoc allergies can play with all of the body systems. For the asthmatic patient, I cannot overemphasize the role of allergies in the disease process. The complementary model clearly shows that our first suspect in the body's biochemistry is the allergic process. The complementary physician will start his or her evaluation of a patient by testing for allergies, then expand the analysis to other biochemical, hormonal, and immune breakdowns. The emphasis on allergies saves the patient much time and discomfort. It also leads to significant success in identifying the allergic culprits and thus helping the patient to avoid relevant allergens.

IT'S TIME TO HELP YOURSELF

The true value of *Asthma: Breathe Again Naturally and Reclaim Your Life* is that it serves as an educational resource. With this book as a guide, asthma patients can begin to make positive lifestyle changes and take preventive measures to control the condition.

My experience with the ideas discussed in these chapters, including elimination diets, vitamin and mineral therapies, and detoxification, has been overwhelmingly positive. As patients begin to experience the benefits for themselves, I believe they will help lead the orthodox medical community toward an acceptance of the complementary approach.

A NEW HOPE

Traditionally, people with asthma have simply had to learn to live with the condition. One of the only hopes for the asthmatic was that one day he or she might "grow out of it." But we now know that most asthmatics don't grow out of the disease. At most, the underlying causes may manifest themselves in another target organ. Same disease, just a new face.

For those patients who don't "grow out of it," the prospects have not been very promising. They must rely on drugs and even emergency-room doctors for their well-being. The fear of the next attack can leave them physically and psychologically spent. It is a constant battle, from episode to episode, that provides no real solutions to the fundamental problem.

It is my belief that the information in this book, and the complementary approach to treatment in general, offers new hope to the countless asthmatic patients who have failed to find optimum relief from orthodox care and are looking for a better way. In many cases, as I have seen with my patients, it is a sincere belief in the health process that puts the individual on the road to recovery.

In *Asthma: Breathe Again Naturally and Reclaim Your Life* Mimi Weisbord provides every asthmatic with the means to reverse the "asthmatic state." The book documents case histories of many people who have battled the disease process. It also drives home the point that the physician can only act as a guide. It is the patient who must implement the treatments, make positive lifestyle changes, and persist in the effort to get better. This book leads the way to more self-awareness and suggests the concrete steps you can take to improve your health. It shows you how to turn hope into action.

Dr. Martin Feldman practices complementary medicine in New York City, with an emphasis on the diagnosis and treatment of allergies. He is the co-author of numerous books on nutrition and allergy, including *Good Food, Good Mood.*

ACKNOWLEDGMENTS

This book began as six pages of notes distributed in my asthma workshops at the New York Open Center, and evolved with the encouragement of my agent, Agnes Birnbaum. Many people helped to make this possible: At the SUNY Health Sciences Library in Syracuse, New York, Dianne Hawkins and other librarians patiently taught me to use Medline and were generous with their time and books. Head librarian Estelle Davis and the Scientific Engineering Division Library of the City College of New York enabled me to find many of the difficult-to-obtain studies. The Library for Medical Consumers, off NYC's Washington Square, gave me a starting place to research asthma. My former student and assistant Shamiza Ally (soon to be a fine M.D.) helped with research, transcription of tapes, and fact-checking the manuscript, as well as offering moral and spiritual support. To all of them, my appreciation and thanks.

Special gratitude goes to Nelson Howe, with whom I've had an "asthma" dialogue for a number of years and who provided inspiration as to how well one could become. Nelson was generous with his time, enthusiasm, and interest, reviewed and commented on a number of sections of the book, and provided his input particularly in the chapters on the mind and exercise.

And special gratitude to Deborah Valentine Smith, with whom I processed everything during nurturing, therapeutic, and stress-relieving acupressure sessions, and who patiently guided me through the shoals of Chinese Medicine. Many of Nelson's and Deborah's words inform this book.

To Katherine Keenan, Ph.D., thanks for friendship and for expertise in interpreting medical lingo and journal studies, and for reading and offering suggestions for a number of chapters, especially that of the endocrine system. And thanks to Suellen Rubinstein for friendship and humor in reviewing several chapters and offering expert editorial advice. Thanks to Irvin Moelis, Ph.D., for reading and making suggestions for the psychological chapter.

Special thanks to Martin Feldman, M.D., who reviewed the entire manuscript, wrote the foreword, and guided me through chapters on the immune system and allergies. And to Warren Levin, M.D., who was generous with time, instruction, and input from the beginning of the project and who reviewed the chapter on steroids. Also thanks to Serafina Corsello, M.D., F.A.C.A.M., executive medical director of the Corsello Centers for Nutritional-Complementary Medicine, who added her expertise on women's hormones, and to Leo Galland, M.D., who was helpful with the digestion and candida. Alfred V. Zamm, M.D., read the manuscript and was always at the other end of the telephone line with sound advice, humor, and kind words. I would also like to thank Drs. Harold E. Buttram, Irvin Caplin, William Crook, Gerald Epstein, David A. Greenspan, Robert Lin, Reed Moskowitz, Gerald Poesnecker, William Rea, and Sherry Rogers.

To Iona Marsaa Teeguarden, thanks for creating and teaching Jin Shin Do®, and for a supportive correspondence. And thanks to yoga teachers Ravi Singh and Ellen Saltonstall, and to Nancy Vinik, who introduced me to Jin Shin Do. Thanks also to the Sivananda Yoga camps, where I practiced yoga and destressed; to the Kripalu Institute, where I recovered after one terrible hospitalization; and to the Swedish Institute for wonderful shiatsu sessions.

Thanks to Timothy J. Aitken for input and recipes in the cooking chapter and to Edward Espe Brown, for his recipes and for his skill in sharing his knowledge of using food and Chinese herbs for healing. Special thanks to chef Robert Appleton for introducing me to Chinese food energetics, contributing recipes, and reviewing that chapter.

Monona Rossol, founder of Arts, Crafts and Theater Safety, has been leading me through the technical world of chemicals and artist materials and toxins for over ten years. Thanks to her for her steady support and for reviewing the chapter on the studio, office, and schools. Also thanks to Irene Wilkenfeld for her input on the schools.

Heartfelt thanks to Dianne Connelly, cofounder of the Traditional Acupuncture Institute of Columbia, Maryland, for her wonderful contribution and loving correspondence; to my nephew, acupuncturist Bob Weisbord, for inspiring late-night conversation; to my brother Marvin Weisbord, who reviewed several chapters and made valuable suggestions; and to all the other family members who lent support.

Many thanks to Babette Bloch, Bill Bishop, Bob Brophy, Ph.D., Jay Danilczyk, Diana Domoracki, Gerry Del Basso, Drew Di Vittorio, Andy Futterman, Nancy Ghirilikis, Gail Graves, Howard Lerner, Mona Herrera, David and Helen Jamison of *Asthma Update,* Jane Poehler, Robyn Pollins, Kathryn Shafer, Ph.D., Jonathan Star, and Michael Winn for their various contributions. And to Donna Barkman, Joan Larkin, Nancy and Jerry Weiss, Judy Beeber, and Marion Lerner Levin for encouragement. And to Doron Shalom for his music.

Thanks to Stanley Myerson of NEEDS, who has been unfailingly supportive from the beginning of my newsletter, *Healthy Home and Workplace.* And to Joy Rothenberg of New York Heal, who has been generous with helpful information and support.

Thanks to the former Macrobiotic Center of New York, where I studied macrobiotic cooking. I learned much about a kaleidoscope of subjects at the New York Open Center which then enabled me to give back what I know about asthma. Many, many thanks to all of those with asthma who came to my workshops looking for a better way—from whom I learned so much. And thanks to all those who shared their stories with me. The stories are true although some names and details have been changed.

To Dr. John Shen and to Robert Atkins, M.D., and the staff at the Atkins Centers for Complementary Medicine particular thanks for helping me get well.

Thanks again to my agent, Agnes Birnbaum, and to editor Jennifer Weis, who believed in this book.

Thanks to my children—Orrin, who calmly helped me through computer crises, and Eliza, for inspiring and encouraging words.

Love and thanks to Alma Bond, Ph.D., who gave me the courage of my convictions and more.

And to Irv, who stood by me through both the illness and the book— my love, devotion, and thanks.

MIMI WEISBORD
New York City 1997

CHAPTER 1

ASTHMA: AN INTRODUCTION

AN ODYSSEY

I had asthma twice. In 1970, my then husband and I bought a country house which had once been occupied by sixteen cats. When we moved in for the summer the last three cats, we were told, had been gone for over a year. While removing wallpaper and pulling up old linoleum, I inhaled mold and mildew in addition to the leftover dander.

This was my first experience with suffocation. The summer was one long asthma attack. There were no inhalers. I was given an injection of steroids to "tide me over" until I got home. I went back a week later for a second. At home I went to an allergist for shots since I obviously had a cat allergy. I also took a pill (Quadrenol) four times a day.

Two years later, after I made some profound changes in my life (including moving out of the house in Brooklyn I had lived in for seven years), my asthma went away.

Exertion left me breathless for a while, but I soon forgot all about asthma. I was rudely reminded on a couple of occasions, though, when spending weekends with friends who had cats at their houses in the country. I would end up getting a shot of adrenaline at a local hospital or leaving the "cat" house, and I would be fine again within an hour. Apart from these two or three instances I was perfectly well for thirteen years. I had no idea that asthma is considered to be a chronic illness.

Because of that experience I was unprepared for the virulence of my next bout with asthma, both the severity and the duration. I was extremely ill for three years in the late 1980s. But because of my recovery from the first encounter, I never gave up looking for a way out of the "chronic" suffering. Having gotten rid of asthma once, I was sure I could do it again.

The Second Round

This time I was living in an artists' building where my fifth floor loft was accumulating vapors from other floors. However, I was too "brain-fogged" at the time, my mind too fuzzy from toxins to figure it out. What I thought was the flu, a severe drop in temperature, and a freshly spray-painted ceiling below sent me over the top. Although I was fortunate in that the doctors I visited immediately afterward told me to "look to the materials in the building," I, unfortunately, didn't believe them. Not at the beginning. No one mentioned an environmental physician, let alone an allergist. Because I hadn't been to a doctor in many years, I didn't even understand that "pulmonology" and "allergy" were different specialties.

So began my odyssey of doctors and emergency-room visits, paramedics wheeling me out of my loft in the middle of the night and lengthy hospital stays. Luckily, I was already in therapy, so I had psychological support.

I learned about macrobiotics and cried when I was told to stick to the diet for two years. I had heard about people who got well in that time by using the diet in conjunction with acupuncture and herbs. But by the time I began acupuncture I was also dependent on a number of drugs, due to the great "advances" that had been made in pharmaceuticals. So I was waiting it out, trying alternatives, and using my medications. These drugs, though they sometimes relieved the asthma symptoms, seemed to be making me worse. Often I felt too weak to get from the bed or the couch, where I spent most of my time, to the kitchen to cook my food. And I couldn't take drugs such as theophylline unless I had something in my stomach. It was the lowest point in my life.

One night I passed out in the emergency room and awoke to find a machine breathing for me. My wrists were tied to the sides of the bed so that I would stop trying to pull the tube from my throat. Doctors told me that I had almost died, and having been intubated, I was now at greater risk for serious episodes.

But there were also periods that felt like "wellness." Each time I got out of the hospital, symptom-free, denial would set in. I thought I was better. Then I would catch a cold and there would be a downhill spiral. Each time I left the hospital I was weaker than ever before.

My two years were up and I was still ill and I started to panic. I was weak and exhausted. I felt I had no life and I needed answers. I didn't know it then but my version of a macrobiotic diet left a lot to be desired; and I had no idea I was now allergic to some of the food I ate regularly. A number of the environmental problems where I lived had finally been taken care of, but the situation was far from perfect. I could only afford acupuncture twice a month and that was not enough. I had taken out a loan but now I was running out of money for herbs and other treatments. My choices were limited to treatment from practitioners paid for by my medical insurance—I could either see doctors who prescribed stronger and stronger medications or end up in the hospital, where everything was covered. I didn't know that there were medical doctors who practiced a different kind of medicine, and that living here in New York City I had other alternatives.

I started going to a neighborhood health library, tentatively looking for anything that would help me know what to do about this condition I hated so much. I made the discovery that the best information about asthma was not to be found under that heading—much of it is to be found in unexpected places. Asthma has to be addressed on every level— physically, emotionally, spiritually, and environmentally—and I discovered that there was a lot more that I could do for myself. Little by little my "brain fog" began to clear. I talked to other people who were dealing with asthma and read countless books, periodicals, and medical journals; but it wasn't until I had endured three scary hospitalizations that I found a doctor who understood the biochemistry of the body in a different way and began to make some sense of the whole terrible experience. It was about time. I wanted my life back.

When one is so ill and isolated with asthma there is a tremendous amount of skepticism and hopelessness, and putting together information can be difficult. I tried to find the meaning in this illness; as I started to recover I felt a need to share my newfound information so that others would not have to go through what I had been through. Friends asked if I couldn't just put this illness behind me and go on with my painting. No, I could not. I began to write my newsletter, *Healthy Home and Workplace,* and do workshops for people with asthma.

Researching my newsletter and this book, I learned even more to explain what I was struggling with then. And although there is better information on asthma available now than there was ten years ago, it is still difficult to put together. This is the important discovery that propelled me to turn my life around and begin to share information with others with asthma: the great discrepancy between the useful, helpful, and healing treatments that are available, and the drug treatment that is the established route. I didn't see anyone recovering who was relying solely on drugs. But I found a number of practitioners helping people recover their health. And lifestyle modifications can make all the difference. You *can* learn to scale down your medications, manage your asthma naturally, recover your health, and live a fuller and happier life. You can even become medication-free.

There are a lot of changes to be made as you wend your way to health. People with asthma need more options and information about how to get well. I am fortunate to be living where I am, having access to wonderful people and sources of information. There are many natural healing methods available and some will be more compatible with your understanding and value system than others. The healing methods described in this book are those with which I have had personal experience. There are many others of great value that I would have tried had I not recovered.

It's been quite an odyssey. I wrote this book to share the result of my search with you now.

ASTHMA: A PUZZLE?

An asthma attack isn't something that "just happens." It is not fate playing dirty tricks. To have an asthma attack a number of things are working together other than, or in addition to, your negative thoughts, your unresolved resentments, or life in the big city. To rid oneself of asthma or to get it under good control with as little medication as possible, a number of paths may have to be explored. There is no magic pill. Your wish to improve and some excellent sleuthing can lead to changes in your life that will make a difference. Learn to pay attention to and trust your body.

You Are Not Just Your Lungs

Most days when you are short of breath, tight in the chest, or just can't breathe, it is very hard to focus on anything else. But the reality is that you are a whole person, and all those organs—brain, heart, lungs, liver, kidneys, stomach, glands—are connected. The total organism that is you lives in the world, interacting with its environment every moment of the day—breathing in oxygen, breathing out carbon dioxide, taking in nutrients and excreting waste, and interacting emotionally with others. Everything you breathe, eat, touch, see, think, and feel affects this organism.

Disharmony creates the imbalances that lead to illness. This is a long process and the symptom (in this case the inability to breathe) is the end point of the process. Are you living in harmony with your environment?

We Know What Happens During an Attack

No one who has ever suffered from asthma needs to be told what happens during an attack. *Asthma* is a Greek word meaning "gasping for breath" or not being able to take a deep breath. The verb "asthmaino" means "I pant" or "I gasp" like an exhausted runner. Current asthma literature looking for a definition characterizes asthma as a narrowing of the bronchial airways, with wheezing, an overproduction of mucus, and shortness of breath. In an asthma attack these conditions lead to a panting for oxygen as the airways fill with stale air which cannot easily be expelled. But the wheezing and shortness of breath of what we call asthma could also be caused by other ailments: a bad cold or flu, heart disease, or emphysema, a disease in which the air sacs have actually been damaged. So there is another definition of asthma: a bronchial condition that can be completely reversed—with drugs or, inexplicably, by itself.[1]

"Asthma poses special definition challenges," writes Dr. Kenneth Moser, a professor of medicine at the University of California, "but seekers after truth about 'what asthma is' ultimately must face the reality that there are no absolutes; rather, there are a variety of truths." He goes on to say that there is "one accepted fact about asthma; namely that airway dysfunction appears to be the final expressive pathway of a number of inciting events—some recognized and some obscure, some persistent and some transient."[2] Although the symptoms everyone experiences during an asthma attack might be similar, physicians sense that the causes may be different. Hence we find categories such as "intrinsic" asthma, "extrinsic" asthma, and "mixed" asthma.

The Poor Treatment of Asthma Is the Puzzle

Not only does orthodox medicine have a problem defining exactly what asthma is, but as you and I may have experienced, it has had a bigger problem in trying to treat it. Look at the statistics of the growing numbers of deaths from asthma. Fatalities have tripled since 1977.[3] The headlines in the 1980s proclaimed "A Puzzling Increase in Asthma Deaths," "U.S. Asthma Mortality Rising," "Asthma Doctors Puzzled As the Death Rate Rises Despite Improved Drugs" and "Are Asthma Drugs a Cure That Kills?" In the 1990s they are resigned to "Asthma Common and on the Rise. . . ."

The way in which orthodox medicine is practiced in relation to asthma *is* puzzling, and the problem has as many parts as the etiology of the illness. Let's look at the established way of treating asthma.

Much time and money is spent in research geared toward understanding the mechanism of the asthmatic response or allergic reaction. This research is usually carried out specifically to formulate newer and "better" pharmaceuticals.

The treatment of asthma is based entirely on treating the *symptoms* with these drugs, rather than looking for and treating underlying conditions.

Drugs that temporarily seem to improve the quality of life eventually create their own problems. Sometimes they actually *worsen* the quality of life at the same time they seem to be resolving symptoms.

Because most doctors have no other tools to use, drugs play an important, actually crucial, part in the management of asthma. (Whole books have been written about this!) But often doctors do not listen to or educate their patients. They do not explain what the drugs do or how the inhalers work. Drugs sometimes help keep people out of the hospital and may be needed to save lives. However, it seems that many people do not understand what the asthma literature would call the "safe" and "proper" use of medication.

In 1991, in response to the rise in publicity about the prevalence and possible deadliness of asthma, the National Heart, Lung and Blood Institute published comprehensive guidelines for treating asthma. Here they state that asthma is characterized by inflammation, and recommend that treating the inflammation should come before regular use of bronchodilating drugs. They also suggest that many need to be desensitized to allergens.[4] But pulmonary specialists are still not sending asthmatics to allergists. Dr. Robert Y. Lin, Chief of Allergy and Immunology at St. Vincent's Hospital in New York City, says that triggers need to be recognized, identified, and eliminated. Dr. Lin says, "There is a lot of variability as to how asthma is being treated and a lack of coordination between pulmonologists and allergists."[5]

Pulmonologists rarely educate patients about lifestyle changes that would improve their condition. And regular use of bronchodilators is still being prescribed over safer and more effective treatments.

Most importantly, orthodox physicians—allergists and pulmonologists—don't use nutrition or vitamins or any of the modalities with which complementary doctors have been helping their patients to a healthier life. There are reasons why we have the allergy or inflammation. Without acknowledging that one can uncreate the conditions that brought about illness, all emphasis is on drugs. The goal is to "manage" the symptoms with a prescription.

ASTHMA ON THE RISE

Federal health officials say that asthma is the only chronic disease, besides AIDS and tuberculosis, that is on the rise throughout the world. Ten million Americans had asthma in 1990, and fifteen million have it now—a 66 percent increase over 1980. Even though over five thousand people died in 1994 we are told that Americans still have one of the lowest death rates, below that of New Zealand and that of England,[6] where drugs can cost up to 80 percent *less!*[7]

Can We Call Allopathic or Orthodox Medicine "Traditional"?

The word *allopathic* comes from the Greek *allo* meaning "other," and from *pathos* meaning "suffering." Allopathic or orthodox medicine opposes disease. It is sometimes spoken of as "traditional" medicine. But one dictionary defines *traditional* as "the handing down of knowledge, beliefs and customs from one generation to another . . . anything handed down from the past and so strongly rooted as to be as inviolable as law."[8] Can we call a practice "traditional" whose drugs and applications are constantly changing?

Alternative medicine is defined as anything that is not allopathic. Many of today's alternatives were traditional healing methods: homeopathy, acupuncture, massage, and the use of herbs. We are fortunate they are being reclaimed. Today there is great interest in alternative treatments, which the National Institutes of Health has duly noted by creating an Office of Alternative Medicine. Dr. Gerald Epstein had a 1993 grant from this office to study mental imagery for healing asthma with what he calls "waking dream therapy." Dr. Epstein has this to say about what happened when traditional healing gave way to science:

"My work carries on a traditional Western medicine that's been here for five thousand years. It was thrown away four hundred years ago or so with the advent of the new science and medicine, the Industrial Revolution, the rise of capitalism and split of the mind and body. That's when they threw away the spiritual, mystical, religious tradition. The mindbody connection was lost, the channel of communication between the invisible and visible realities was severed. This traditional medicine was an integrative mindbody one. The medicine that grew up in the last four hundred years I call 'alternative medicine.' The alternative to the traditional. But they cleverly call *this* the 'traditional medicine' and all the other ones alternative and complementary. So **we're** doing the real traditional medicine, which employed not only herbs and the natural remedies of the earth, but also the mind as a central piece in the healing process."[9]

According to a recent study, one in three adults surveyed has turned to alternative therapies, perhaps because the allopathic treatments just didn't work. However, many alternative or "complementary" doctors may also use drugs, judiciously, while they rebuild the immune system. And today there are allopathic doctors who are keeping an open mind and beginning to incorporate alternative therapies into their practice. Complementary physician Robert Atkins, M.D., feels that the more valid systems used, the greater the probability of success.[10]

Unfortunately, most of us have been so bombarded with television commercials that we are brainwashed to expect a quick fix. In TV Land there's a pill for whatever ails you. Never mind that the headaches, stomachaches, coughs, arthritis, and asthma may be warnings that something else is wrong.

Alternative medicine is not another quick fix. If you are seeking alternative and natural healing as a way to get better, ask yourself how much you are willing to participate in this process. Unfortunately, there are no quick fixes. Although alternative therapies have much to offer, ultimately we are the ones who have to take responsibility for our own healing.

Now is the time to ask yourself:

Am I willing to engage in constructive activity for wellness?

Am I willing to take responsibility for my state of health?

Am I willing to exchange debilitating habits for productive ones?

Am I willing to be active instead of reactive?

Asthma is an illness of many parts which must be dealt with on many levels. Developing a healthier lifestyle can affect every area of your life, making you stronger, slimmer, sleeker, more clearheaded, and more creative, with a sense of empowerment and peace of mind.

Although bronchodilators and anti-inflammatories are useful in allaying or repressing symptoms, they are not really enhancing wellness, changing the direction of the illness for the better, balancing or nourishing the body, or helping the immune system to heal. They can, however, be used judiciously as an adjunct to other, safer modalities that will support the integrity of the body. If we must, we can make use of these drugs at the same time that we are nourishing, exercising, resting, and detoxifying the body to regain health. While we are using positive methods for enhancing wellness, our minds and spirits can be engaged in constructive activity which is empowering, rather than engaged in passive dependency on drugs.

The information in this book is offered as a starting point. Everyone's condition is different and that has to be taken into consideration as you read the book. Find one area in which you feel you can work; start with one idea you can use. It is up to you to decide what you want and how far to go. If you can incorporate only one new healthful change in your life, it will be for the better. No one can do this for you as well as you can for yourself. The information here can help you develop awareness and give you tools with which to begin.

It took us a long time to become ill and it will take some time to get well. Have patience. As the Chinese say, "A long journey begins with a first step." And the journey will be an exciting one. It's time to start down that road to recovery.

CHAPTER 2

ORIENTAL MEDICINE

TRADITIONAL CHINESE MEDICINE

Oriental medicine developed over many thousands of years. It is rooted in the natural world and emphasizes the connection between human beings and the environment. In traditional Chinese medicine, nothing can be understood except in its relation to the whole. "Its unity and soundness form the real base of Chinese medicine, in which all functioning constituents interconnect as parts of a cosmic whole," writes Leon Hammer, M.D., psychoanalyst and acupuncturist, in *Dragon Rises, Red Bird Flies*.[1] For over four thousand years health has been seen as a harmonious balance of energies that can be maintained or restored through herbs and acupuncture, diet and other aspects of lifestyle.

A Western Experience with Chinese Healing

David, a college student, had asthma for most of his life. He took medication for sixteen years and thinks he was "addicted." He reports having used a bronchodilator inhaler (Proventil) for eight or nine years, in recent years four times a day, plus Slophylline and then Theo-Dur. In addition, he sometimes used Intal, and occasionally was given a course of steroids. He thought that a lot of his problem was exercise-induced, but he complained of a constant chest tightness when he wasn't using the medication.

After college David went to China for a year to study. He laughed when he told how he brought with him a year's supply of medication, only to find he could buy the inhalers there "for a tenth of the price."

"After I had been there for six months I decided to try acupuncture for asthma, but I didn't know how to find the right person. A friend of mine was getting massage from a woman who had just graduated from the College of Traditional Chinese Medicine in Beijing. We were introduced and she was happy to have a willing, real live patient on whom to practice while she was waiting for her accreditation. She also wanted to learn some English and so we traded skills.

"I had acupuncture for a grand total of four months, between once or twice a week—maybe thirty times. She put the needles mostly in my back, for about forty-five minutes. At the same time she would do moxibustion (heating an herb over the acupuncture needle), which was unbelievable. There were times I would go there and my chest would be a little tight, and she would put the moxibustion sticks over two points in my back and light them, and my chest would be clear in about two minutes. Now I'm a very skeptical person but that stuff offered instant relief. Very impressive.

"She explained to me the whole concept of how in the West the asthma medicine they were giving me dealt with the symptoms, but was not going to where the real problem was in my body. She said that according to Chinese medicine, asthma meant a weak kidney and weak lungs. But the kidney in Chinese medicine is not really how we think of it. She felt I had asthma because those two areas in my body were weak. On the one hand the acupuncture was used to strengthen those areas and treat the root cause of the asthma; on the other hand she said you need to eat certain kinds of foods to strengthen.

"After about a month I started to reduce the amount of inhaler I was taking and at one point, when I didn't take it for one day it sort of felt weird, but I got up the next day and I just stopped."

David says that there were several factors involved in his getting well. "I think the acupuncture did something and I think I was overmedicated and was addicted. I do feel like I was cheated . . . the fact that I would go into these doctor's offices and they would charge me seventy-five dollars for a breathing test to tell me that my chest was tight, when I could have told them that without taking a breathing test.

"As it turned out, after about three and a half, four months, I was fine. It's been twenty months now and I've probably taken my inhaler maybe three times since then, when I've gotten a really nasty cold and had a tight chest. I've mentioned to my family doctor, 'Hey my asthma doesn't seem to be around anymore,' and he said, 'It must just be in remission,' but it's been in remission for a while and I really do attribute it to the acupuncture."

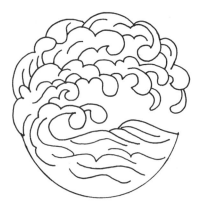

"HIGH TIDE FOR THE LUNG"

As for other aspects of lifestyle, David also gave up milk in China because it was expensive and hard to get. And he did not resume drinking milk when he returned to the United States.

The Tide of Qi

In Chinese medicine the *Qi* (pronounced chee, sometimes written as ch'i or chi) the life force, moves through the body-clock, through each organ meridian, like waves at high tide, for two hours during the twenty-four-hour cycle. Qi moves through the lungs between 3 A.M. and 5 A.M. This means that our biological clock at this time is focused more on the lung meridian; in a normal person there would be a fuller lung energetic, high tide for the lung. But if there is too little (deficient) lung energy, the lungs might not be able to meet this demand. And if there is already too much lung energy, the addition could create stagnation and blockage.

This early-morning time is when many people find their asthma worsens.

In an article on pulmonary function published in Great Britain, N. B. Pride writes, "Airway narrowing in asthma is frequently at its worst in the early hours of the morning." He goes on to say that researchers have postulated that this may be due to circadian rhythms, dust mite exposure, a late response to allergen exposure, mucus obstruction, or sleeping postures. "The underlying causes," writes Pride, "remain uncertain despite extensive investigation."[2]

Eight Pillars

Chinese medicine originally had eight pillars and included practices of meditation, exercise, balanced diet (including culinary herbs and spices), astrology (including the I Ching), geomancy (Feng Shui, the science of the placement of objects), massage, herbology, and acupuncture.

It is based on a theory of yin and yang, that everything in the universe has an opposite: dark and light, night and day, passive and active, cold and warm, contraction and expansion.

In Chinese traditional medicine each yin organ is paired with a yang organ. The lung is paired with the large intestine. It's the balance and equilibrium between these opposites that creates harmony and health.

The Qi

Energy or *Qi* is the central concept of Chinese medicine. Qi is life force, in yogic practice it's called *prana*, the idea that all living matter contains energy.

Qi Gong (pronounced chi kung) is a way of learning to master the flow of energy in your body through meditation and movement. Michael Winn is a Qi Gong therapist who uses a variety of forms of Qi Gong to help people move the flow of Qi at a physical, emotional, mental, and spiritual level. As Michael explains the concept of Qi:

"There is pulsation in every atom, molecule, and every cell in your body. And not just the organs and cells in your body, but everything is literally pulsating. Everything is made out of Qi, vibrating, pulsating at different rates. Some of it looks more solid, some might look like empty space, but there's always some energy field. And a human being, from the Chinese point of view, is a condensation or crystallization of certain patterns of this energy.

"Chinese medicine works because it alters the flow of patterns of energy. Western medicine says, 'Let's zero in on the specific thing we need to fight off here. You've got this virus, this bacteria, this chemical toxin coming in— we'll put up a barrier and beat it.' Chinese medicine is exactly the opposite. It says basically that you want to have complete Qi, full Qi and balanced flow of energy. It's the point of view of the whole being, the whole person."

How Chinese Medicine Views the Lung and Asthma

When the Chinese talk about an organ such as the lung, they mean the whole complex, the energetic meridian and the energetic field. They are not talking about just the physical lung. The problem of asthma may not originate in the lung. In Western medicine we don't describe energetic states such as those defined by Oriental medicine. There is no model of the energy flow between the different organs. "The Western model," says Winn, "is that of the body as a perfectly functioning machine.

"In Chinese medicine it's the energetic functions of the lung that we are talking about, some of which are invisible, some of which you cannot dissect and find and see. It's the energy, it's multidimensional, it is not just in the physical dimension. That's what a human being is. We're not just this solid physical body, we are this energy field, the lower layers of which we call the mind, the part that has thoughts and feelings."[3]

WHAT ASTHMA IS

"We have to define what asthma is," says Drew Di Vittorio, a practitioner of classical Taoist herbalism. "According to our school of thought there are many different reasons why one would have what Western medicine terms "asthma." Many people whom I see have been told that they have asthma, but it is not what we consider asthma. 'True' asthma is inflammation and dampness.

"The herbal formulas that we use treat inflammation as well as strengthen the energy of the lungs. Someone who has an asthma condition has a yin or weak condition. That means it's long term, it's in the organs themselves, so it takes a long time to actually heal. If we just cleanse the lungs of someone who is in a yin state they may not get well, they may just get weaker and weaker."

RED POINTS

"We can tell if it's inflammation from the pulses. This also shows up on the tongue in the form of red points. These little red points are from what we call an air disease—an external wind invasion that is remaining dormant inside the body. They change according to what we're breathing in. If we're getting a cold they'll raise up and move back. If we're not really getting a cold but we know something's in our body that hasn't come to a head, they'll also raise up and move back a little bit. As the cold gets better they'll come forward. It's kind of a barometer of the actual air disease inside the body.

"Mucus is sometimes sent to our lungs as a way of being expelled from other parts of our body. Mucus is also sent there to help expel any germs that might be present. So if your body is too weak to expel the mucus, the mucus builds up and gets hard, and as your body gets weak, it causes inflammation. The bronchi then have difficulty expanding, and they go into spasm."

"Sometimes the lungs are just weak. This could cause asthmalike symptoms. We say, 'The kidneys can't grasp the Qi.' This means that the final product of Qi is made inside our lungs and sent down into the kidneys and when the lungs and kidneys are both weak, they can't make that connection. This causes breathlessness. Asthma can mean weakened kidneys or a weakened pair of lungs. Weakened energy or a weakened Qi."[4]

The Meridians and Three Kinds of Asthma in Chinese Medicine

Deborah Valentine Smith, a senior teacher of Jin Shin Do® acupressure, explains that each person with asthma is different and must be treated differently. It's important to keep in mind that meridian function includes not only the function of the organ but its related functions.

Although the asthma problems and imbalances may be different for each person, Deborah Smith says that basically there are three kinds of asthma:

1. **Spleen/Pancreas meridian–related asthma.** This is characterized by a phlegm condition, but don't confuse phlegm with mucous, which is the normal discharge of the mucous membranes. The spleen meridian moves fluids. Phlegm results when the spleen is not functioning properly. This can result in edema or congestion of the lungs. The emotion connected with the spleen is worry.

2. **Kidney meridian–related asthma.** When there is a low reserve of energy, the kidney energetic can't receive energy from the lungs. This results in shortness of breath. The kidney meridian regulates the bone marrow, and weakening kidneys can result in fatigue. The emotions associated with the kidneys are fear and anxiety.

3. **Liver meridian–related asthma.** The liver meridian is responsible for the balance between control and movement in the body. It nourishes muscles and tendons. If the liver meridian is imbalanced, these can overcontract or be too flaccid. The emotions associated with the liver meridian are anger, guilt, and resentment, but also self-assertion. In liver meridian–related asthma, the bronchioles go into spasm.

Smith says that people usually have a bit of all of these weaknesses. The inhalers make kidney weakness worse by further weakening the kidney, which has to filter toxins. The adrenals are part of the kidney energetic that helps to nourish the bones. Prednisone can hasten osteoporosis by further depleting the adrenals.[5]

HEALING METHODS

There are a number of healing methods that came out of Chinese concepts of balance of yin and yang, and moving energy. These include acupuncture, acupressure, herbalism, medicinal or nutritional cooking, medical massage, Tai Ji Chuan, and Qi Gong.

Winn says, "Qi Gong means practicing with your energy or mastering your energy. Tai Chi, martial arts, and meditation are branches of Qi Gong. They are all different applications of ways of managing your energy. I would say that acupuncture is an external branch of managing energy. The martial arts are ways of doing it directly. Acupuncture evolved out of this science as people's way of moving their energy declined and they started using needles to try to move it."

Acupuncture

We might not know much about either acupuncture or Chinese medicine here in the West if the late *New York Times* columnist James Reston hadn't developed appendicitis on a trip to China (he was covering Nixon's 1971 visit) and had not been treated with acupuncture and moxibustion for the pain. Luckily for us, he returned home and wrote about his experience. That incident created so much interest that subsequently there was an exodus of young people to China, Japan, and India, as well as to Great Britain, where acupuncture was already being taught. When these "New Age" students returned to the United States, a number of them went on to write the books that we are reading today.

HOW ACUPUNCTURE IS PRACTICED

At present some believe that acupuncture is only effective for pain, not understanding that the Chinese see illness as an energy dysfunction and that acupuncture is used to regulate and enhance this flow of energy. Acupuncturists also use traditional methods of Chinese diagnosis, which include observation of face and tongue, and pulse reading.

The Tongue

Although doctors in the West used to look at tongues, the Chinese have a more sophisticated method that allows them to determine the health of an internal organ by the condition, color, texture, coating, thickness, and markings on the tongue. A healthy tongue will be pink and moist with no markings and a very thin coating.

Pulses

While Western doctors count only the speed of the pulse, a practitioner of traditional Chinese medicine will be looking for six pulses on each wrist, three superficial and three deep, each related to imbalances in a different organ. In an earlier age, Western doctors were also interested in the qualities of the pulse. Back in the second century, Galen, a Greek physician, described over a hundred different qualities of pulses in his writings. He also wrote about excesses or imbalances which produce disease, such as too much phlegm creating asthma or pneumonia. Many of his theories resemble those of Eastern medicine.

WHAT NEEDS ATTENDING

"The theme of acupuncture is that the Qi, the life force, is flowing," says Dianne Connelly, cofounder of the Traditional Acupuncture Institute in Columbia, Maryland.

"The Qi flows through these different pathways, these 'bowing servants.' There are twelve main pathways or meridians; one is the great lung. From the Chinese perspective, that flowing Qi is animating the capacity to breathe."

Connelly says that to the Chinese, the word *asthma* doesn't mean anything until you actually find out what it means to each person, what is the anatomy of the experience. "People might come to you with the label 'asthma,' but the experience for each of them is really personal, a unique phenomenon.

"The only way I know to investigate or inquire as to how that Qi is flowing is to go in deeply with a person, to take their pulses, to find out what actually is their lived body experience, and to be able to say, 'It's not that something is wrong and needs to be fixed. It's because something is happening as a possibility in the kingdom and needs support. How can we listen? How can we smell, hear, feel, touch, and use our senses to be able to be present in such a way as to see what is the call here? What wants attending? What needs supporting?' Once we bring that balance present, then that symptom can just disappear because it wasn't something that needed to be fixed in itself. It was like a crying child that says, 'Pay attention here, something is happening and we need some balance and some ease,' which is the opposite of disease."[6]

THE ACUPUNCTURE POINTS

There are 365 acupuncture points along the twelve meridians. An acupuncturist will insert very fine needles into points considered therapeutic, usually a combination of points, to rebalance disharmonies in the body. The acupuncturist will determine where the needles go by listening to the patient speak as well as examining the pulses, face, and tongue.

The needles are very fine and not particularly painful although there is usually some sensation for a moment. Some practitioners may turn or adjust the needles until a kind of "electrical charge" is felt. Sometimes moxibustion treatment is also used. The moxa, an herb called mugwort (*Artemesia vulgaris*), is heated at the acupuncture point. This will affect the Qi and blood in the meridian. There are usually five to fifteen needles in a treatment and points are chosen to correspond to individual disharmony.

Connelly compares the points to little gates and locks. "The acupuncture needles go into little doors and gates: 'Open up now, we need a bit more flowing here.' To the Chinese, life is movement. If there's no movement, we get stuck, then there's a squawk that tells us that something is not in balance and easy-flowing.

"The moxa tends to act as a kind of support for what is done with the needles and is the builder of the Qi. From a physiological Western point of view, no one knows for sure how it works; it's just been found to have this healing property. It's used on the acupuncture point on a bed of ginger or garlic or salt, depending on the location, or even directly on the skin. You light the herb and when it gets hot you take it off. It helps build that Qi, it helps build the strength and that internal flowing."

WHAT WILL I EXPERIENCE?

Because asthma is the name of a symptom of many different conditions, people with asthma may have diverse experiences with acupuncture treatment. Also, practitioners work in different ways, and the relationship between the patient and the practitioner may make a difference. Several people have told of acupuncture experiences in which they are breathless and "feel worse" after the treatment and never return for another treatment. One explanation for feeling worse could be that they are in a weakened condition and the movement of the energy is too much. But usually there is improvement after the worsening.

By the time I got to an acupuncturist, I was too weak for acupuncture. Every two weeks my back was massaged using Chinese massage. Sometimes "cupping" was performed to draw out the cold that the doctor explained had gone deep inside my body. In this procedure, a vacuum is created in a glass cup with a match, and the heated cup is placed over the acupuncture point. The cupping relieved the symptoms temporarily, and helped with the cold. Later, after acupuncture treatment began, the doctor placed the cups over the needles and I experienced an intense relaxation and euphoria.

I was told that one could feel worse after treatment because everything that is inside is being brought out. I felt very weak and tired for about twenty-four hours after acupuncture because my body was so depleted. So I planned my appointments for days when I could rest.

Acupuncture did not "cure" my asthma but it began to address some of the underlying problems. And it made me more aware of what was happening in my body. Today when I go for acupuncture for whatever reason I understand that it's a process, and I feel more attuned to that process. I stay with it longer and I better understand the effects. Appointments are scheduled closer together as this seems to work best for me. Acupuncture and herbs undoubtedly set the stage for my success later on.

JIN SHIN DO ACUPRESSURE

After being treated with acupuncture on and off for several years I unfortunately had to stop my treatments. But in my quest for relief from asthma I accidentally found one of the best treatment methods that I could study, and even use to work on myself. It became very important for relief of my asthma symptoms and gave me an increased sense of well-being.

My yoga teacher had mentioned that she gave acupressure treatments and I decided to give it a try—I was feeling so tight in the chest and debilitated that it was difficult to do the standing postures in yoga class.

The "massage" was not what I expected. Instead of working all over, she pressed lightly on one spot of my fully clothed body with one hand, while she held another spot with a couple of fingers of the other hand. She was completely still and became very meditative, and in what seemed like a few seconds I was in a trance and incredible state of relaxation. *"What is that?"* I asked. And that's how I became a student of Jin Shin Do.

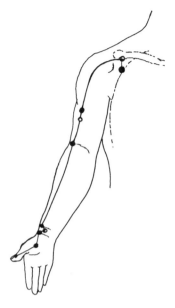

THE LUNG MERIDIAN

Acu-Points

Jin Shin Do® Acupressure was created by Iona Marsaa Teeguarden, M.A., L.M.F.C.C., who derived this technique by combining the Japanese method of Jin Shin Jitsu with traditional acupuncture patterns and Taoist philosophy. At the basic level, Jin Shin Do uses 55 of the 365 acupuncture points to develop and maintain well-being rather than just for relief of symptoms.[7]

Acu-points are not really magic buttons to push to achieve a certain effect. Some will be useful sometimes and others will help at other times depending on the state of the different organ systems of the body at the time of discomfort. However, the practice of finding and stimulating these points can give you a powerful tool which may help a lot when you need it. Here we are learning some points for symptom relief.

My teacher and Jin Shin Do practitioner, Deborah Valentine Smith, also had asthma. It was her positive experience with acupuncture that led her to study this related practice. Acupressure, like acupuncture, works on the theory that our problems come from a blockage in the flow of Qi, leading to deficient or excessive function. Jin Shin Do acupressure works to release chronic muscular tension or "armoring" so that energy can move through. Two points are held at the same time, creating a flow of Qi or energy between them. The main (local) point can be held with one hand while the other hand moves from one related (distal) point to another.

You will produce a greater effect if you use local- and distal-point combinations, working with visualization to see the energy flowing from point to point in the body. In Jin Shin Do, you have to be able to focus awareness and be willing to experience the physical sensations of what you are feeling.

The acu-points will feel a little tense or tender to the touch. Sometimes they are painful. But holding or gently massaging the point will soon ease the pain and make it soften. Give equal time to both right and left sides of the body, beginning with the side that feels most painful and tight.

Get comfortable, sitting or lying down so that you can fully relax while holding the points. Points are usually held for one to three minutes or until they soften. For those familiar with acupuncture, the number of the acupuncture point is given first; the Jin Shin Do number is in parentheses.

Point Combinations

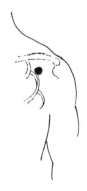

Lung 1 (JSD #30)

This is the main point for lung meridian–involved problems. It helps energy to move through the lungs, balancing their function.

To find: Massage from midpoint of chest under collarbone to the outside of rib cage. At about two fingers' width below the collarbone pressing toward the rib cage you will feel the tenderness or resistance of Lung 1. Don't forget the other side. You can hold each point separately or cross arms and hold both points at the same time.

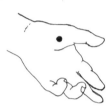

LUNG 10 (JSD #36)

In the center of the fleshy part of the base of the thumb, you will feel the pain as you press up toward the metacarpal bone. I found this point most helpful first thing in the morning to loosen mucus.

Lung 1 and Lung 10 can be held together this way:

Left side: Hold Lung 1 with the middle finger of the right hand while pressing the little finger of the right hand onto Lung 10 at the base of the left thumb. Concentrate on the flow of Qi down the left arm between those two points. Reverse for the other side.

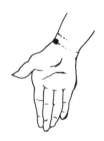

LUNG 9 (JSD SOURCE PT.)

This point is in a little indentation located on the wrist fold just below the base of the thumb. This is a good point to hold for the balance of the lung meridian especially if you have difficulty holding the two points together.

22

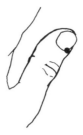

LUNG 11 (JSD THUMBNAIL POINT)

This is the last point on the lung meridian at the lower corner of the thumbnail toward the outside of the hand.

The Lung Source point and Lung 11 combination may help smokers stop smoking.

The Lung Source point and Lung 11 can be held together in this way:

On the left hand: With the right thumb hold the source point on the left hand while the right index finger holds Lung 11 at the base of the thumbnail of the left hand. Reverse for other side.

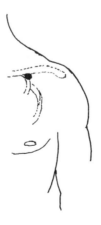

STOMACH 13 (JSD #3)

You can find this point under and at the midpoint of the collarbone above the nipple. A very good general point for releasing the chest and shoulders.

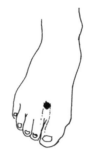

LIVER 3 (JSD #42)

To find this point: Massage up between the first and second toes, at the junction of the first and second metatarsals. This is helpful where there is tightness in the bronchioles and difficulty breathing in the absence of phlegm or mucus congestion. This can be powerful for wheezing associated with cramping or tightening of bronchioles because it's the source point of the liver meridian. It allows the flow of Qi through the sinews, which are responsible for muscular contraction and relaxation. Therefore, it helps release muscular tissue in spasm.

Hold JSD #42 with any chest point for chest tightness. It may also help with liver-related allergic reactions.

Both feet could be done at once. Hold points for one to three minutes.

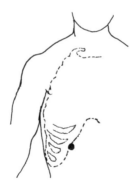

LIVER 14 (JSD #5)

This point is called "Gate of Hope" and is the point where Qi leaves the liver meridian to enter the lung meridian. It can be a powerful point for releasing the diaphragm, which gives us more room to breathe.

To find this point: Run your index finger down along the bottom edge of the rib cage to the tender point just inside the nipple line.

Hold JSD #42 with JSD #5 in the diaphragm area to help with breath.

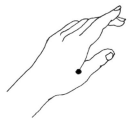

LARGE INTESTINE 4 (JSD #35) (*Not to be used in pregnancy*)

This is what the Japanese call the "hoku" point. It is in the same place on the hand where Liver 3 (JSD #42) was on the foot, in the webbing between the thumb and index finger a little below the junction of bones. Press toward the bone of the index finger.

This point can be very relaxing. It helps energy to move down and so is good for elimination. Because it's the source point for the large intestine meridian, it helps to balance the function of that organ. The bowels should move regularly because there is a connection between respiratory problems and toxicity in the large intestine. If there is congestion of Qi in the upper body, activating this point helps it to move down. This makes it useful also for colds and headaches.

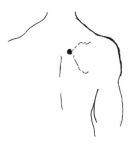

BLADDER 38 (JSD #18)

This point is in the muscles between the inside edge of the shoulder blade and the spine. Let someone you trust work up the muscles on either side of the spine an inch at a time up to the inside of the shoulder blade. You will probably recognize fast that that's the place to be, as tension and often phlegm are released there.

To work on yourself, lie down with two little rubber balls under those points and relax your shoulders back. You can hold the JSD #5 on the rib cage or the JSD #30 points at the same time.

Work that whole area along the inner edge of the shoulder blades—all the points along there are associated with meridians which influence the chest and so will help it to open.

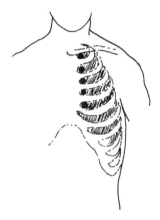

KIDNEY 27, (JSD #3 area) K 26, K 25, K 24, K 23, K 22

These are the kidney meridian points in the area in between the ribs, right up against the breastbone on either side. These can be very helpful for chest tightness, anxiety, and to relieve the armoring in the chest.

Put all five fingers in between the ribs, under the collarbone, on the side of the breastbone. Do one side at a time. Hold or massage points.

In addition you can work from each point in between the ribs, toward the outer edge of the rib cage for lymphatic drainage.

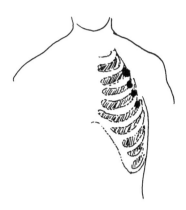

SPLEEN-RELATED POINTS
SP 17, SP 18, SP 19, SP 20

On the outside of the rib cage go down the rib cage with fingers in between the ribs. You can accomplish this by crossing arms in front of your chest to do opposite sides. Or do one side at a time. The outside of the rib cage is spleen and gall bladder meridian–related.

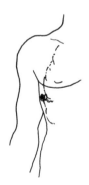

SPLEEN 21
THE GRAND LUO

This is a point on the outside of the rib cage, between two ribs, almost two hands down from the armpit about halfway between front and back. This is a painful point on everyone, so you will know it when you find it.

TO STOP ASTHMA ATTACKS BEFORE THEY START

Here's a point combination to help people on the verge of an asthma attack.[8] The Kidney 27 (JSD #3:K) point described above, right up under the collarbone; the Bladder 42 (JSD #17) point halfway up the back, in the muscle on either side of the rib cage; and the Large Intestine 11 (JSD #25), which is just above the bend in the arm on the outside edge.

You can hold the JSD #17 by putting your fist behind your back (or lying on a small rubber ball) while holding JSD #3 with the other hand. Then move to and hold the JSD #25.

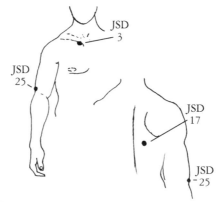

STOP AN ASTHMA ATTACK BEFORE IT STARTS
(JSD#25) (JSD#3:K)   (JSD#17) (JSD#25)

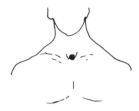

CONCEPTION VESSEL POINT

This point at the top of the sternum (at the notch) will also help for heading off asthma attacks. The nerve that goes to the diaphragm goes under the collarbone close to that spot. By crossing your arms, resting your right elbow on the left arm, and resting your chin on your hand (in think position) and thumb on this point, you could hold it surreptitiously during conversation without anyone knowing what you're doing! Be sure to press toward your toes, not in toward your windpipe!

Working with Jin Shin Do

Pay attention to the first awareness of a respiratory problem or an attack coming on, notice what's happening, and breathe.

"Working with people as a Jin Shin Do therapist," says Deborah Smith, "I have often found that a problem for some kinds of asthma is a spasm which makes it difficult to exhale the breath fully. I will hold points on the chest and ask the person to breathe into those areas so that they push my fingers up, and as they exhale, I'll push into those points and ask them to release more than they think they can. That often opens up the breath and gives people a sense of how much more there is."

Thinking of illness as an imbalance in the energy or Qi flowing through the meridians of the body gives us a new way to view our asthma, and enlarges our understanding of ways we can help ourselves. Trying some of these pressure points to relieve symptoms is simple and cost-free and has proven for many to be an effective method of self-treatment. Practice some of the easy-to-reach points and breathe deeply into them as you hold them. Try this when you are relaxing and not having an emergency and soon you will have a repertoire of points you can count on when you need them.

CHAPTER 3

IS IT ALL IN YOUR HEAD?

THE PERCEPTION OF ASTHMA

Many people who struggle with asthma today have internalized the old notion that asthma is a strictly psychological condition. We do know that the body and the mind are connected, a concept that is being utilized more and more in the practice of medicine.

Although your mind did not give you asthma, once you are ill the mind can play a role in exacerbating the illness. And the mind can be enlisted to play a part in recovery. Your belief system will also determine the extent to which you are willing to participate in what it takes to get well.

Is Asthma Simply the Result of Stress?

Some people say that their asthma was caused by stress. But can stress alone cause asthma? Of course stress, usually a combination of chemical, physical, and emotional stressors, can deplete the adrenals and compromise the immune system. But most people, when they think of stress, think simply about the emotions. Is emotional stress responsible for your asthma? Maybe.

Do you think asthma is an emotional or psychological illness? According to "The American Asthma Report II," a national survey conducted by Glaxo, approximately 28 percent of the 5 percent of all American adults who have asthma say yes.

Sir William Osler, an influential world-renowned Canadian-born physician, wrote around the turn of the century that "there is, in a majority of cases of bronchial asthma, a strong neurotic element." Written a hundred

30

years ago, this proclamation captured the popular imagination and never let go.

Many asthmatics are still suffering from the perception on the part of unallergic and unknowledgeable people that asthma is self-created. With fifteen million asthma sufferers in the United States alone, that's a lot of people to blame. Asthma seems to be thought of by many as a psychological aberration, an illness that's not really respectable. Many asthmatics feel they are to blame for their illness and the accompanying debilitation. Along with the physical suffering there are feelings of helplessness, fear, and isolation. This feeling of loss of control over one's life often leads to shame and secretiveness which prohibit those with asthma from seeking out useful information and sharing their feelings with others.

Sometimes it is embarrassing to be perceived as asthmatic. When an illness comes and goes, with periods of feeling perfectly fine, how do you explain why one minute you are all right and the next you are gasping for breath? Mark, a fifty-four-year-old professor at a prestigious private college, feels that asthma is very depressing. "It's depressing walking around not being able to breathe. I would feel rotten going to work. But because I didn't want to be seen by the students as asthmatic, I would work to overcome it during class. As soon as the classes were over I felt rotten again."

A forty-year-old professional woman recounted, "For a couple of years I didn't work at all. I had the sensation of suffocating all the time, but without any mucus. I had central nervous system symptoms—irregular heartbeat and others. My immune system was way off. Every time I went out I couldn't breathe. I was wheezing from plastic, ballpoint pens, pillows, even moving air. I had to give up my spontaneity and a big chunk of my life. Everyone said it was psychological."

Although asthma sufferers may be stigmatized for their psychological problems, no one blames them for their lifestyles, which may include overwork, poor eating, and/or polluted working and living environments—the aspects that make major contributions to their illness. They do get blamed, however, for what is perceived as their anger, their negative thoughts, or their neurosis. One Boston woman, a young dancer, developed asthma while on tour performing in badly polluted cities in Eastern Europe. Her colleagues, who blamed her bad attitude for the hard time she had breathing, told her to pull herself together! Because the filthy air was affecting her and not them, they felt that it must be her fault.

Nancy Hogshead, the Olympic swimmer, tells how this "tough it out" attitude may have played a part in the lateness of her asthma diagnosis:
"While my teammates were concentrating on stroke technique, kicking

off the wall, and pacing, I was focused on getting air in and out. About once a year I would even lose consciousness from lack of oxygen. My coaches praised my toughness for 'pushing the limits.' "

Hogshead feels that her asthma wasn't diagnosed because she was an Olympic gold medalist, not the stereotypical asthmatic, "a hopeless and passive individual, a hypochondriac. . . .

"There is the prevailing notion that the asthmatic can be cured with the force of their personality. If they could just 'BE TOUGH.' "[2]

Everything Isn't Psychological

Because asthma can be triggered by so many uncontrollable elements—viruses, a change in the weather, pollen count, smoke, cat dander in malls and schools where there is no cat, chemicals outgassing from every kind of man-made object—it is easier for the uneducated public to lash out at the asthmatic with accusations of being neurotic, controlling, guilt-inducing, and manipulative, than to try to understand the complexity of the illness.

Stress and Distress

Reed Moscowitz, M.D., a psychiatrist and the founder and medical director of the Stress Disorders Medical Services at New York University Medical Center, says, "I think what happens in these situations is that the individual has a vulnerability, an Achilles' heel that is the first spot in their system that will give when you put strain on it. And for asthma it's the breathing system which registers physically that stress is too much. It varies with the genetic predisposition of the individual. Although I think that the prime cause is the predisposition, there's always a balance of forces. If the stressful forces are greater than our coping abilities, and we have a predisposition to a certain kind of illness, that could push us over the edge into clinical symptomatology."[3]

And Asthma Causes Stress

"The disease itself brings out many emotional factors which would not be present if it were not for the disease," writes Dr. Irvin Caplin in *The Allergic Asthmatic*. As for emotional factors making asthma worse, he says, "There is certainly no question at all that this can and does occur. In my opinion, however, this is not nearly as common as most patients are led to believe. A doctor who cares for asthmatics on this premise assumes that he has no failures but that his patients' emotional problems are to blame for their asthma. The overall problem is usually a combination of many factors."[4] Accepting the fact that it can work both ways, doctors should look at the patient as a whole and be eclectic in their approach.

Secondary Gain

There is also the problem of secondary gain. As adults, we might ask ourselves:

Now that I have asthma, am I gaining anything by staying sick?

Do I have an attack before I have to speak in public or before an event I perceive as stressful? (We may be intimidated by demands we don't feel we can meet, by others' expectations, or by the need to be assertive.)

Do I suffer the perception of not being safe?

Do I enjoy being taken care of and am I not ready to give that up?

Do I really need a vacation from work?

Although this kind of "secondary gain" may not play a part in your asthma, it may help to assess how much it affects your resistance to doing what you know could make you well again. It may be that the perception of a situation creates the stress that triggers the asthma that keeps you from doing what you want to do. A professional psychologist, a marriage counselor, or a therapist who deals with the fear could be of help here.

There's another kind of secondary gain. The asthmatic child or adult may be the symptomatological member of a dysfunctional family. Things may go better for the family if one member's illness distracts the others from looking at what's really wrong. Although the asthmatic may be accused of using symptoms to get attention, sometimes the family needs to keep this person ill and dependent on them for their own reasons. Family therapy could be of help here.

Denial

Many people who have asthma deny it. Some doctors feel that *denial* is the asthmatic's major psychological problem. In studies in four different countries, only half of the people who doctors diagnosed as asthmatic thought that they had asthma. And doctors are more likely to label women asthmatic than men. So more people may actually have asthma than is known.[5]

Patients who had suffered life-threatening attacks of asthma, according to another study, not only had high levels of anxiety afterward but increased levels of denial.[6] Because asthma is so unpredictable it is easy to deny. It is very hard to admit that you are not in control of your life. Children want to play and be like their peers, and so do adults. It is especially difficult for adults living a "normal" life one minute and short of breath the next to understand this isn't going to disappear on its own.

Dr. Robert Lin says that because of tremendous denial, asthmatics inadequately assess their own conditions. "The reason that asthma doesn't have more advocacy is that the public perceives it as trivial. Even asthmatics talk about their asthma as if it's just a nuisance. 'My asthma flared up a little today'—like someone might complain that their arthritis gets worse in rainy weather. This lack of understanding prevents people with asthma from avoiding triggers, assessing how they feel, and getting help."[7]

My Way of Coping

I vividly remember sitting at home with my medications, sick and weak, my chest so tight I couldn't breathe. I couldn't go anywhere or do anything and was too exhausted to cope with my special diet. I really could have just died there because my "coping mechanism" was, If you don't move you don't need any breath. Besides, I felt that my asthma could change for the better at any moment—it might clear up by itself. Sometimes it seemed to. Then for a couple of hours I would run around and clean, cook, or do the laundry. So sometimes it did temporarily change for the better and sometimes it did not. And when it did not I ended up in the emergency room and I was lucky if there was someone here who could get me there, because with this attitude you can end up not being able to take care of a crisis.

When there is such a disparity between what you tell yourself and what you are experiencing, you must really acknowledge that, respect it, and begin to find the courage to ask "How do I change it?"

What We Can Do

- Imagine life without asthma. What is the difference between my life now and how I imagine it could be, asthma-free?
- Ask "Do I want that?" You really have to recognize your situation to begin to change it. Puffing the inhaler helps give the illusion that all is well. But it should be a sign that things have to change.
- Ask "How can I change this?"

34

- Read on and check off one item in each chapter that you can begin to use to make a difference.
- As you go from chapter to chapter, check off areas of possible interest in which you can begin to work.
- Turn awareness into action.
- Expand your awareness to other areas as you master one new part of your life.
- Take a course in Tai Chi, yoga, or martial arts for learning a different way to work with the body.
- Don't be pessimistic about your prognosis. One Japanese study found that severe asthmatics had compliance problems due to unenthusiam about their therapy.[8] Choose a therapy about which you can feel enthusiatic.

Coping with the Blow of Illness

Each person has a different propensity for what will best help deal with the stress of asthma. For some people visualization is a powerful tool. For others, meditation. Many people need to learn to relax the tension in the neck, shoulders, and back. Dr. Moscowitz says: "An asthmatic attack is the final culmination of stress having built up. So you need help to break the stress at an earlier level before it builds up to the point where you're symptomatic."

THE ROLE OF STRESS IN THEIR LIVES

Nelson Howe is a creative arts therapist who uses movement, art, and the martial arts as part of his therapeutic practice. Howe, a lifetime asthmatic who has been medication-free for several years, says that psychological therapy increased considerably his feeling of being in control of his life, and this helped his asthma. "Each return of my asthma was connected with the stress of not feeling in control of my life. When I work with people with asthma they feel that the body has betrayed them. Learning proper breathing is one way we begin to reverse that. Then the emotional piece of despair and panic needs to be reversed. The third part is to reverse that learned helplessness through the empowerment process. All three need to be operative for healing. It's also important for people with asthma to understand their experience is common to other asthmatics. When you have asthma you feel completely alone; we become isolated and feel it's unique to us. It's important to be able to share the experience of the illness without shame. Asthmatics don't share much because of the old psychological implications."

TAKE STEPS TO COPE WITH STRESS

Dr. Moscowitz uses a three-step process for coping with stress:

1. **Awareness**. Take a moment to do a mind-body scan. Take a moment to focus on feelings. Are my feelings negative or positive? If they are negative, make a note of the negative feeling and what's causing it, because you're going to come back and take a problem-solving approach. And be aware of what your body is feeling. Do you feel anxious? Are you already breathing rapidly and shallowly?
2. **Acting on the awareness**. The first thing to do always is to shift gears quickly through breathing, through that slow, rhythmic yoga-type stomach breathing, because that turns off the adrenaline response and gets us back to normal physiology. Then we can begin, if we are emotionally upset, to take a problem-solving approach to deal with the situation.
3. **Take a problem-solving approach**. If we notice that our muscles are tense, that we have been under a lot of strain, we can do a muscle-relaxation exercise, or we can meditate, or do a visualization exercise.

Dr. Moskowitz feels that quiet pleasures that bring happiness and peace of mind are healing. "Anything that engages our positive emotions, our feelings of mastery, competence, and enjoyment, that enable us to feel good about being alive."

Another Treatment Model—Taoist Healing

Iona Marsaa Teeguarden has combined her knowledge of psychotherapy and acupressure with Taoist philosophy. In her 1987 book *The Joy of Feeling* she talks about stress from the viewpoint of both Eastern philosophies and Western psychology. Her approach is based on an "emotional kaleidoscope"—a five-element model that relates dozens of emotional polarities to particular "elements" and their related meridians and points.

She writes that chronic distressed feelings, in general, negatively affect our physical condition. And although negative emotions are natural, they "must be constantly eliminated. Toxic, destructive thoughts and feelings must be encountered and let go to make room for healing, creative thoughts and feelings."[9]

Iona Teeguarden writes that with illness there may be a "sudden awakening to what is important. . . . Illness can make it very important to let go of that which is destructive and let in that which is creative."[10] "Clinging to old feelings requires physical tension. Prolonged physical and emotional tension is distress."[11]

LETTING COME AND LETTING GO

These concepts come from her study of Taoism and Chinese, Japanese, and Korean ancient healing systems. In Chinese medicine the organs are paired. The lung is paired with the large intestine and one will be affected by the other. Emotions are connected with each organ. The lung holds grief, sorrow, loss, and anxiety. To breathe we must be able to "let in" (air, prana, Qi, oxygen) and "let go" (carbon dioxide, sorrowful emotions). Iona Teeguarden writes, "Difficulty in letting go can manifest in depressed breathing and respiratory problems or in problems of the colon (the Lung's partner organ)."[12] People with respiratory problems may have difficulty in reaching out to other people and letting people come and go in their lives.

CRYING HELPS

In a "Joy of Feeling" workshop, Iona told us that crying is therapeutic for asthma, because the lungs are connected with sorrow. When you feel like crying, let yourself go and cry as much as possible.

Dr. Gerald Epstein also feels that crying has to do with the meaning of asthma—"a crying for freedom, a fight for liberation, a crying over separation and a crying over the loss. The crying is also a demand for autonomy."[13]

MEDITATE AND VISUALIZE HEALTH AND BREATH

Meditation slows the breath and regulates the vibration of the whole body. The Taoists recommended listening to the breath until it is light and quiet as a technique for meditation.[14] People in various parts of the world have been meditating for centuries. The yogis and the Taoists are just some of the people who have understood that meditation and breathing techniques can affect or influence all of the internal organs.

Yogis in India have demonstrated amazing control of their respiratory, digestive, and circulatory systems through years of discipline and practice of mental and physical exercises, in particular the practice of regulating the breath. "Breathing," writes Andrew Weil, a Harvard-trained physician, in his book *Health and Healing,* "is unique in being under the control of both voluntary and involuntary nerves. Possibly, yogic breathing exercises provide a bridge between these two systems, giving the will access to nerves and functions ordinarily closed to it."[15]

In our speeded-up modern life, in which we always feel we must be doing something, it is often hard to take time out and just be quiet. But it is in that silence that we can access and be aware of the deepest and truest part of ourselves, and it is here that healing can begin.

Learning to Meditate

We all know how to concentrate on an external task. Meditation requires that we get used to focusing the mind inward and deepening the experience of perfect concentration. The meditative state transcends concepts of past, present, and future. In meditation there is only "I" consciousness or God consciousness. In meditation we concentrate on *now* and everything else drops away. And right *now* is the right time to begin to learn to meditate:

1. Sit up straight in a comfortable position in a chair with both feet flat on the ground. If you are flexible or already practice yoga, you can sit on a rug or blanket on the floor in a cross-legged position. Sometimes it is most comfortable to sit on the edge of a cushion, allowing the knees to open toward the floor. Maybe at this moment you are curled up on a couch as you read. You may simply sit up cross-legged in the comfort of the cushions for this meditation.

2. Make sure your back is straight without too much strain so that the energy can flow freely up the spine. If you are sitting in a chair, use the back for support and place your feet flat on the floor. If you are sitting on the floor you can use a wall for support. Place your hands on your lap, palms up or down, thumb and forefinger together.

3. Close your eyes and in the stillness listen to your breath. Concentrate on the quiet inhalation and exhalation of air through the nostrils. Keep your shoulders still and breathe gently into your abdomen.

4. Take a neutral position toward your thoughts. Don't work at emptying your mind. When thoughts come, let them go. Don't judge them, or

charge them with any feeling whatsoever. You can meditate on the spaces between your thoughts.

Try to make a special time of day and find five minutes to practice this. Eventually you can increase your time and work up to half an hour or even an hour. The morning on awakening is best. Just sit up in bed and meditate before you get up. You can meditate when you finish the wake-up stretches in chapter 5.

CONTEMPLATION

Quiet contemplation is a good way to relax, destress, and become peaceful. You can sit in your meditation posture and follow the steps for meditation. But instead of meditating between thoughts, you could contemplate one aspect of your life in which you need help. You could ask a question of your inner self as to how to proceed and in the silence deep within, you may find the answer.

CONTEMPLATE NATURE

Those lucky enough to have mountains, water, seashore, gardens, grass, or trees to contemplate can quietly focus on one aspect of these. The rest of us can create little respites in our lives by using bowls of seashells, pebbles, beautiful stones, plants, dried leaves, or fresh flowers to contemplate. These create a link for us with the natural world.

Visualization

Ideas you visualize can affect you emotionally, spiritually, and physically. Most religions use visualization as a basic technique to help people realize their spiritual goals, say Mike Samuels, M.D., and Nancy Samuels in their fascinating book *Seeing with the Mind's Eye.* But ancient peoples also used visualizations for healing the body. "The shaman, or healer often visualized himself going on a journey, finding the sick person's soul, and returning it to him. The shamanistic philosophy of healing sees the cause of illness as a disharmony in the sick person's world."[16]

This idea that imagination could affect the body's functions predated Aristotle, although it was his ideas that were embraced in the Renaissance. Writing about illness and the role of the imagination in a 1976 article in *The Journal of Psychological Medicine,* Carol McMahon says, "Imagination was believed so powerful in inducing physiological changes that it was said to imprint characteristics on embryos in utero."[17]

HEALING THROUGH MENTAL IMAGERY

Dr. Gerald Epstein, psychiatrist and author of *Healing Visualizations: Creating Health through Imagery,* says that for twenty-three years he has worked with mental imagery in many diseases and has had good results with most of them. His work, he says, "is a purely Western-based work; it comes from Western tradition and carries on a traditional Western medicine. In the West until four hundred years ago the mind was a major way of healing."

Dr. Epstein says that the mind is a channel between the invisible and visible worlds. All illness comes from the invisible into visible manifestation. He feels that all the remedies for the mind are in the mind, and that there are three functions of the mind that create these remedies: voluntary will, imagination, and memory. These three functions of the mind can reverse doubt, expectation, and denial, the tendencies of the mind that create all illness. "That's essentially the basis, the pillars on which the Western spiritual medical tradition was constructed. The way of the West was always described as a way of transcendence and as a way of treatment. Waking dream work is a way of transcendence. Short imagery exercise work is a way of treatment."[18]

Yogic philosophy says that in order to have something you must first be able to visualize yourself having it. So let's learn to visualize that "something"—our health!

TECHNIQUES FOR VISUALIZATION

1. Choose a time of day and a place where you can take some time undisturbed.
2. Loosen clothing.
3. Begin "hara" breathing, that is, breathing your attention slowly into the abdomen, using long, complete exhalations.
4. If you lack experience visualizing, try some practice visualizations such as visualizing a circle or a triangle or a three-dimensional object such as a favorite flower. Try to see it in color. Or you could imagine your childhood room and try to see it in detail.
5. When you feel you have mastered the simple visualizations you can move on: Imagine a safe and peaceful place. Try to feel the sensation of really being there in your whole body, in all of your senses. What season is it? What is the temperature? How does it smell?

6. Relax deeply, exhaling completely and soundlessly. Forget about what you think you should be seeing and accept what you see. Feel receptive to your image and experience yourself as calm, peaceful, and in a perfect state of health.

To prepare for visualization, imagine your limbs getting heavy or feeling light and floating. One woman imagines lightness as "falling like a baby." You can start counting backward from ten to one. Tape your visualization and play it back when you sit down to visualize. Researchers working with positive imagery have found that it enhances immune function by producing a rise in T lymphocyte cells.[19]

SOME SAMPLE VISUALIZATIONS

Guided visualization can be very powerful, but some people prefer meditation or making up their own visualizations. People who do best at visualization may be those who can clearly picture objects, a room, or a color easily at will. You need to find an image that is natural to you, deeply meaningful to you, that's really yours.

To get you started, here are some sample visualizations.

A Time Before Asthma Was Learned

Nelson Howe has used guided imagery both in his practice for stress-reduction and for his own asthma. "There were occasions when I used imagery when I'd wake up unable to breathe at four or five in the morning, the worst time. Using imagery, I didn't have to use an inhaler or anything else. I could just lie there and it was as though my body could go backward from that attack to literally experience the time before asthma had been learned."

Here is one of the visualizations he found in a hypnosis workshop:

"I got some incredible images there but one of them proved really important. It felt so real that I had absolutely the experience of flying. Being an eagle. Being way up above clouds that had an ugly gray-and-yellow cast. I was far above, where the air seemed crystalline clear. And I had no problem at all breathing as I floated around up there. In that experience I repeatedly came back to a cliff that seemed to be high up above the clouds. There was a kind of a mountain that projected way up and I could settle there to rest between flights. There was a tactile quality of gripping that rock and breathing that wonderfully clear air. And after a while I would feel that I could push off and soar above those clouds."

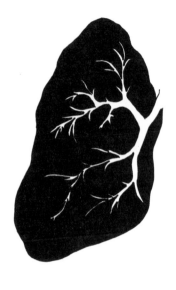

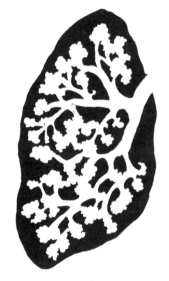

A. Tree in Winter   B. Tree in Summer

The Tree in Summer

Examine carefully figures a and b. The airways of a person with asthma are said to resemble the Tree in Winter (fig. a). The bronchi are the tree trunks; the bronchioles are the branches—small, narrowed, few, and bare of leaves. We can change this and bring first springtime, renewed life, and then the full bloom of summer to our bronchial tree (fig. b).

Slowly breathing into the abdomen (not the upper chest), imagine the white light energy being inhaled into the trunk (the bronchus). Continue slowly and peacefully for as long as it takes to visualize the trunk being filled with light. Then breathe deeper into the main branches (the bronchioles) and see them beginning to fill with light. When the branches are glowing with white light, breathe into the smaller branches (the alveolar ducts) and the tiny blossoms (the alveoli). With each inhalation inhale the light, filling all of the branches with new shoots and twigs of light, and finally, millions of little blossoms filled with light that radiates throughout the lungs.

Begin to inhale more deeply. Inhale the light and exhale all darkness and constriction. Do this until you experience the lungs radiating white light and air. Soon you will see your bronchial tree blooming like the Tree in Summer (fig. b).

The Exorcism

In his 1989 book *Healing Visualizations: Creating Health through Imagery,* Dr. Epstein gives us a visualization called "Exorcism" to heal asthmatic lungs. This can be used, he says, if your asthma is not of recent origin and parental influence or family discordance is a problem. It should be done for three minutes every morning for seven days, or anytime you experience wheezing.

"Close your eyes. Breathe out three times. See yourself taking off your clothes. See yourself in a mirror nude from the neck down. In the mirror, with your right forefinger (left forefinger if you are right-handed), touch on and into your upper chest area from the front all the way around to the back, making a complete circle. Now touch the area of greatest discomfort and *see to whom you can't breathe—that is, see whose face appears in the area.* Who is restricting your breathing, and what color appears there? Breathe that color out via long, slow exhalations while removing from the area whomever you've seen, at first as gently as you can. If the person does not leave easily, use increasing force, going from the gentle to the vigorous, perhaps eventually going so far as to use a golden scalpel to cut out the person. As you are removing this person, tell him/her that he/she has to leave and to stay at a far distance from your body; that he/she will no longer be welcome in you body and will never be allowed to enter your body again. After the removal, see yourself becoming very, very tall and reaching your arms far up into the sky, all the way to the sun. Take a piece of the sun in your palms and place it in the space just vacated. See the area healing, and see how you look and feel. Then, put your clothes back on, breathe out once, and open your eyes, knowing that you are breathing easily."[20]

Kathy is a thirty-eight-year-old psychotherapist who has had asthma since she was a toddler. She says she was never symptom-free until four years ago, when she began the imagery exercises. "I used to be in and out of the hospital all the time. The last time I was hospitalized about eight years ago I almost died. They kept me in the hospital for four days filling me up with steroids. I didn't know there was any other way until I found Dr. Epstein's book and then found him. I did his work and here I am, asthma-free for four years.

"My first step was to do the 'Exorcism' and then to try to use the imagery instead of the inhalers. At first I was very fearful, but one day I decided to try an imagery exercise instead of taking my inhaler, and it worked. I didn't believe this simple exercise could be so effective."

Kathy is now symptom- and medication-free, and if she feels any tightness, she uses the imagery. "The experience of getting better after so many years of being told I wouldn't be able to made me feel that I'm supposed to teach others. But most people are as skeptical as I was of the visualization exercises. They either don't believe it or they say that their asthma is different than mine—they always come up with some reason why they can't cure themselves. I think the big challenge for asthmatics is to let themselves think that they can possibly live without their medication."

CONTACTING YOUR LUNGS THROUGH TAOIST VISUALIZATION

Michael Winn, my Taoist friend and Qi Gong therapist, says there are several levels for making contact with your lungs through visualization. He suggests practicing this and then combining it with the healing hissing sound in chapter 5.

First level is physical. Inhale through the nose and exhale a *hsssssss* and go inside and imagine you are the lungs and you feel what they're like. Dry and spongy, expanding and contracting. Feel them fill with air. Identify with what it's like to be a lung. Notice all the characteristics in as detailed a way as possible—the bronchioles and alveoli, all the little things that are taking in air and energy and passing them on to the bloodstream.

Second level is feeding the lungs color. Inhale through the nose and exhale with a hissing sound but this time add another level, feeding them the color white. As you do, imagine there's a beautiful white cloud all around you and that the cloud is highly charged with electromagnetic energy. Life force is crackling—and you start breathing this in. On the inhale, breathe in this pure white cloud, white light, feeling it charging, cleaning out the lungs; and on the exhale, release any toxins, any dark colors, anything that's blocking them or preventing them from functioning properly. Do this repeatedly—charging your breathing with the white cloud all around you and releasing out.

Third level is contacting the emotional level of the lung function. Inhale and then release all the trapped air. This time imagine that your lungs are two of your own children and you're hugging them. They're a little sad and a little depressed and not feeling very good. You want to go in and hold them and hug them and give them the love that nobody else did. You just noticed that you've been ignoring them all this time or maybe even blaming them for not being healthy. Remember—they are totally innocent children and not to blame. So this is a good time to ask their forgiveness. They've been wounded in some way and they want to be healed. Acceptance, love, and support are ultimately the only things that they need. So tell them you are going to give them all the love they need for the rest of their lives. Thoughts and painful feelings may come up. It's important to accept them, to thank them, and to let them go.

Fourth level is whole body skin breathing. This time you are breathing in and out through the nose because it helps connect the brain to the feelings. The skin is the outer organ of the lungs. You need to let the pores breathe because the skin is releasing all the time. But this is a little more radical—it's these energy fields that are around you all the time that you're not letting in. The life force is trying to pulsate into the rest of you. It's really emotionally coming in, through the skin, into the organs and bones and bloodstream: the direct, primary eating of Qi. Do the healing sound again to release, relax, and see the white cloud but this time breathe in the white cloud, not just into your nose or lungs but through every pore. You're breathing in this white cloud, these charged particles of energy and you feel the whole body breathing in the white light and then breathing out. This is not just a visualization. In Taoism you are actually experiencing this. At first you may not notice much, but eventually you will become conscious that you are moving energy fields in and out of your body. You start to pulsate your skin. You feel a little tingling and you'll feel a little vibration coming into your skin and then as you do it longer it goes deeper into your body. By bringing your awareness to the process you are amplifying it.

Once you do that you have taken a big load off your lungs, because you now have the skin breathing more efficiently and eating Qi directly. The primary source. So you don't need to take as much from air. If you practice this a lot, your whole life just gets more effortless.

CLOSE YOUR EYES AND DREAM

Try one of the guided visualizations or create one of your own. Soon you will know which is best for you. Your needs may change. Accustom yourself to having access to this powerful form of relaxation and self-awareness so it can better serve you when you need it. With practice, meditation, contemplation, and visualization can calm the breath, relax the body, and dispel feelings of panic. Your mind really can affect all of the organs of the body.

A Positive Attitude

Keep a positive attitude! Serafina Corsello, M.D., trained as a psychiatrist and now a complementary doctor in the New York City area, says:

"Patients need constant reinforcement. Changing habits is most difficult. There has to be a change of attitude. People are stuck in a self-destructive mode that they think is the only mode. Pessimism and diffidence are the

greatest nemesis of humanity. Optimism and love are important to living."
She says that attitude plays an important role in getting well and staying
well. "Too many people live with the image of the half-empty glass. It is
far better to see the glass as half-full."[21]

And then we can begin to visualize it filling completely!

CHAPTER 4

GHOSTS OF THE PAST

OUR FAULTY IMMUNE SYSTEMS

Remember all those motherly warnings we were given as kids to "dress warm," "go out to play," "eat your vegetables," and "get to sleep"? We hated hearing them and often didn't heed them, but they turned out to be great advice after all. At one of my asthma workshops a group of people in their thirties asked, "Why us?" They told how they had spent their twenties having such a great time—drinking, eating whatever they pleased, working late at the office, and carousing in clubs until the wee hours. They never considered that their former lifestyles could actually have something to do with those breathing problems that are tormenting them now and ruining the party.

When we start having symptoms of asthma—shortness of breath, wheezing, and chest tightness—we immediately think of going to a doctor to "fix" our lungs. But our lungs and airways are affected only because our particular weakness is there. The reality is that all of the organs and organ systems of our body are interrelated, including the mind, and depend on each other in a miraculously complex series of events.

So if we want to know "why us?" we have to look at how and where we have conducted our lives. "But," you may ask, "isn't there a strong genetic component?" Of course as babies and young children we may have developed asthma through no fault of our own. Let's take a moment to look at this. Let's start with our ancestors.

Is It Genetic?

A doctor once told me that if you want to predict what diseases are in store for you, you must look to your parents and grandparents. Researchers are now trying to find the gene for just about every disease imaginable, and they may someday find the gene for asthma. The good news is that just because asthma may have a genetic component doesn't mean we must manifest this illness. The bad news is that if asthma or allergies are part of your family history you are more likely to be susceptible yourself.

The Allergic Component

You may have been born with allergies because your mother unknowingly ingested food and perhaps milk to which she was allergic during her pregnancy. Babies who are nursed the first year of life are said to have stronger immunity and be less likely to be allergic than those given baby formula. But that may only hold true if your mother herself ate a nutritious diet and not if she continued to ingest allergens while nursing. Foreign proteins can be found in breast milk. A 1931 British researcher explained that this is how "infants may be sensitized to foods with which, to all appearances, they have never come in contact."[1] And women who smoke during pregnancy may give birth to babies who are twice as likely to develop asthma or early respiratory disease.[2] So your immune state and digestive strength during your first year of life might have depended, to some extent, on your mother's diet during pregnancy and breast-feeding.

There can also be a chemical component to a baby's weakened immune system. Your father or mother may have inhaled, ingested, or absorbed toxins from a workplace or living situation. This can also lead to immune deficiency in the not-yet-born infant.[3]

In Chinese medicine they talk about "Prenatal" or "Original Essence." This Essence, the amount and kind of energy you were born with, is determined by the constitution of the parents.[4] We are all born with a certain amount of Prenatal Essence or *Jing*, a basic savings account. Some have a greater vitality and others are weaker. Whatever your Prenatal Essence, whether a weak or strong constitution, you have to conserve what you have. It can be affected for the better through proper nutrition and healthful living, but what is lost can't be replaced.

From the moment of birth the environment can conspire to weaken our immune systems. Chemicals play an increasingly large role, as do molds in the house, poor eating habits, poor digestion, and lack of sleep. As our bodies develop, lots of sweets, sodas, and fast foods can cause lots of problems, including nutritional deficiencies. Other factors such as emotional stress, parasites, candida, bacteria, and viral infections all wear down the body. Our airways may have become symptomatic because there is an underlying genetic weakness, but these other problems are not being addressed by symptomatic relief of the swelling, inflammation, and mucus production of asthma.

Viral infections can provoke acute asthma attacks. One-half of the subjects in a study of adult-onset asthma were found to have developed it following a respiratory infection.[5] Viral infections and colds may also temporarily increase bronchial response to histamine.

BALANCE THE IMMUNE SYSTEM AND IDENTIFY THE ALLERGENS

The quicker that asthma is diagnosed, the quicker a natural intervention can be considered and the easier it is to reverse the process provoking the asthmatic condition, explains Martin Feldman, M.D., a New York City complementary doctor. "This is especially important in children, where, the sooner we can intervene, the more rapid the reversal and more lasting the correction."[6] He finds that with an asthmatic patient there are three basic issues:

1. Allergies have to be analyzed. Overwhelmingly, asthmatics have allergy to dust, dust mites, cats, dogs, molds, pollens, grasses, weeds, and trees, and many also have chemical, formaldehyde, and other allergies.
2. The toxins and the allergens in the food and environment must be controlled so that there is less allergy and immune burden.
3. Third is to test or analyze the immune system function, which almost always needs rebalancing.

REBALANCE THE IMMUNE SYSTEM

Your immune system is made up of a complex network that defends the body against infections and attacks by foreign invaders such as bacteria and viruses. When the immune system is in balance you will not get frequent colds, flu, and allergic reactions.

To rebalance the immune system Dr. Feldman tests the thymus, the lymphatic system, the spleen, and the bone marrow. It is also important to test levels of major immune nutrients: vitamins A, B$_6$, C, and E, as well as bioflavonoids, gamma-linolenic acid (GLA), essential fatty acids (EFA), zinc, and selenium. He does this through kinesiology, but it can also be done through the blood. Foods must be considered as part of the allergy complex. Usually there is heavy environmental or inhalant allergy and as your immunity gets worse and worse, you tend to get more sensitized. That's why you have to do all three: identify the allergens, correct them, and rebalance the immune function.

Dr. Feldman also believes that the body must be detoxified. He writes, "In many instances where I tested the immune system status before and after a one-week juice-and-food cleansing program, the immune system was in better balance and the patient had fewer and less-severe symptoms. Whereas juice and food cleansing programs are generalized body cleansers, more specific programs are available that target the removal of toxins such as heavy metals, including copper or mercury, pesticides, herbicides, and chemicals. There is no question that toxins impair immune system function and thus enhance the problems of immune sensitivity or allergy."[7]

IMMUNE SYSTEM BREAKDOWN

An asthma attack involves many factors that ultimately come about because of immune system breakdown. "In general asthma is an overactivity of the immune system," says Dr. Feldman. "A number of conditions are well known to be related to a diminished or weakened immune state, such as recurrent infections or a lingering cold. In its most extreme state we have what is called the AIDS illness—a very, very severe breakdown of immune function. Asthma is the other side of the immune coin, an imbalance whereby the system is overactive. It's poorly modulated, so instead of doing its job with moderation, it does its job with excess."

For example, a person with a normal immune system would be able to deal with dust entering the body through the eyes, nose, or mouth. But the person with an asthmatic condition and dust allergy has a poorly modulated immune function and the dust will be reacted to in an extreme manner.

A Key Issue

The overactive immune function of the asthmatic requires the exact same nutritional correction as the underactive immune system. Dr. Feldman feels that this is the key to the whole nutritional issue. "The way that we treat this imbalance nutritionally is to use the same building blocks of immune nutrients which are well known to form the essential ingredients of proper immune system function. The nutrients which will help the depletion of immune function found in severe conditions of low immunity are the same nutrients which will help to rebalance the condition found in overactivity of immune function in the asthmatic condition."[8]

WHAT ARE THE IMMUNE NUTRIENTS AND HOW DO THEY WORK?

The nutrients involved in a balanced immune function are:

Vitamin A. Best used as beta-carotene, a precursor of vitamin A and best used for childbearing years because it allows the body to make what A it needs, not the excess A which could hurt the fetus. One of the many functions of both vitamins is to better the body's immune response and resistance to infection.[9]

Vitamin B_6. The most important of all the B vitamins for a healthy immune system. If B_6 is deficient, hormonal activity of the thymus is reduced.[10]

Vitamin B_{12}. Vital for every cell of the body. Vegetarians especially need B_{12}.[11]

Vitamin C. Probably the best-known and most used vitamin. It is a powerful antioxidant and helps the immune system destroy free radicals.[12]

Bioflavonoids. Boost the effects of vitamin C. In the form of quercitin, bioflavonoids are antioxidant and antihistamine.[13]

Vitamin E. High vitamin E levels correlate with optimum immunity.[14]

Essential fatty acid (EFA). Omega-3 oils such as linseed oil or flaxseed oil can produce a significant antiallergy and anti-inflammatory effect.[15]

Gamma linolenic acid (GLA). Found in evening primrose, borage, and black currant seed oil, this has been shown to have a positive effect in immune disorders.[16]

Zinc. A major building block as it works with other vitamins to protect the immune system.[17]

Selenium. Stimulates the immune system and protects against infection. It also works to protect the macrophages' DNA, RNA, and membranes.[18]

Guidance with your vitamin and mineral program by an experienced complementary physician or qualified health professional is advisable in order to tailor your doses to your specific body biochemistry. A therapeutic trial with moderate doses of these nutrients can then be attempted to assess the effect.

How Do We Test for Immune System Nutrients?

Nutrient levels can be tested, but testing for minerals such as zinc and selenium is easier and more accurate than testing vitamins. "Take vitamin B_{12}, for example," says Dr. Feldman. "The blood level of vitamin B_{12} at any one moment does not give the whole picture about vitamin B_{12} metabolism since the vitamin B_{12} that is in transit in the blood doesn't tell us about the entire amount in the body, nor does it tell us the effects of vitamin B_{12} or the body's handling of vitamin B_{12} in a general way. To test for B_{12}, methylmalonic acid is looked for in the urine or homocysteine in the blood."[19]

Another method of testing is through energy medicine, a method of testing the energies of the body's biochemical status by either electrical machines, such as electro-acupuncture machines, or via a shortcut of the same analysis with what is called "muscle testing" (kinesiology).

It's important to know the status of the immune function nutrients because people with immune system problems of any kind, whether over- or underfunctioning, may have a deficiency.

For a Better Immune Response

We can enhance our thymus and lymph glands.

- The thymus gives us the ability to develop an immune response but it is susceptible to stress from many sources including chronic illness. Antioxidants are important for thymic hormone function.[20]
- Vitamin A (used with caution), zinc, vitamin E, beta-carotene, vitamin C, and selenium may be recommended by a nutritional doctor for the health of the thymus gland. Vitamin A and beta-carotene help it produce more T cells.[21]

We can stimulate the lymphatic system.

- Goldenseal, echinacea, and Panex ginseng are herbs recommended to improve lymph function by stimulating macrophages.[22]
- Vitamin B_6 is necessary for the integrity of lymph tissue.[23]
- Sea vegetables are lymphatic cleansers that also detoxify.

The skin, part of the lymphatic system, is another path of detoxification.

- Skin brushing in the morning helps lymphatic function. Use a dry natural-bristle long-handled brush that isn't used for anything else. Michael Alatriste created the Ibiki-Ken method, in which you brush in long strokes starting at the feet, up the legs, from the hands up the arms into the body. The abdomen and buttocks are brushed clockwise, the left chest clockwise, the right chest counterclockwise. Brush the neck up from the clavical to the chin, and the back of the head downward toward the shoulders. This encourages toxins to be released energetically and physically.
- You can also rub the entire body with a damp, hot washcloth before bedtime.
- Swedish massage and chiropractic are helpful for the proper lymphatic flow.
- Exercise such as fast walking, jogging, and aerobics will also increase lymph flow.
- Root herbs such as burdock, echinacea, and licorice are good lymph cleansers. Red clover tea with lemon helps the lymph and is also a good blood cleanser and tonic.[24]
- Additional ways to enhance immune function include slow, sustained breathing exercises, good nutrition, and meditation.
- Poor nutrition and overexercise can deprive the body of nutrients.

The Digestion

Many stomach and intestinal conditions can compromise your immune system by leading to faulty digestion and malabsorption of food. Gastroesophageal reflux and esophageal dysfunction are conditions associated with asthma that are discussed in asthma literature.[25] Gastroesophageal reflux is caused by food being brought up into the esophagus. It is characterized by the heartburn, belching, and burping of indigestion and it occurs more often at night when the person is lying down. "Management" is suggested, which includes eating small but frequent meals, avoiding food or drink between dinner and bedtime (a good idea for everyone), elevating the head of the bed six to eight inches, and avoiding theophylline, caffeine, and fatty and spicy foods.

However, you may not be aware of other digestive problems that may affect your asthma.

Phlegm and the Spleen/Pancreas

We have seen that the asthmatic condition characterized by phlegm in Chinese medicine is thought to be related to the spleen–pancreas meridian. While Prenatal Qi transmitted by the parents determines to some extent our constitution, a second source of Qi comes from digestion of food. This is called "Grain Qi," and its source is the spleen/pancreas—in Chinese medicine the primary organ of digestion, "the foundation of postnatal existence."[26] The digestive system (Earth) is the creator of mucus and the respiratory system (Metal) is the receptor of mucus, explains Taoist herbal practitioner Drew Di Vittorio. He adds that the Metal (respiratory) system includes the large intestine and the skin. So mucus and the accumulation of mucus, the biggest factor in allergies, is directly related to these systems.

A seventeenth-century physician, John Floyer, also felt that defects of digestion and what he called "mucilaginous slime in the stomach" were "the immediate cause of asthma."[27]

Are You Absorbing What You Eat?

Today a small but growing number of alternative and complementary doctors are interested in the digestive process in treating asthma and allergies. They find that children under the age of sixteen and sometimes adults with asthma have a much higher probability of low stomach acid, low pancreatic enzymes, or a combination of both. These conditions create a greater likelihood of malabsorption. Combined with problems of the food supply, it is all the more likely that there are nutrient deficiencies. Absorption and assimilation have to be optimized.

Orthodox medicine does not always recognize the problem of faulty digestion until it's severe. Doctors recognize the malabsorptive process when there are states of extreme depletion of the body, with weight loss and major breakdown of absorption, but not when absorption is sluggish or inefficient.

Too little hydrochloric acid will result in food not being digested properly. And needed nourishment from food and/or supplements will not be absorbed. If you have low stomach acid you may experience belching, burping, bloating, undigested food in the stool, weak or cracked fingernails, indigestion, and possible yeast overgrowth.

Testing the Digestion

There are several laboratory tests that can determine the amount of hydrochloric acid in the stomach, including the gastrogram, developed at the

University of Heidelberg. These tests are widely used in Europe but uncommon in the United States.

PANCREATIC ENZYMES

Most absorption of food takes place in the small intestine and for this process to be effective we need proper pancreatic enzymes and bile. Enzymes produced by the pancreas are critical for digestion. For those who are deficient, pancreatic enzymes can be taken as supplements with a meal. A good combination pancreatic enzyme supplement might include amylase, protease, and lipase. Your complementary physician has several ways to test for pancreatic enzymes depending on your condition.

STOOL ANALYSIS

Digestive deficiency can be tested by analysis of the stool. The Great Smokies Laboratory is the leader in stool testing (see Resources). Any physician can order this test, which determines how well the digestive system breaks down and assimilates the components of the meal. Yeast overgrowth, as well as the presence or absence of friendly or pathogenic bacteria and parasites, can also be tested. All asthma patients could benefit from this test.

OTHER ASPECTS OF THE LOW ACID STATE

Stomach acid is one of the major acids of the body. If sufficiently low it may create an imbalance of the body's acid base, perhaps tipping it toward an alkaline state. So the constant interplay between acid production and the rest of the body's acid/alkaline balance should always be considered.

LEAKY GUT SYNDROME

Another digestive problem to consider is leaky gut. A hydrochloric acid deficiency can lead to bacterial overgrowth says immunologist Leo Galland, M.D., and not uncommonly is one of the things that contributes to the "leaky gut syndrome."

You may not have heard of leaky gut syndrome, a disorder that leads to increased permeability of the intestines. Viruses, bacteria, and nonsteroidal anti-inflammatory drugs such as aspirin are common triggers or mediators that can damage the mucosa that protects the functioning of our intestines. Food allergies can also create intestinal permeability, but leaky gut syndrome more commonly creates food allergies.

Dr. Galland says, "Any disorder associated with food allergy is associated with leaky gut. In people whose asthma is food allergic, leaky gut may be part of what's going on." There are several aspects of the leaky gut problem. If there is malabsorption, then nutritional supplementation, if needed, will not be well absorbed. If there is bacterial overgrowth, then nutritional supplements may not be well tolerated.[28] In some cases malnutrition can develop. Dr. Galland suggests a nutrient-rich, allergen-free diet, and because hyperpermeability can affect the function of the pancreas, pancreatic enzymes may be required.[29]

THE LIVER

The liver in those with leaky gut syndrome has to work overtime. To help repair the mucosa and support the liver, Dr. Galland suggests basic vitamin and mineral supplementation, including all the B vitamins, retinol, ascorbate, tocopherol, zinc, selenium, molybdenum, manganese, and magnesium. Additionally, lactobacillus GG, glutathione (GSH), and N-acetyl cysteine might be used. Flavonoids such as quercetin, plus essential fatty acids and fiber supplements are also sometimes recommended.[30]

MORE NATURAL LIVER SUPPORT

Digestion and elimination and detoxification of the body are major tasks of the liver. If the liver is congested and not functioning properly these processes go awry.

Christopher Hobbs, a fourth-generation herbalist and practitioner of traditional Chinese medicine, has written a fascinating book about the liver entitled *Foundations of Health: The Liver and Digestive Herbal* in which he explains the herbs, tonics, and bitters that provide nutrients to help strengthen and stimulate the processes of the body. His recommendations include:

- "Bitters," the tonics that contain bitter herbs such as artichoke (which in Italy is used as a digestive).
- Bitter greens to activate the immune system and help activate the secretion of hydrochloric acid, bile, and other digestive enzymes.
- Raw fruits and vegetables, which act as cleansers.
- Foods like cabbage, broccoli, nuts, and seeds containing sulfur, which help build enzymes.
- Antioxidants, minerals, amino acids, and flavonoids, all of which help protect the liver.[31]

Hobbs explains that when high levels of toxins and pathogens such as *Candida albicans* burden the liver, it can't do its job of breaking down and eliminating bacteria, toxic chemicals, and other debris. In the following section we are going to learn about *Candida albicans*, a yeast which can result from poor immune function, and find out how it may adversely affect our asthma.

THE YEAST CONNECTION

I had noticed the half dozen books on the subject of candida in the health food stores but never dreamed it had anything to do with my asthma.

In the days when things like this were not widely discussed, I had "yeast" problems. Nowadays everyone who watches TV knows about women and their yeast problems, as pharmaceutical companies battle it out, promoting products over the counter that used to be had only with a doctor's prescription. Anyway, I would never have connected that with my asthma.

One rough New York winter, between semesters, I went south to yoga camp to work on my breathing and shape up. I was enjoying a cabin all to myself until one day, returning from lunch, I found a smiling, bright-eyed roommate. "I may wheeze all night," I told her, to warn of my breathing difficulties. "I know what's wrong with you," she said, "and I'm going to make you all better!"

And that's how I learned about candida. So how could a yeast problem affect my breathing? It was explained to me how you can start out with yeast in one part of your body and it can very quietly move to another part, such as the respiratory tract. She told me how she had suffered from exhaustion for two years, some days not being able to get out of bed. Finding a doctor to treat her candida had turned her into this energetic, smiling person with whom I was now speaking.

It was a fascinating story—but, I thought, a little far-fetched and highly unlikely. I tucked it into a corner of my mind with all the other strange information I was collecting and didn't do anything about it until I got out of the hospital a month later—after my third and last visit—breathing, but weaker than ever. This time I promptly went to the health food store and bought a few of those books about candida.

So What's the Connection?

Candida albicans's connection to a variety of illnesses has been controversial since Dr. William Crook's book *The Yeast Connection and the Woman* hit the bookstores over a dozen years ago. Because candida overgrowth is not easily determined by laboratory tests or physical examination, many doctors don't feel certain about a diagnosis. And conventional medicine still doesn't believe that a yeast found in all healthy bodies can be giving anyone a problem.

Yeasts, says Dr. Crook, are single-cell living organisms that live on the surface of all livings things. Yeast is a kind of fungus, and one family of yeasts, *Candida albicans*, normally lives on the inner warm creases and crevices of your digestive tract and vagina. But, he says, it's a kind of Dr. Jekyll and Mr. Hyde because "it can branch from a single cell yeast form into a branching fungal form. And these branches can burrow beneath the surfaces of your mucous membranes."[32]

Candida doesn't cause everyone problems. But when the body is weak or compromised by certain drugs, candida can run wild and an overgrowth can occur. Dr. Crook has found that most, if not all, of the people who develop a candida problem have a history of taking antibiotics, especially broad-spectrum antibiotics, birth control pills, and/or steroids for extended periods of time. So in the case of asthma, those of us who have had to use prednisone, for instance, are going to be susceptible even if we had no yeast problem before the asthma. Antibiotics which kill off friendly yeast organisms include amoxicillin, ampicillin, Ceclor, and tetracycline. Antiulcer medications such as Zantac (ranitidine) and Tagamet (cimetidine) also encourage candida overgrowth in the stomach.[33] In addition, substances such as sweets, alcoholic beverages, environmental molds, and yeast-containing foods are on the list of items to avoid for people who develop candida.

Candida can also develop from hormonal imbalances during pregnancy, or from birth control pills. And while a weakened immune system can cause candida to take over, it also works the other way around—an overgrowth of yeast can interfere with a cell's ability to protect itself and so the candida can suppress immune function.[34]

Respiratory problems like asthma, sensitivity to chemicals (which may trigger an attack), and eczema can also can be yeast-related.

Can We Have an Allergy to Candida?

Candida plays a central role in many, many allergies, says New York City complementary physician Warren Levin, M.D. Although it's possible to be asthmatic without having candida, if you have it for a long time, he says, you become allergic to it. "Then there is usually a gradual spreading of the allergy phenomenon and with that spreading some trigger comes along and then asthma can certainly come into the picture. The combination of steroids and antibiotics is a major player in the development of candida."[35]

Dr. Leo Galland also feels that an allergy to candida aggravates asthma. "Some asthmatics will have candida not only in the stool, in the gut, but also in the bronchial tubes, because they have used a lot of cortisone and had a lot of antibiotics. Especially if you use cortisone inhalers. So you could start out with a small yeast problem and have asthma and end up with a big yeast problem as a result of the drugs used to treat you because you were sick. One of the official side effects of the inhaled steroids include a yeast infection in the throat (thrush) or even the bronchi, because you are inhaling them down into the bronchi. These inhaled steroids are thought to be the drug of choice, with the least side effects, but what are they comparing them with? All steroids or with bronchodilators?"

Is Yeast Playing a Role in Your Health Problems?

Dr. Crook writes that you may be able to tell if yeast plays a role in causing your health problems if you have had several of these experiences:

1. Feel "sick all over" but causes haven't been found.
2. Have taken prolonged courses of broad-spectrum antibiotic drugs.
3. Have been pregnant.
4. Have taken birth control pills and/or steroids.
5. Are troubled by fatigue and muscle aches.
6. Symptoms are worse on damp days and in moldy places.
7. Crave sugar.
8. Feel spaced out or suffer memory or concentration problems.
9. Are bothered by depression, irritability, headaches, and/or digestive problems.
10. Are sensitive to tobacco, smoke, perfume, and other chemicals.
11. Have been bothered by recurrent vaginal, prostate, or urinary infections.
12. Have been bothered by hormone disturbances, including PMS, menstrual irregularities, sexual dysfunction, and low body temperature.
13. Suffer from constipation, diarrhea, bloating, or abdominal pain.
14. Are bothered by chronic fungus infections of the skin or nails.[36]

Dr. Crook believes that asthma is a yeast-related disorder which affects men and women equally.

What Steps Can We Take to Get Rid of the Yeast?

- Try a yeast-free, mold-free diet, and eliminate all items that might encourage yeast. Two of the most important points:
  a. Avoidance of sugar and simple carbohydrates. Candida multiplies in the presence of sugar, so some diets even suggest removing all carbohydrates for the first several weeks or months.
  b. Avoidance of allergy-provoking foods.
- *Lactobacillus acidophilus* is often taken before meals to help repopulate the gut with friendly bacteria.[37] Some people need lactose-free acidophilus.
- Good digestion is important for preventing and recovering from candida overgrowth.
- Caprylic acid or citrus seed extracts (ParaMicrocidin) are nonprescription antifungals which some doctors recommend either alone or combined with medication.
- A couple of drops of tea tree oil in hot water makes an antifungal tea recommended by herbalist Letha Hadady.
- Garlic and green plants rich in chlorophyll, such as barley and wheat grass, are also recommended.
- A complementary doctor can confirm candida and prescribe more potent drugs for difficult problems if necessary. But medication alone won't rid the body of candida, so the antiyeast diet is very important.

Serafina Corsello, M.D., finds that yeasts are a big problem because they produce a lot of toxic by-products. She feels that antibiotics such as nystatin should not be taken all the time because the yeasts become resistant to it. Instead, she tries to build up the immune system, put the intestines in good order, do allergy desensitization, and give antioxidants for immunological reserve. "Patients have to watch their diet and watch their stress."[38]

Everything Plays a Part in a Weakened Immune System

In addition to yeasts, says Dr. Crook, nutritional deficiencies, viral infections, environmental chemicals, emotional stress, parasites, and environmental molds all play a part in weakening the immune system. To restore immune function Dr. Crook recommends selenium and other antioxidants as well as identifying additional vitamin, mineral, amino acid, and fatty acid deficiencies. He recommends staying on your yeast and gluten-free diet, exercising, and avoiding chemicals.

Parasites

Parasites and candida may go together. In a series of patients who had candida, Dr. Levin found that 50 percent of them also had parasites. Parasites, he says, are associated with a high eosinophil count because people are allergic to the parasites they're infected with, just as with candida you become allergic to the candida. "However, I do not normally see elevated eosinophils in people with uncomplicated candida problems. Even if they're severe they don't raise the eosinophil count, whereas parasites have a tendency to raise the count even when they're mild."

Dr. Rea's Rain Barrel Total Load

William J. Rea, M.D, well-known author, researcher, and director of the Environmental Health Center of Dallas, Texas, has been instrumental in helping us understand the effect that our environment has upon our immune systems.

According to his theory of "the total load," your resistance is like a rain barrel filling up at each exposure to pollutants that enter through air, food, and water. As we are chronically or acutely exposed to toxins, allergens, and bacteria, the barrel fills until it can hold no more and spills over into illness. Along the way, an infection can make it "spring a leak."

Dr. Levin says that the concept of the total body load is important to understand. "In that diagram Dr. Rea is saying that each person can be represented by the rain barrel, which is a different size for different people. What you were born with, to some degree; what you did with what you were born with; what nature and other things did; how many illnesses you've had; and nutritional deficiencies and toxicities all have to do with the size of the rain barrel. And then you put a bucket of this, and a bucket of that— the rain barrel is capable of holding up to a certain point and when it finally spills over you have symptoms. The tendency is to look at the last bucket that went in and say 'I'm allergic to this' and ignore all the other stuff."

Infection Lowers the Threshold

"Infection is shown as a spike which lowers the threshold. Everybody knows that if you get a cold or sinusitis your asthma can be worse. But that's acute infection and I think chronic infection is more likely to load up the barrel. When people have chronic infection—dental infection, sinus infection, prostate infection, pelvic infection, but most important, intestinal infection with candida and parasites—they become allergic to what they are carrying as an infection organism that is there twenty-four hours a day, 365 days a year. It's an unremitting nudge against the immune system, whereas most allergy is intermittent. There are breaks in your exposure to most environmental substances but not to what's inside. The immune system gets worn down and exhausted; it has deployed all its troops just trying to hold the line against these things, and when something else comes along it can't handle it."

Your Yeast-Free Diet

Many candida sufferers are allergic to the yeast and molds in foods, and eating foods to which you are allergic will weaken your immune system. Some products acquire yeast and molds through manufacture and storage. Anticandida diets usually call for the elimination of these yeast-containing foods:

- Leavened products such as breads, rolls, muffins, bagels, cakes, cookies, crackers, pretzels, croutons, and bread crumbs
- Grains that are enriched, processed, or bleached
- Most dairy products containing lactose or milk sugar such as cheese, cream cheese, light creams, milk, skimmed milk, sour cream, buttermilk, sour milk products, and most yogurts
- Artificial dairy substitutes (rice and oat milk are fine but are not sources of calcium)
- Flours that are white, bleached, enriched, or processed
- All malted products, such as malts and malt syrup
- Fermented beverages, beer, wine, cider and ginger ale, miso, and soy sauce
- All mushrooms and truffles
- Boxed and canned soups containing MSG
- Coffees and teas (which unfortunately have molds) except Taheebo tea (also called Pau D'Arco or Lapacho)

- Condiments, sauces, and foods containing vinegar: MSG, barbecue and other commercial sauces, ketchup, green olives, horseradish, mayonnaise, mustard, pickles, pickled foods, relishes, salad dressing, sauerkraut, soy sauce, etc.
- Fruit juices and fruit drinks, canned, bottled, and frozen
- Peanuts, cashews, and pistachios and their butters
- Pickled and smoked meats
- No vitamins that are not labeled yeast-free
- Yeasts: baker's yeast, brewer's yeast, citric acid, hydrolyzed vegetable protein, MSG, torula yeast

Also:

- Sugar in all forms should also be eliminated.
- High-gluten foods should be minimized.
- Antibiotics, birth control pills, and steroids should be eliminated along with over-the-counter drugs that contain sugar. Liquid theophyllines are in this category.
- Eat a nourishing diet. A doctor interested in discovering and treating your candida can also help you restore immune function with a proper diet and nutrients.
- Some people confronted with the antiyeast diet feel that there's nothing left to eat. But there's plenty of wonderful eating yet to come. And the substitutions you'll be making will definitely be to your advantage.

SUBSTITUTE YEAST-FREE GRAIN PRODUCTS

There are now many products in health food stores that are yeast-free. Read labels carefully.

Look for rice cakes, puffed rice cereal, hot rice cereal, brown rice snaps, rice noodles, Rudolph's rye bread, sourdough breads, Mana bread, Kavli rye crackers in the red box, Wasa *lite* rye crackers, whole wheat matzo, yeastless spelt bread, DeBoles pasta products, Udon and Soba noodles, Chinese cellophane noodles, tortillas, taco shells.

Taheebo tea comes from the bark of a Brazilian tree on which mold doesn't grow. Anti-fungal, -viral, and -bacterial, it helps to keep candida in check.

I've encountered a number of women as well as men who have improved remarkably from the yeast-free diet. Jenny, a thirty-six-year-old teacher, for instance, was in the hospital for a week after her first asthma attack in 1990. "They gave me aminophylline intravenously which gave me heart palpitations and almost led to cardiac arrest. I felt I had gotten sick because of my period but no one would listen. They also gave me Asmacort, Ventolin, and Proventil pills. The very first time I found out about yeast was when I came to your workshop and I went straight to the doctor and got it treated. He said it is the yeast that makes the asthma worse before my period. The gynecologists said that my period had nothing to do with it. My biggest problem now is food. If I stop eating fermented foods or yeast-related products and foods that contain gluten, my asthma goes away! I'm the picture of health in two weeks."

Dana, a forty-two-year-old office manager, became ill in 1989 and went to a number of doctors, internists, and pulmonary specialists who diagnosed asthma and prescribed a number of medications but didn't discuss allergies, although she had had severe eczema as a child. "Then I went to an allergist and found that I was allergic to molds and grasses. The shots didn't always help and when I started to get reactions to them I stopped.

"There were a lot of things from your workshop that I started doing. It helped to realize that more of the problems were allergy-related. I started cutting out white refined sugar, wheat, and yeast, and I sensed a swelling up when I tried using them again. I started to notice which foods were bothering me. I think that yeast made the biggest difference. If I cut out yeast I'm in good shape."

How a Yeast-Free Diet Helped Me

Learning about candida was crucial to my own progress in recovering from asthma. Although my macrobiotic diet had some excellent features, the seitan (a wheat product) and tempeh and other fermented foods were not doing me any good. When I eliminated them along with other ferments and allergens, (such as barley malt and sunflower seeds and oils), my improvement was great.

Today I can eat fermented food occasionally. But if I find myself eating too many yeasty products in restaurants or while traveling (I don't have the stuff otherwise), I go right back to a strict yeast-free diet and improve fast.

OUTSIDE INFLUENCES

We are bombarded by toxic substances in our environment—in our food, in our air, and in our water. Toxins permeate products with which we wash our clothes, personal products we use on our bodies, and products with which we furnish our houses. The ability of our bodies to rid themselves of these toxins largely determines our health.

The Food

While our ancestors enjoyed the fruits of farming with rich topsoil and non-pesticide-treated seeds, modern agricultural processes have resulted in foods depleted in nutrients and saturated with a variety of chemicals. In the first half of the century, consumers in this country enjoyed locally grown seasonal fruits and vegetables that did not have a long lag time traveling from farm to supermarket (where they may be sprayed again with fungicides). They were not grown specifically to "hold up" while they lingered on shelves waiting for someone to buy them.

When I was a child, a farmer went door to door several times a week in our Philadelphia neighborhood, selling fresh eggs, milk, and chicken. Animals were not fed with hormone- and antibiotic-laden feed. It was exciting to eat fruits and vegetables only when in season. Today a whole generation is used to seeing every kind of edible available any time of year from anywhere in the world. But unless they grow their own produce, buy it from a farm stand or farmer's market, or travel abroad, they have no idea how wonderful food can taste.

Then there is fake (but fat-free) food, and additives, dyes, preservatives, and artificial sweeteners. Soon we will be seeing the results of irradiated and genetically engineered seeds.

Even with the huge array of products available, including whole and organic foods, most people seem to be too busy or too indifferent to make good choices. Fast food, always popular, is on the rise. And so in this land of plenty, people are probably more nutrient-deficient than ever before. Supposedly we are living longer these days than previous generations—but it seems to me, when it comes to eating well, my parents' and grandparents' generations did a lot better.

Most American cities do not have clean air, and according to Dr. Morton Lippman, a professor of environmental studies at New York University, pollution today is often even higher in rural areas.[39] Today the amount of available oxygen in the air is almost 50 percent less than it was a few hundred years ago.[40]

Dr. William J. Rea is one of the doctors who has shown how exposure to chemicals can have an adverse effect on your immune system. In a lecture in 1994 in New York City he spoke about chemical pollution and its consequences:

"Thirty years ago in Dallas, we had 360 days of crystal blue sky; now there are about six days of it. We have a city that has no industry—all we have are cars. So what's in the air? Nothing much—Two hundred and forty-eight tons of acetone to dissolve your nervous system. One hundred and eighty-nine tons of bichloroethylene to degrease you. It will remove spots in your nervous system, remove your neuro-sheaths. Tylene? Another solvent that will screw up your blood vessels. We've got sixty-nine tons of freon, a fluoride compound. You've all heard about fluoridation in drinking water. Well, we breathe the stuff. We've got solvents—xylene, hydrochloric acid and ammonia in the air—about seventeen tons of it, but we neutralize it with sodium hydroxide. And we could go on and on because this is true of most city air. You're breathing that all the time, so just to get up in the morning you have to be able to counteract these kinds of substances."[41]

OZONE AND THE "SPREADING EFFECT"

Ozone is the most harmful ingredient in smog and is found in all large urban areas at unhealthy levels. Ozone is also found in unexpected places such as outgassing from copy machines, color laser printers, and electrostatic precipitating air "purifiers." According to the American Lung Association, not only is ozone linked to emergency-room admissions and hospitalizations for respiratory problems; it also affects millions of otherwise healthy people who are sensitive to it. A study at the University of Toronto found that patients who inhaled air with what the EPA set as a safe level of ozone became twice as sensitive to ragweed and grasses as when they inhaled clean air.[42] Dr. Noe Zamel, director of the pulmonary function labs at the university, suggested in an interview in the *New York Times* that ozone may increase permeability of the airways, allowing more allergen to enter.

Because of our perception of the seemingly endless ability of the streams, lakes, rivers, and oceans to renew themselves, and because water is such a good solvent for so many organic materials, we have just about finished off the pure water on this planet by employing the liquid two-thirds of the earth's surface as our own personal dumping ground.

NOT A DROP TO DRINK

Unfortunately, municipal water-treatment plants, constructed mostly in the early part of the century, were made to kill bacteria and disinfect rather than to detect and remove chemicals, radioactive wastes, and other contaminants. Even if these plants could purify water, it would probably be fouled again before it reached your glass by chemicals leaching from city plumbing or even from your own household pipes, which may be made of lead or copper.

CHLORINE

Municipal water supplies are treated to deactivate microbiological contaminants, which consist of bacteria, protozoa, and viruses. The chemical most commonly used to kill these microorganisms is chlorine. Chlorine was first added to drinking water in the United States in 1908 to kill typhoid and cholera germs.

Two Tucson physicians cited chlorinated water as a cause of asthma back in 1934.[43] Dr. Alfred Zamm writes: "For a chlorine-sensitive person, a shower with chlorine-treated water can trigger all manner of problems, because the heating and splashing of the water aerosolizes chlorine-infused droplets and liberates quantities of gas, both to be breathed in the confines of the shower stall. The dissolved gas is also released when heated in the laundry, for example, or in a swimming pool, or even in a closed bathroom from a hot tub of water."[44]

Heavy Metals

Heavy metals also play a part in the destruction of immune function, through ingestion, absorption, and inhalation of fumes. Let's take a look at where some of these metals are coming from.

THE TOOTH CONNECTION—MERCURY FILLINGS

People with asthma, says Dr. Zamm, are immunologically impaired and do not tolerate the environment. And mercury control, he says, is the "ultimate" in environmental control.[45] Dr. Zamm feels strongly about two ways to go about "fixing what's broken." One is through the nutrient selenium, which enhances the patient's ability to withstand petrochemical onslaught; the other is through the removal of silver dental amalgams, because they contain mercury. This filling removal doesn't work for everyone and there is no test to find out if it is going to work for you. However, many doctors and dentists conclude that mercury is a toxin and we are slowly being poisoned by having this stuff in our mouths. Dr. Zamm feels that root-canal teeth should be pulled as there are many toxic chemicals such as chlorothymol and iodothymol put into root canals. (Pulling these teeth is the subject of some controversy.) He says his asthma patients begin to recover when their mercury fillings and root-canal problems are taken care of. "First things first," says Dr. Zamm. "First get out the toxins, the mercury fillings and root canals, and then talk philosophy." In *The Journal of Orthomolecular Medicine* Dr. Zamm writes: "Mercury poisoning is the greatest masquerader of our time. Dentists are not in a position to see the cause and effect relationship of the insertion of the mercury and the development of illness three to 10 years later. Even the patient himself does not connect the illness to the original dental process."[46]

In addition to selenium, Dr. Zamm recommends taking zinc because it competes with mercury and may be protective to some extent. He recommends his patients take 50 mcg of yeast-free selenium twice a day, because it binds with mercury to "render it biologically inert in some respects," and 15 mg of zinc once a day, both after eating.[47]

(Dr. Zamm's protocol for safer dentist visits is in Appendix II.)

Nina, a magazine editor, developed asthma in the winter of 1992 when she was thirty-six years old. "I'm all better now. I believe the immediate cause was mold and I think the primary reason I got asthma was because I had candida. I was treated through the antiyeast diet and an elimination diet; finally Dr. Zamm made me get the fillings out and I've never had asthma since. I had six enormous mercury fillings, so big that they had to cap the teeth. They were capped with gold and porcelain. I can't remember a time when I didn't have fillings in every single one of my molars and other teeth as well.

"When I got sick I didn't really understand that it was asthma; I experienced it as shortness of breath. When I found out I was allergic to mold, an allergist prescribed inhalers and shots but I felt that this was not getting to why I had the asthma. I was a very sick person at that point. I had Epstein-Barr and mononucleosis, which I had gotten in the fall of 1989, and had never recovered. I couldn't stay awake, I never had any energy, my memory was affected, my digestive system was affected. Earlier I had had vaginal yeast infections, bladder and urinary infections. I had taken birth control pills for five years, and antibiotics since childhood. Asthma was the last thing on the list. At that point I had never been to any alternative doctors, but regular doctors were totally unable to help me; they never understood that all of my symptoms were related and that they were all allergic. Dr. Zamm understood this and got rid of them. I know he saved my life."

OTHER SOURCES OF MERCURY

Mercury can be found in many everyday products, sometimes as a preservative. Look for mercury in water-based outdoor paints, artist paints, pesticides, antiseptics, chemical fertilizer, treated seed, fish, cosmetics, fabric softeners, floor waxes and polishes, pharmaceuticals, wood preservative, fluorescent lamps, furniture polish, air-conditioner filters, cellulose sponges, calomel, body powders and talcs, thermometers, adhesives, and Mercurochrome.

What We Can Do

- Avoid exposure by reading product labels carefully.
- Avoid silver amalgams when having teeth filled.
- Clean up broken fluorescents or thermometers immediately. Wear disposable dust mask and gloves. Damp mop so that vapor will not be dispersed throughout the house.
- Provide plenty of fresh air for painting and renovation.
- Limit fish consumption and buy fish from different sources. Watch out for tuna and swordfish, which tend to absorb more mercury.

ALUMINUM

Some of the many sources of aluminum exposure are pots and pans, dental crowns and amalgams, baking powder, antacids, deodorants, construction materials, aluminum cans and foil, pesticides, toothpaste, ceramics, food color additives, table salt, cigarette filters, animal feed, and bleached flour. Alum is used to kill bacteria in drinking water.[48]

- Avoid aluminum exposure through cooking by using pots made of stainless steel, glass, or Corning Ware.
- Read labels carefully.
- Wear proper masks for dusty procedures in the workplace.
- Air home and workplace thoroughly no matter the weather.

COPPER

Although copper is an essential element, there are situations in which it can become a toxin. Copper excess disturbs the body's copper/zinc balance and leads to zinc deficiency.[49]

What We Can Do

- Check water for copper levels if you have copper pipes and plumbing. This is a major source of too much copper in the body.
- Tin-lined copper cookware wears out fast. Use for decorative purposes only.
- Don't use fungicides containing copper in swimming pools.
- Avoid copper intrauterine birth control devices.

LEAD

Lead is well known for its toxicity because of its prevalence in house paint and industry. Lead can enter the body through ingestion and through inhalation of dusts and absorption through broken skin. There is no safe level for lead.

We may still be exposed to lead from house paint, which was legal for use until 1977; stocks in warehouses were being used up well into the eighties. Other lead exposures come through auto exhaust fumes, lead plumbing, drinking water, heavy crystal glassware, pottery, cheap ceramic and fine china dishes, pesticides, hand-painted glassware and dishes, canned juices, and evaporated milk.

What We Can Do

- Hire a professional to test paint at work or at home.
- Test with lead check swabs—use lead check swabs on walls and to check dishes, mugs, and cups for lead in glazes.
- Use only a HEPA filter vacuum such as the Nilfisk to clean. Otherwise damp mop.

- Do not renovate or repaint unless lead is first abated.
- Encapsulating existing lead paint is safer than removal.
- Run tap water until it's cold, especially if it hasn't been run for at least six hours. Save the runoff for washing dishes or watering plants.
- Don't use hot water, which is more likely to contain lead, for cooking, drinking, or making infant formula.

TESTING FOR HEAVY METALS

Mainstream doctors don't usually test for heavy metals unless there is an "occupational" hazard. However, many hazardous exposures occur in the home. You can be tested by hair analysis, blood, or urine, depending on the doctor, laboratory, and what you are being tested for. Follow the advice of a knowledgeable environmental doctor for this.

Other Immune Suppressors

POSITIVE IONS, ANOTHER NEGATIVE OUTSIDE INFLUENCE

Ever wonder why on certain days you feel exhilarated and other days you feel awful? Air is made up of molecules that are positively or negatively charged, and when the air is fresh and well balanced there is a ratio of five positive ions to four negative ions. Both are necessary for human life.[50]

After a thunderstorm people usually feel great. But in certain locations and weather situations (dry winds, siroccos, mistrals) the balance is upset by too many positive ions. This also occurs in pressurized airplane cabins, cars, air-conditioned offices full of computer terminals and other machinery, and in homes with sheets, carpets, and couches made with synthetics, as well as by wearing synthetic materials. Any electrical environment will be imbalanced in this way.

This is especially pertinent for those with asthma because too many positive ions actually affect the ability to breathe. According to a 1991 study, researchers found that the cilia, the microscopic hairs that line the lower part of the throat and sweep out the dusts and pollens, are stimulated by negative ions and depressed by positive ones. Positive ions slow the delivery of oxygen while negative ions facilitate it.[51]

What We Can Do for Ion Balance

- Take a "breather" during the day and get out of the house for at least a half an hour.
- A trip to the seashore provides air rich in negative ions.

- Wear natural fabrics, especially cotton, which is neutral. Make sure bed-clothes and night clothes are cotton.
- Don't redecorate with synthetic materials. Get rid of synthetic carpets and drapes.
- Open windows every day.
- Ionizers are not the answer, as they put ozone in the air, and this can actually destroy lung tissue.

DETOXIFICATION

All of the chemicals and pollutants we have discussed here, says Jeffrey S. Bland, Ph.D., a noted researcher and nutritionist, plus the substances we produce in our own intestinal tracts, can be put in one word: *xenobiotics*. Dr. Bland says, "Over millions of years of evolution, our bodies developed a mechanism to resist exposure to toxins which would otherwise jeopardize the function of our nervous, immune, endocrine, cardiovascular, pulmonary, musculoskeletal, hepatobiliary and renal systems. The mechanisms by which our bodies protect themselves from xenobiotic exposures are related to detoxification processes which are influenced by diet and nutrients."

Dr. Bland goes on to describe how this detoxification is controlled by the enzyme systems. Several organs such as the liver, kidneys, and intestines work together to turn the toxic materials into nontoxic ones that can be excreted from the body. If your "total load" of xenobiotics is greater than your body's ability to do this, "subtle signs and symptoms of toxicity, initially affecting primarily the immune, endocrine and gastrointestinal systems, may result."[52]

The absorption of proper nutrients, as we have seen, depends on proper digestion. This is of major importance, as is an optimum diet. These factors will affect how well your body detoxifies xenobiotics.

Fasting

Various kinds of fasts have gained in popularity but recent research suggests that fasting can have the opposite effect than the one desired. Bland says that in many cases fasting can impair detoxification. A long-term fast can deplete the body's detoxification systems and increase susceptibility to toxicities. Fasting can deplete the nutrients the body needs in order to detoxify. Researchers have found that fasting or a poor diet can reduce antioxidants and "significantly increase stress, and this xenobiotic exposure can damage the immune, endocrine, cardiovascular and nervous systems."[53] Fasting has also been shown to increase hyperoxic lung damage in mice due to decreased glutathione levels.[54] Dr. Bland suggests that for optimum management of true toxicity symptoms doctors should do the following:

1. Use a low-allergy diet program.
2. Enhance the intake of specific nutrients necessary for supporting the detoxification pathways and reducing oxidative stress.
3. Deliver macro- and micronutrients in a food program which optimizes nutrient digestion and absorption.
4. Provide the diet and its nutrients in a form resulting in high compliance.
5. Control overall diet quality, including protein, carbohydrate, and fat sources, for improved metabolic control.

FASTING WITH ASTHMA?

"Is there a true toxicity?" asks Dr. Martin Feldman. Before you start fasting it is important to find out if there is a true toxicity. With asthma, the body is working hard to remodulate the immune system and is burning up immune system–related nutrients. So asthmatics have a very high probability of deficiencies of immune nutrients and other basic substances such as protein. A person with asthma could be deficient for many reasons: malabsorption, low stomach acid, or an absorption problem from low pancreatic enzymes.

IS JUICE FASTING A GOOD IDEA?

You may get a certain amount of initial relief from juice fasting because you are not eating those foods to which you are allergic. But if you are only drinking juices, they can actually make your deficiencies worse. Juice fasting must be done with skill to have enough nutrients to keep the body in balance for that day or that week. With carrot juice, for instance, you get a sugar overload.

"So what is the answer?" asks Dr. Feldman. "It is to have not just a juice fast but a metabolic clearing fast. There are cleansing fast products available that are nutritional powdered blended drinks and can be used in addition to just simple juices. Some of these products support liver function, digestive function, and support the body with nutrients, while the cleansing, fasting process is being undergone. One of the best, and low in allergens, is called Ultra-Clear.

"Even with these nutrient drinks I would advise anyone with asthma considering a fast to have enough protein during the fasting process. But not a protein to which they are allergic, such as soy if soy is an allergen. Before embarking on a fast, the nutrient formula should be tested for allergy intolerance."

Water

Many people who are ill don't drink enough water for proper bodily function. With asthma the need for water is usually increased. Mucus and other aspects of the asthmatic process are helped and not hurt by more fluid. For those with chest tightness, thick mucus, and the yellow and green mucus of infection, increasing fluid intake, especially plain water, helps considerably. Bottled spring water, pure well water, or water purified by reverse osmosis and a charcoal filter are the kinds you will want to drink. Drinking water should be room temperature.

Labored breathing, fever, and sweating all contribute to dehydration. And when you are busy trying to breathe you may forget to drink liquids. As tissues become dry and mucus gluey and difficult to cough up, a more serious condition can result.

Scott Gerson, M.D., a practitioner of Ayurveda, a medical science from India, suggests carrying a thermos of hot water and sipping from it during the day (until about 8:00 P.M.) for optimal health.

Curing Patients with Water

In a very interesting book, *Your Body's Many Cries for Water,* F. Batmanghelidj, M.D., describes the process whereby he claims to have cured patients with asthma and other illnesses with plain water and a little salt. Dr. Batmanghelidj says that dehydration increases histamine release. "It has been shown in animal models that histamine production in histamine-generating cells will decrease with an increase in the daily water intake. On average, these conditions respond after one to four weeks of water regulation of the body."[55]

For those of us who spent years drinking orange juice instead of water, Dr. Batmanghelidj says that the high levels of potassium in orange juice can promote "more than usual histamine production."[56] And histamines, as we know, cause allergy problems.

Dr. Batmanghelidj cautions: "Don't treat thirst with medications."

SOAK BATHS

The skin, says herbalist Carolyne Cesari, is the largest organ of elimination. For detoxification she suggests soak baths every other day with baking soda or Epsom salt added to the water. She recommends a once-a-year regimen of four rounds of eight baths each, over a six-week period, every other day, followed by a cold shower to close the pores. She advises taking pancreatic enzymes if you take soak baths.[57]

Help the Body Detoxify

WITH VITAMINS

For lead. Vitamin C and B complex vitamins protect against toxic effects.[58] Selenium, zinc, and cysteine also help.[59]

For aluminum. Magnesium, vitamin C and zinc, and calcium help counteract toxic effects.[60]

For mercury. Dr. Zamm recommends selenium and zinc.

For copper. Manganese and molybdenum as well as vitamin C and zinc.[61]

WITH AMINO ACIDS

Cysteine, glutamine, glycine, methionine, taurine, and tyrosine play a role in detoxification processes as well as in building the immune system.[62] Cysteine helps glutathione, a powerful antioxidant and detoxifying agent, to detoxify carcinogens and other dangerous chemicals in the liver.[63] (More about this important amino acid and how it helps asthma in chapter 9.)

WITH EDIBLES

All the sea vegetables help with the detoxification process (see chapter 8).

Sulfur-rich foods such as kale, brussels sprouts and cauliflower, raspberries, the onion family, and watercress.

Aduki beans and purslane also detoxify.

Dandelion, rich in potassium, is an excellent detoxifier, helping the body rid itself of wastes. Eat the greens or make a tea.[64]

Tumeric can help detoxify from exposure to cigarette smoke.[65]

Burdock, yellow dock, and Oregon grape root are good liver cleansers.[66]

Another way to detoxify and also to balance and strengthen the body is through exercise. Exercise may also provide more enjoyment. We will learn a number of beneficial exercises as well as better breathing in the next chapter.

CHAPTER 5

EXERCISE, YOGA, AND OTHER KEYS TO BETTER BREATHING

BREATHING IN AND BREATHING OUT

When I first began to study yoga, pre-asthma, I ambitiously got up and out to Kundalini Yoga class every morning at 7:00 A.M. One night I wasn't so sure about rising early the next morning so I telephoned the teacher and asked, "What are we doing tomorrow? What part of the body will we be working on?" "In the old days," he answered, "you would have had to climb a mountain and sweep out some holy person's hut for a year before they might have shown you even one breathing meditation. Everything we do is fantastic." And it is.

Learning to Exhale

To most people breathing comes naturally, but for those of us with asthma, learning to observe the breath and exhaling properly may be a matter of life or death. Learning to exhale is a key element in unlearning the asthmatic response. Breath is life. We simply can't live without it. Yoga breathing exercises help clear the lungs of mucus, increase lung capacity, and oxygenate the cells. They help balance the mind and body and promote better health by not only oxygenating body and mind but also by unblocking channels of energy.

THE SECRET IS IN THE EXHALE

Exhaling is the part of breathing that many people with asthma find most difficult. But exhaling completely may be the key to unlearning the asthmatic response.

Those awful times when I was in the midst of an asthma attack, I couldn't remember what it felt like to breathe normally. I had a dim recollection that I really didn't have to think about it when I was breathing normally. When my breathing quieted down I wondered why I could not always keep it quiet and calm like that. So I tried to analyze the difference. That's when I found out about trapped air.

When there is chest tightness and airways start to close, there is often a reaction of panic that leads to an abbreviated exhale as you inhale quicker in the struggle to get more oxygen. When it happened to me I would be afraid to exhale, afraid that I wouldn't be able to take the next breath, that breath I needed so badly. But the shorter and shorter exhales and the gasping for oxygen lead to stale air being trapped deep in the airways and less and less *room* to put fresh air. Now there is a full-fledged asthma attack.

What's really needed here is to expel as much stale air as possible so that fresh oxygenated air can be inhaled. The asthmatic response can be unlearned. How to do it? The secret is in learning to exhale! Let's try a few exercises that help.

PRACTICING THE EXHALATION

A good time to practice exhaling is when you are not having an attack. By practicing when you are feeling fine you are rehearsing what to do when you feel the approach of a crisis. A kind of fire drill for avoiding an asthma attack.

So let's run through some everyday ways we replace stale air with fresh air without thinking about it.

Sighing

Let's try a few good sighs and think about the process. A brief inhale and a long forceful exhale as we making that sighing vocalization. *Aaaaaaaaaaaaaaaaahhhhhhhhhhhh.*

Stretching

Now let's do some stretching along with the sighing and see what happens to the sigh. Ah, ahh, *aahhhhhhhhhhhhhhhh.* Louder, wasn't it?

Yawning

To have a really good yawn you open your mouth really wide, stretch your arms, take a very deep, noisy inhale and let it out with kind of a long noisy *haaaaaaaaaaaaaaaaaa*. Do another yawn and stretch as you let it out as far as you can go.

Laughing

What's the first thing you have to do to laugh? Have a sharp intake of air. Then what happens? It comes out in stages as *hah, hah, hah, hah, hah*. Have a really good laugh. See how many *hahs* you can make. In my asthma workshops we start out forcing ourselves to laugh, as everyone is a little embarrassed by it. But hearing all that silly forced laughter makes everyone really laugh. It's pretty funny.

Whistling

Inhale slowly through pursed lips (into the belly), whistle slowly as you exhale all the air out. Try it again a few more times.

Now whistle as you inhale, and exhale slowly through pursed lips all the way to the end of the exhale. Try that a few times. You may be able to increase the number of whistles by one or two each time you practice. See how slowly you can do each part.

Hissing

Simply inhale through the nose and slowly hiss all the air out through the teeth. By this time you should be getting the idea—the *exhale* is twice as long as the *inhale*!

A Taoist Exercise for Stopping an Asthma Attack

THE LUNG SOUND

In this exercise a hissing sound is used to expel stale air and push your asthma out and away.

Stand erect, hands at your sides. Slowly raise your arms in front of you to waist level. Imagine that you have your arms around a large beach ball in front of you, and as you very gently lift it up, inhaling and filling the lungs, turn the palms out right about third-eye level, forehead level. Then, looking off far away in the distance, put your teeth together and vibrate this hissing sound which vibrates the lungs. *Hsssssssssssssssssssssssssssssss*. Look far into the distance, slowly push your palms out in front of you while straightening your arms, and then push them out to the sides and down, all the time making this hissing sound *hisssssssss*. Like air escaping from an inner tube. Let that energy leak out, release it, and project it into the distance. As you release the sound you're signaling to the life force trapped in your lungs to move out the stagnant, trapped Qi in the lungs. Then relax your arms down. Cross your arms over your heart and put your hands over your lungs and hug them. Close your eyes and go inside and smile into the lungs. Contemplate the feeling for a minute before you start again.

You can coordinate this exercise with the four levels of making contact with the lungs through visualization given in chapter 3.

A Few More Practical Breathing Strategies

We can use breath control when we get into difficult situations out in the real world. We've probably all had trouble at one time or another with stairs. Especially going up.

For going up the stairs: Inhale for two stairs and exhale for two stairs. You will be breathing harder than usual but you will be getting more oxygen. If that breath is too quick, try inhaling for four steps and exhaling for four. Count any footsteps on landings as steps.

On crowded trains and subways: No need to panic—just relax. Exhale a long exhale and do slow stomach breathing.

For trafficky street corners: Relax by letting facial muscles go and shoulders drop and very slowly exhale completely through your mouth. Then begin quiet stomach breathing. Do this as you wait for the light to change.

Our impulse in these situations is to protect ourselves by contracting the chest and not breathing. It doesn't work. Breathe breathe breathe.

VOCALIZE!

Vocalization has been used for centuries as a way to strengthen the lungs and promote health. The Greeks advocated singing, reading aloud, crying, loud speaking, and oratory for the health of the lungs.[1] Through the centuries vocalization was an accepted part of physical exercise.

Sing

Inhale and see if you can increase the number of phrases you can sing before you have to grab a breath.

Read aloud

You might enjoy reading a poem out loud and seeing how expressive you can be. Practice a speech in front of the mirror.

Regulating the Breath — the Basic Breathing Exercises

Now that we have learned the value of emptying the lungs we are ready to learn some important basic yoga breathing exercises that are especially useful for respiratory problems. Yogic breathing is called *pranayama* ("control of the breath"), controlling the motion of prana in the lungs. Every form of energy is derived from prana. The deeper your breathing is, the more life-giving energy you can get from the air. Regulating the breath is one of the secrets of yoga, health, and long life.

In yoga each movement is coordinated with a breath to derive the greatest benefit. But breathing exercises themselves are very powerful and centering. It's best to practice early in the morning, but anytime is better than none as long as you don't practice on a full stomach.

These are some basic yoga breathing sets that are recommended for everyone. And yoga masters claim that a steady daily practice of alternate nostril breathing and three-part breathing will keep the asthma away.

ALTERNATE NOSTRIL BREATHING

In this breathing the exhalation is always twice as long as the inhalation, making it perfect for overcoming the asthmatic response. Incomplete exhalation doesn't allow all the stale, stagnant air to be expelled. With the long, complete exhalation, stale air is expelled and room is made for the lungs to be replenished with fresh air.

1. Sit in an erect position, keeping the spine straight. Tuck the second and third fingers of your right hand under the base of the thumb (to keep them out of the way) and extend the last two fingers straight up, as you cover the right nostril with your right thumb.
2. Begin by exhaling slowly and completely for eight counts through the left nostril. Then inhale deeply for four counts.
3. Close the left nostril with the fourth finger, keeping the thumb over the right nostril and hold the breath for sixteen counts.
4. Release the thumb and exhale slowly and completely through the right nostril to the count of eight. Do not force the exhalation. It should be completely quiet.

5. Inhale deeply through the right nostril for four counts and hold the breath with both nostrils closed for sixteen counts.
6. Release the left nostril and exhale to the count of eight.

That is one complete set. Try to continue for several minutes, working up to five minutes a sitting. This breathing calms and balances all of the systems of the body. It steadies the breath and increases lung power. It is also good for balancing the left and right sides of the brain.

BREATH IS LIFE

"Breath is life," says Kundalini Yoga teacher Ravi Singh; "the more you breathe consciously the greater your longevity and vitality. Breath is a conveyance for life-force. The ancients called it prana—a link to infinity. The source of breath is the source of all energy, which is infinity, or God, or whatever you call it. Breath is the best medicine."[2]

THREE-PART YOGA BREATHING

Three-part breathing is also called the full yogic breath. You begin with belly breathing, then bring the breath up into the diaphragm and finally into the chest. The shoulders don't move, but stay quiet and relaxed. The full yogic breath increases oxygen to the lungs, blood, heart, and brain.

Try to learn one part of this breathing technique before you go on to the next. It may take a little time to perfect, but it will be well worth it. You can do three-part breathing in the morning on awakening, before you fall asleep at night, or anytime you want to destress and relax. The full yogic breath will help clear congestion in the lungs and increase lung power.

1. Abdominal Breathing

1. Lie on your back, arms six inches from your sides, palms up, feet a shoulder width apart. Or sit comfortably in a chair, feet flat on the floor.
2. Rest your hands lightly on the *hara,* the area just below the navel. Exhale slowly and completely, as your abdomen contracts. Relax your back muscles as you continue to slowly finish the exhale. This will allow the release of the stale air deep down in the airways.

3. Inhale slowly. Feel your abdomen expand.
4. Repeat for several minutes.

2. *Diaphragmatic Breathing*

Continue to lie on the floor. With hands lightly touching the bottom of your rib cage, continue to inhale slowly, this time expanding the rib cage, and relaxing it as you slowly exhale. Shoulders and chest should not move.

3. *Three-Part Breathing*

Inhalation

Imagine that the abdomen, rib cage, and chest are three round, connected balloons. We're going to inflate all three, one at a time, starting at the bottom.

1. Inhale your abdominal breath.
2. Continue bringing this breath up into and expanding the rib cage.
3. Continue the inhale right up into the upper chest, keeping shoulders down and relaxed.

Exhalation

1. Exhale the air from the abdomen.
2. Exhale the air from the rib cage.
3. Exhale the breath from the chest. This takes some practice to coordinate properly. When you get it going, it should roll like a wave, rising and falling. Make sure the exhale is long, relaxed, and complete before inhaling the next breath. This exercise is great for relaxation and for loosening mucus. All of these exercises will help increase your lung capacity.

If any of the breathing exercises seem to take more time than you would like to give them, try to do a few minutes rather than none at all. When you start feeling better you might want to increase the time because breathing *feels so good*. Pick the ones that feel right for you and work on doing those; when they become easy, go on and add to or vary your repertoire. Then try to practice every day.

EXPERIENCE THE BENEFITS OF EXERCISE

In the old days doctors warned mothers that their asthmatic children should not exercise because getting out of breath could bring on an attack. But now that we've watched so many asthmatic medal-winning Olympic athletes on TV, we know better. Although we may know better, it's hard to put that perception into practice, because with asthma, even the simplest things can be an effort and often painfully difficult.

Right now you may be working with your doctor to cut down your medication, but it's going to be worth it to premedicate if that's the only way you will be able to work out. But if you have a cold or flu, it's best to take it easy. Rest and do the long, slow, deep breathing.

Doris, who has been struggling with asthma for many of her fifty-nine years, says, "I exercise a lot. I walk, jog, and work out with weights and the machines at the gym. Between the exercise and the inhaled steroids"—she had been taking prednisone—"my forced expiratory volume (FEV) went back up from about 20 percent to 70 percent. Before I exercise I medicate so I make sure I can get a good workout. I can't say that my asthma is completely under control but I'm much better than I was."

What, Me Exercise?

Nelson Howe, who has asthma plus a Black Belt in the Korean martial art Tai Kwon Do, says that asking an asthmatic to exercise is almost like asking the impossible. Nelson has a private therapy practice in which he has incorporated martial art strategies for working with fear. The whole point of asthma, he says, is that you can't breathe. "So," the asthmatic asks, "how could I possibly exercise?" When we feel like we're suffocating and having a problem walking even the shortest distance, thinking about exercise is what Howe calls "absolutely contraindicated."

"Many asthmatics are almost exercise-phobic. If you look at asthma as a chronic condition, what happens is you learn all kinds of strategies to deal with it, and one of these strategies is to immobilize, to cut down the activity level. With asthma, it feels like you can't get enough oxygen, so when you become as immobile as possible, the oxygen demand goes down and you don't feel quite so desperate to get the next breath. The problem is that if you experience that over and over, cutting down movement gets deeply learned. As an asthmatic you're likely to learn to walk slowly even if you're not in the midst of an asthma attack; even if the medications work, you don't tend to push to a fast pace. Unfortunately, it's not even in the vocabulary anymore."

But there are important reasons to get your body moving again:

- Although exercise may initially create stress on the body (if you are unused to exercising or don't have a regular program), exercise eventually helps the body deal with stress.
- Exercise brings nutrients and increased oxygen to the cells and helps the body rid itself of carbon dioxide and waste products.
- Exercise enhances the cardiovascular system as well as the respiratory system.
- Bilateral exercise keeps the body in balance since it exercises both sides of the body equally. Swimming, yoga, walking, bicycling, running, and dancing are practical bilateral exercises for people with asthma. Virtually all the martial arts are bilateral.
- People who exercise regularly have an increased feeling of well-being, reduced stress, and less anxiety.

Howe says that those of us with asthma need to improve our body's efficiency in utilizing oxygen, and exercise until our natural hormonal system kicks in. Because it takes some time to strengthen the system without relying on external crutches, the best time to start is now.

Just remember: Too much exercise with sweating can deplete the body of precious minerals; therefore, exercising strenuously without taking extra nutrients is not a prudent thing to do. There is evidence that the stress of chronic or excessive exercise may be counterproductive for the immune system.[3]

EXERCISE-INDUCED ASTHMA

Although the importance of exercise cannot be overstated, some people, including a number of athletes, seem to have asthmatic reactions only when they exercise. This can happen because breathing harder, and cooling the airways, triggers an attack through the autonomic nervous system. Cold itself can trigger an asthma attack. Mast cells may be activated in exercise-induced bronchoconstriction and studies indicate that leukotriene release may make a major contribution to exercise-induced asthma.[4] However, it is important to keep exercising. Premedication with Intal is often helpful for exercise-induced asthma.

Get Up to a Good Start

In the practice of yoga many of the *asanas* or yoga postures are done lying on the back or sitting on the floor where you don't have to fight gravity. This makes them perfect for us! If you are unused to exercise, a beginner's yoga class will help your body stretch, balance your internal organs, help to reduce stress, and teach you to focus on what your body is feeling. Even if you have never stretched in your life, you can incorporate the following into your daily routine.

Getting Up in the Morning Exercises

You can do these while you are still lying quietly on your back in bed. If your bed isn't firm it might be better to move to a mat on the floor.

Stomach Breathing

We start with hara breathing. This is a slow breath into the hara, your center, the place about two fingers below your navel. Start with a long, slow exhale as your belly flattens. As you inhale, your belly expands. Smile into that place and feel that it is breathing. Breathe in deeply and exhale slowly and completely. Your chest and shoulders should be still. Focus your mind on relaxation. Continue for several minutes.

Stretching to the Left, Stretching to the Right

Still lying down, raise your arms over your head and stretch arms and legs, rolling to the left and then to the right.

Stretching Up

Clasp your hands, interlock your fingers, and turn the palms upward as you raise them overhead, inhaling. Stretch, stretch, stretch. Then exhale your hands down. Let's try that one more time.

Pressing Fingers

With your right hand, pull back each finger of the left hand and press back a little, then squeeze each finger tightly. Don't forget the thumb. Then let your left hand do the right. Then pull back on all the fingers at the same time. Do the other hand. Rub both hands together to warm up.

Hugging Knees and Squeezing Toes

Bring your right knee up toward your chest, wrap your hands around the knee, and hug toward the chest. Keep your back and shoulders down and flat as possible on the bed. Hold that a little longer. Then grab your toes and squeeze one at a time and all together. Do the same with the left knee and toes. End by giving yourself a good foot massage. Both feet of course.

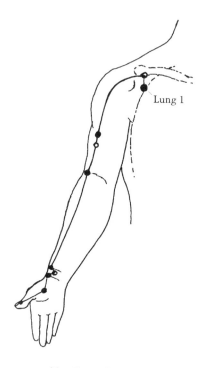

THE LUNG MERIDIAN

Lung Meridian Massage

The lung meridian is a channel for energy flow that starts at Lung 1 just above the armpit and moves down the top edge of the arm to the outer corner of the thumbnail.

We can give ourselves a lung-meridian massage in this way: Relax your left arm in your lap, and with the right hand grab your arm just below the left shoulder. Squeeze gently with your thumb in the indentation just above the armpit. Then move down the top of the arm, squeezing the muscle gently as you work slowly down the arm to the wrist, hand, and thumbnail. Repeat on other side.

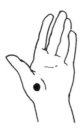

LUNG 10

Thumb Pressure for Bringing Up Mucus

Press and hold the pad (Lung 10) of your thumb, the fatty part at the base, closing your eyes and taking a few more slow hara breaths. Hold for two minutes. Repeat on the other side.

Knee Drop

Wrap your arms around the knees as you bring them in close to the chest. Then straighten your arms out to the sides and let your knees drop to the right—while your head relaxes to the left. Hold for a while as you focus your attention and relaxation at your waist and torso. Then let your knees drop to the left while head relaxes to the right. Hold and relax into the stretch.

Time to Sit Up for Neck Stretches

Put your hands on your shoulders on either side of your neck for support and let your head drop slowly and carefully to your chest. Slowly raise your chin. Keep sitting up tall so that when you carefully drop your head back, your chest is also lifted. Return to upright head position, drop your arms, and slowly and with care drop left ear to left shoulder and right ear to right shoulder. Keep the shoulders down and relaxed.

Now is a good time to meditate on your breath. Do your hara breathing. Hara breathing will help restore your "essence" and revitalize your body. It is also the essential breathing to begin *immediately* if you feel you are having an asthma attack. The great thing about this powerful, restorative breath is that you can take it with you wherever you go. Practice in the office, in your car, waiting for the traffic light to turn green, on the bus, or at home watching TV. The best way, of course, is in a quiet, peaceful place where you can focus and not be interrupted.

Relax with your eyes closed, and do a little more long, deep breathing. A few yawns and it's time to get out of bed. And look how much you've accomplished already!

EIGHT SILKEN MOVEMENTS OR PAL DAN GUM

This is a powerful and beneficial set that can be done in about ten minutes. These are great to do when you get out of bed to get a good start for the day!

Pal Dan Gum are Taoist exercises that recharge the energy centers and have been used for thousands of years in China and Korea to

* release blockages in all twelve organ meridians
* release tension and stress
* recharge the inner organs
* promote improved blood circulation
* make muscles and joints more flexible and resilient
* promote radiant health

Focus your attention on the breath and the effect of the stretch on each part of the body you are working on. Inhale through the nose and exhale through the mouth. Unless otherwise noted you will be inhaling as you open the arms and body and exhaling as you contract or close. The breath can be a powerful way to reduce stress and promote physical and emotional well-being. Repeat each exercise twice or as many times as is comfortable.

Iona Marsaa Teeguarden, from whom I learned these exercises in a Joy of Feeling workshop, says, "Just by concentrating your attention on the blocked places and sending your breath into them, you will find yourself gradually moving away from the *fear of feeling,* and towards the *joy of feeling.*"[5]

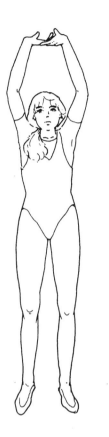
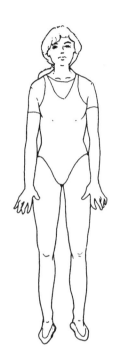

1. Upholding Heaven With Two Hands
(Improves circulation)

Inhale slowly while raising arms (palms up) above the head, interlocking fingers and pushing upward with palms while you rise up on toes. Look up toward your upstretched hands. Hold for a few seconds. Exhale while lowering heels and bringing arms back to sides.

Illustrations from *The Joy of Feeling*, Bodymind Acupressure,™ Jin Shin Do,® Iona Marsaa Teeguarden. Courtesy of Japan Publications, Inc. Tokyo/New York, 1987.

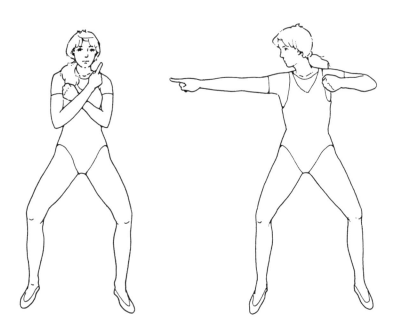

2. *Opening the Bow*
(Stimulates the Lung Meridian, expands the chest, and increases lung capacity)

Legs apart, bend knees into horse-riding position, arms crossed in front of chest, left arm on outside. Inhale while reaching left arm out at shoulder, fists clenched, index finger extended. Look to the left over left arm while right elbow pulls back imaginary bow at shoulder height. Exhale arms back to hands-crossed position with right arm outside. Turn to the right and repeat with right arm out.

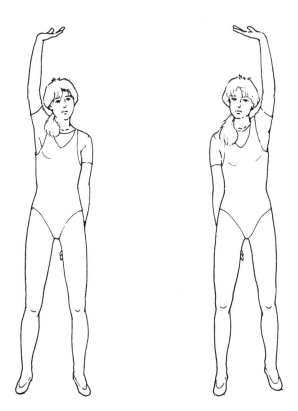

3. *Raising Hands Separately*
(Strengthens digestion)

Begin with left hand below and right hand above an imaginary ball. Inhale while pushing up with right hand above head and left hand pushing down (hands flexed parallel to the ground, palms facing out), exhale, returning hands to ball. Turn imaginary ball so hands are reversed and repeat.

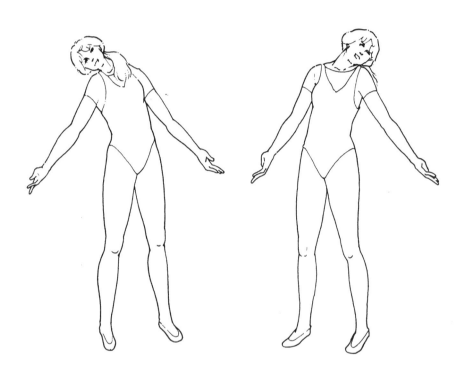

4. *Looking Backward (Strengthens and tones the muscles of the chest and upper back, stretches muscles in the sides of the neck; can relieve fatigue in lungs and other organs)*

Starting with arms crossed in front of chest, right arm in front, inhale, pressing hands and arms out and back while turning head to one side and looking over right shoulder. Arms should be straight and back with palms facing forward. Exhale, returning hands to crossed position in front of chest with left hand in front. Repeat turning to other side. Then repeat both sides two more times.

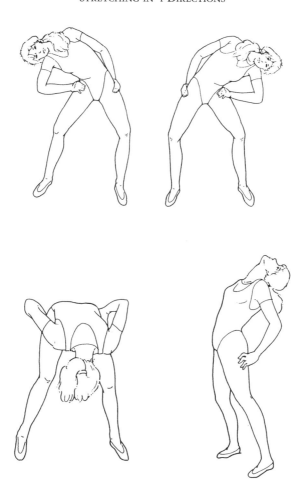

5. *Stretching in Four Directions*
(Benefits circulation, digestion, and the nervous system)

Hands on hips, inhale while upright and exhale while stretching forward, backward, and to each side. Inhale when you return to starting position.

Inhale while circling hips back and exhale circling forward.

Gently let head touch right shoulder, then left shoulder. Breathe into the tense places in the neck. Close eyes and focus on the effects of the exercise.

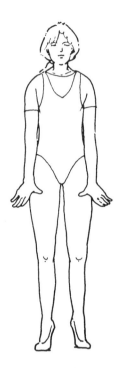

6. *Standing on Toes*
(Strengthens Stomach and Kidney Meridians, good for centering)

Arms lowered in front of body, inhale into hara (two and a half inches below the navel) while rising up on toes and flexing hands parallel to floor. Exhale while lowering heels to the ground. Repeat ten times.

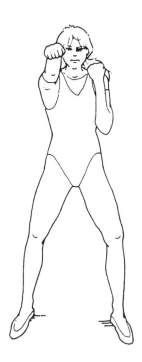

7. *Punching with Angry Eyes*
(Good for Liver Meridian, releases pent-up anger)

Eyes wide, clench fists at waist, palms up. Firmly punch forward eight times as fist is turned facing downward, then to each side, exhaling sound through the mouth.

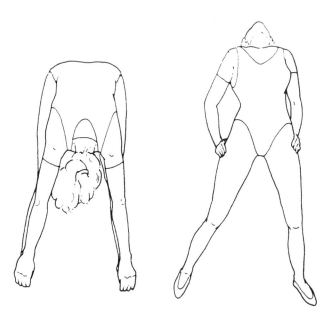

8. *Holding Toes and Stretching Back*
(Improves circulation, helps the body get rid of toxins, and stimulates the kidneys)

Stand erect, feet shoulder width apart. Exhale touching toes, inhale to up-right position, hands on hips, exhale as you stretch back.

Squat, feet flat on floor (if you can) and rest arms on knees. Hold for one minute. Stand very slowly by letting trunk and head hang down and straightening vertebra by vertebra until completely straight.

Shake out arms and legs and close eyes for a minute to concentrate on the effects of the exercises.[6]

- These exercises can be performed in about ten or twelve minutes, so they are easy to fit into your day.
- You can do most of them waiting for the kettle to boil or while waiting for your vegetables to steam.
- Take ten minutes away from your desk and do the whole set in your office at work. Maybe you can get others to join you.
- Use Upholding Heaven with Two Hands whenever you are feeling tight in the chest—it's a perfect break from any activity. It stretches out the hands and arms and provides an excellent breathing benefit by lifting the rib cage up from the lower organs.
- If you are an established couch potato get up right now and try one section. Add one every day and soon you'll be doing them all and feeling great!

LEARNING YOGA

Yoga is a Sanskrit word meaning "union," the union of the individual consciousness with the infinite consciousness. In India, yoga is practiced for mental clarity and to experience the infinite self. Because yoga also helps to release toxins from the body, balances the internal organs, and helps develop flexibilty and strength, yoga is practiced more for health and vitality in the West.

One summer in the Catskills when I was very ill, I took a beginner's class with yoga teacher Ellen Saltonstall. I had actually been practicing yoga for a while but I was so debilitated with asthma, I felt that beginning was all I could do. I loved this class and I benefited from the way that Ellen taught us to be aware of all the small adjustments that can be made in the body to create a new way of experiencing yourself.

There are many poses in Hatha Yoga that Ellen says work well for asthma. All the back-bending yoga poses, such as the cobra pose and the camel, help the chest become more expansive. She also recommends inversions such as the shoulder stand and poses that strengthen the legs.

"When the thighs and the legs are working correctly," Ellen explains, "the breath becomes more free. Anything that energizes the lower part of the body is helpful. When people have distress in the upper body all the subtle energy of the body goes there; we don't have any groundedness, we don't have any connection to the earth. This creates a vicious cycle of more anxiety. So the grounding of the energy which happens through various yogic actions of the legs is tremendously helpful. Strong legs, legs that are used, legs that are aware of the ground, and legs that are aware of the support that they give to the upper body are what we want."

In Ellen's beginner class I learned the fine points that make such a difference, even standing still.

TADASANA—THE MOUNTAIN POSE

Standing still may seem like a strange way to begin to exercise, but standing in the pose called *Tadasana* will help you develop an invaluable awareness of what is happening in your body. The more sensitive you become to what your body is feeling, the more you will be able to utilize everything you are learning in this book.

Tadasana, or the Mountain Pose, helps to align the body into its optimum position so that the energy flows through, the whole body is even and balanced, and you experience yourself as grounded.

Let's pretend we're in class and Ellen is leading us through Tadasana:

"Bring your feet together parallel so that the inner edges of the feet are touching, if possible, toes facing straight forward. You can pretend that each foot is a car with four wheels. Two front wheels on either side of the ball of your foot, and two back wheels on either side of your heel. And all of those points are equally bearing weight. That takes a minute to adjust. So just stand and breathe and see what's going on naturally for you. Perhaps there's a lot more weight on one foot, or the outer edges of both feet and not the inner edges. Most people find some imbalance, so you can work to even it up. And you'll probably find that as you do that the arches naturally lift up. If they don't, if you have flat feet and the arches are kind of dropped, you can lift all your toes up. That will activate the arch muscles and the arches will become more lifted. Then you can stretch your toes out but still feel the activity and strength of the arches.

"Stretch your knees, lifting your kneecaps up and firming the thigh muscles. Press the thighs back into the back of the hip sockets, so instead of hanging forward from the hips as many people do, you actually move your hips back a little bit so that more weight goes onto your heels for a moment until you rebalance again. Then you have a softening in front of the hip joint, and you can be more vertically over your support, as opposed to hinging forward from the hips. That's also good for lengthening the lower back. You can feel your tailbone descending and upper body lifting so that the lower ribs lift away from the waist both in the front and the back. Take a few deep breaths to elongate the lung area all around—in the front, on the sides, and in the back. Fold your shoulders slightly back in toward the spine, so the shoulder blades come flat onto the rib cage and let your head stretch up over the center. Try not to let your head come forward or back, but just be lifted straight up through the center of the top of your head, right over the rest of your spine. The gaze of your eyes and the angle of your chin are parallel to the floor. Not too high or too low.

"Stand this way for a minute with your eyes closed and let your awareness scan the whole body. Feel the expansiveness of your breath from the inside and let the pose be both energized and quiet. Roll the shoulders slightly back so the collarbones become wider and the shoulder blades fit more closely into the ribs and closely toward the spine. That firms the upper back a little bit and opens the front chest. Your arms hang loosely at your sides. Focus now on this new awareness of how your body can feel."

The Mountain Pose has a balance between activity and receptivity, between the earth and the heavens. Like any yoga pose, it has that dynamic quality of being both still and active. This helps us to feel a continuous flow of energy throughout the body which will also allow the spiritual energy to flow.

"EVERYTHING WE DO HERE IS FANTASTIC"

All of the yoga methods I have practiced over the years have been wonderful, each having its own special energy and benefits. But recently I returned to Kundalini Yoga class and talked with my original teacher, Ravi Singh. I was surprised to hear that he had had asthma:

"I was born prematurely and my lungs didn't inflate. They gave me a zero chance of living but I beat the odds. I had asthma, allergies, and lung problems all during my youth. When I was thirteen I asked the doctor about long-distance running and he told me if I did that it would kill me, but being the stubborn person that I am, that's exactly what I started doing. It didn't kill me and that cued me into the fact that doctors weren't infallible. When I first discovered Kundalini Yoga it was a godsend, and I never had an asthma attack again."

In order to address what's wrong, Ravi says, you have to be brave and confront what's hard. Although we often don't want to extend ourselves, in order to make progress we have to do what's difficult. By going through the resistance we are working directly on the problem.

"When you begin to tune in to your body you automatically know that certain habits aren't in your best interest; the evidence will be too compelling to deny. After you tune in to your body it's with you forever. The body gives you signals about what needs to be addressed and if you don't heed them it will keep worsening until you do. Asthma is a symptom of something that's happening in the body that has to be addressed in one's life or one's psyche. The holistic approach is the best because unless you take everything into account you're never going to solve the problem."

THE SALUTE TO THE SUN

Now we're ready for something more aerobic. The sun salutations are probably the most famous of all Hatha Yoga postures. They stretch and tone the muscles and every part of the body, including the internal organs. They also activate energy (prana) in the organ meridians. They can be started very slowly and gently. If you are not in great shape you may want to just do two sets to begin. Pretty soon, with regular practice, you will be able to move on to ten or twelve sets. It is best to practice this in a class with an experienced yoga teacher who will guide you to correct body positions. Then, and only then, the sun salutations can be done faster for a more vigorous workout. Be sure to warm up first and focus carefully on what you are doing with your body.

There are a number of variations for the sun salutations but this is the way they were taught at yoga camp:

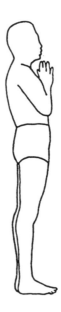

1. Stand up straight with feet together and palms in prayer position at the sternum, the center of the chest. Your weight should be evenly distributed. Inhale and exhale deeply.

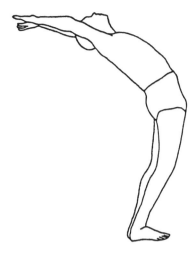

2. Inhale as you stretch your arms up. Lift your chest and look up, arching your upper back.

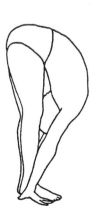

3. Exhale as your arms sweep forward, bending forward and bending the knees until you place your fingertips pointing forward on the floor alongside your feet. Bring your head toward your knees.

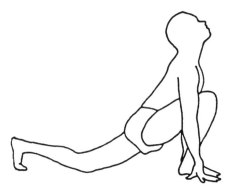

4. Inhale as you stretch the left leg back, toes curled under, knee slightly touching the floor. Hands still pressing down, press your chest forward and look up.

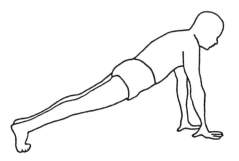

5. Holding the breath, bring the right leg back and pause in the "plank" position. The body should be straight and in line as much as possible.

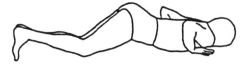

6. Exhale as you first lower the knees to the floor, then lower chest down to the floor near your wrists, and forehead to the floor.

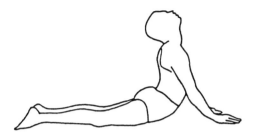

7. Inhale as you lower the hips, point toes, draw the chest forward, and look up. Keep your shoulders down, legs and feet together. Elbows may be bent, hands in line with shoulders.

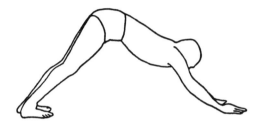

8. Exhale, toes pressed down and curled under, and push hips up into inverted V. Head is down, press heels toward the floor. Shoulders drop away from the ears.

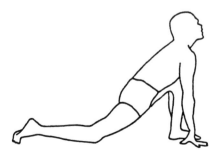

9. Inhale as you bring left foot forward and place between and in line with your hands. Rest the other knee on the floor and stretch your chest forward.

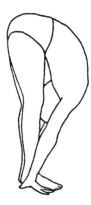

10. Exhale as you bring the right leg forward, bending from the waist, bending knees enough to again place both fingertips on the floor.

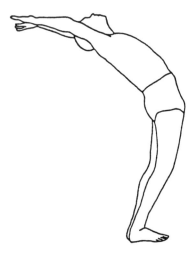

11. Inhale as you stretch your arms forward and up and, arching your upper back, look up (as in #2).

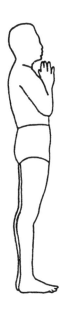

12. Exhale and slowly come back to an upright position and gently lower your arms. Take a slow deep breath and exhale as you bring your hands back to prayer position. Now you are ready to inhale as your arms stretch back and start again, this time with the right leg first.

That is one set. Do two sets today and then rest lying down on your back. Sun salutations may seem difficult at first, but you will appreciate how the chest tightness lessens as you go on.

The beauty of yoga is that while the asanas (the physical exercises) shape and strengthen the body, they do not fatigue like more extreme exercise. Yoga works to help rebalance the internal organs, helps you to attain a clear mental state, and most importantly, helps to maintain flexibility of the spine. When the spine is strengthened and flexible, there is better circulation of blood, nutrients, and oxygen throughout the body, and health is regained. A "side effect"—a flexible spine keeps you young!

The Spiritual Level

Vocalization was used in Western culture for health through the ages. But vocalization has always been used for harmony and balance and spiritual purposes all over the world. People chant, recite, or sing the name of God in church, synagogue, temple, and mosque, in ancient languages, the sounds of which have healing properties. Chanting the ancient syllables or mantra "is the fastest possible vibratory union between ourselves and the Creator."[7]

Ravi Singh says that the spiritual level of Kundalini Yoga is most important, the ultimate cure of any condition regardless of the cause. Along with the breathing and the postures, mantras are used, coded sounds that have a unique vibratory effect on consciousness. The mantra is not like an ordinary sound uttered over and over again; the mantra has certain inherent qualities that relate to the infinite. Ravi explains, "The science of naad yoga—naad meaning 'no beginning'—relates to the sound current, the unstruck sound, the sound current that gave rise to all manifestations—in the beginning was the word. Mantras are thought to be deeper than silence, emanations of silence, and there is nothing more powerful as a healing modality than silence."

THE FINAL RELAXATION

All exercise sessions should end with a final relaxation, bringing awareness to every part of the body, feeling the effects of the exercises and consolidating your gains.

Relax lying down on a mat on the floor, and cover yourself with a blanket (it is important to keep warm). Arms relax to the sides, palms facing up, legs and feet are slightly apart, shoulders are relaxed back, letting the spine retain its natural curve. Now we want to go over the whole body and consolidate the benefits of the breathing and stretching.

With eyes closed and breathing softly into the belly, slowly bring your awareness first to your toes, then your feet, your ankles, your lower legs, your knees, thighs, and hips. Slowly bring awareness to your fingers, your hands, your wrists, your lower arms, upper arms, and shoulders. Then bring awareness into your lower back, middle back, and upper back, up the spine from the bottom to the top, and the nerves and muscles alongside the spine from the bottom to the top of the spine.

Starting with the small intestine, bring awareness to each organ of the body. Then the belly, the waist, the chest, and the neck. Bring awareness to your face, mouth, nose, eyes, and ears and up through the top of the head.

Feel you are breathing white light into each part of your body; breathing in white light and circulating it to where it is needed. Pay special attention to your lungs. Start out with a quiet breath, breathing white light into your lower lungs for a few breaths; then breathe a little deeper and circulate the light into the middle of the lungs. Go slowly. Take your time. Each breath is a little deeper as you bring the white light into the very top of the lungs, filling every part of the airways. (The shoulders are quiet.) Continue to breathe fully and see the light glowing throughout your body and filling your lungs. See yourself floating in the sea of light surrounding you. And relax into the light.

EMPOWERMENT AND THE MARTIAL ARTS

Facing Fear with Tae Kwon Do

Brooklyn-based Nelson Howe, who has a Black Belt in Tae Kwon Do, uses this Korean martial art in his therapy practice for helping people overcome fear. The martial arts are empowering and that's particularly important in the case of asthma. "Because asthma is a chronic condition," says Howe, "people feel more and more helpless and unable to affect the condition—it takes away most of the pleasures of living. They've learned to feel helpless and deprived. The martial arts approach begins to reverse that learning and work on the person's ability to have choices, to do something that is often perceived as very hard to do."

The personal-best aspect of sports is very close to the martial arts approach. Developing the will to enhance one's health is part of the picture in terms of recovery. From Nelson's experience with asthma and his work with others in Tae Kwon Do and Expressive Therapy, he's found that personal empowerment is an important key to overcoming the effects of asthma. And the necessity of dealing with recurrent asthma was important in shaping the direction of his own life. Through this experience he learned to teach others to begin to put their asthma into what he calls "permanent remission."

One way he tries to give a feeling of empowerment is in working with groups developing "tiger energy." This energy is transformational and erases fear. "It's an energy everyone already has but perhaps hasn't been allowed to express. When you make friends with it again, it feels like nothing can stand in your way. Nothing will stop you, not even your asthma."

TIGER ENERGY

This exercise will give you a feeling of that empowerment: the feeling of your energy forming a wave that powerfully erases fear and carries you forward in life. Nelson leads us through this exercise to liberate energy and dissolve fear.

"It's important to be able to do the out breath before we start. It's an out breath in which we begin to vocalize with more and more energy until we are shouting at the top of our lungs. I combine it with Tae Kwon Do punching so each time you punch, you shout. Don't shout anything specific: it's just a wide-open mouth, loud-as-you-can-go shout, hitting with your breath.

"The shouting mobilizes the entire abdominal area. But you also need to mobilize that area the Japanese call *hara,* so that when you contract the muscles to breathe out you are pulling from the bottom of your abdominal cavity, pushing the breath all the way out from the very bottom."

1. The first step is to begin to develop that breath.
2. Then take the horse-riding stance, legs apart, knees slightly bent, as if sitting.
3. Imagine yourself a tiger. With your arms out in front of you your fingers become claws. Become this tiger standing on hind legs with front claws ready to spring.
4. As you enter this position, push your breath out so you can feel your stomach contract. Then relax the stomach so the breath automatically comes back in again. You must feel your stomach way down into your pelvis. It is crucial to force your breath out from way down there using the muscles of your stomach.
5. Once your stomach has pushed the breath out, again let the breath come back in automatically when you relax.
6. Now make a face like a tiger with mouth wide open, upper lip curled and teeth showing. This time push your breath out very fast, partially closing the throat. You want to sound like a ferocious animal making an enormous hissing sound which comes from the air passing through the throat. The sound comes out with such force that it sounds like a steam engine letting out steam or some huge animal making a sound combining a hiss and a growl.
7. As you forcefully expel your breath you will feel all the energy in your body going from your feet through your stomach and out your hands and fingers.
8. To increase your energy in this exercise, you can face a wall and push your fingers against the wall as if to drive your hands through it. As you push, you exhale. Visualize your asthma being pushed away, being defeated with this stream of powerful energy.
9. If there is a person or situation that is frightening, direct that energy at the person or situation you need to conquer. Feeling your power and energy will enable you to protect yourself and move forward in your life. The "tiger energy" can restore your power of choice.

"It's taken me a long time to believe that I could sustain aerobic exercise," says Andy, a social worker from Pennsylvania. "I've had asthma since I was two and was given Tedral and theophylline liquid. As a kid I engaged in sports, and when I would get out of breath I relied on inhalers.

"Later in life I used over-the-counter inhalers. I moved to the country in the summer and got a little worse but used homeopathic remedies and there was some benefit. I really didn't want to use inhalers and I stopped in 1983. I had a few years of rough summers but I felt I had to go through it. And then the first frosts would come and I would be clear. Looking back on it I probably created more scarring and I didn't really help myself by stopping the inhaler. Maybe it led to the bad asthma attack I had five years ago that I couldn't come out of for five days. I was working in a rehab center in an old hotel with old carpets and a lot of molds—there was smoke in the building and my marriage wasn't too good, with stress all around, and the bucket tipped over.

"I took whatever medicine the doctor gave me because I needed to function, but this time when the first frost came, the asthma didn't disappear. About eight months later I met Nelson and started working with him and then I came to the workshop.

"In Nelson's class I worked in Karate and martial arts. I started aerobic activity slowly. I had avoided it for a long time even though I knew I needed to do it to build myself up. I think that a combination of doing his class once a week and taking uphill walks has been good. I might need the inhaler to do the walk but at least I'm doing something; it's only been about a year now that I can do the exercises. I tape aerobics from TV and early morning and after work I play the tapes and do two minutes of aerobic exercises in the house.

"THE TIME OF FEARING VIGOROUS EXERCISE IS OVER"

"I'm not afraid now. It came to a point where something changed and there was a really good balance, a good feeling if I kept doing it. I learned some techniques working with and being guided by Nelson and I sensed what I needed to do to bypass that tightness and focus on the hara. Somehow concentrating all the heat down there, and using all my energy to focus there made the difference.

"I have made a lot of improvements in my life. I'm going to be fifty soon and still I get discouraged. I wonder when I'm going to get off these herbs.

But the herbalist says, 'You are doing very well, people of your age usually get worse and worse.' And I've been getting better and better.

"The most important thing is that I don't avoid the aerobic anymore—I'm getting to like it and it gives me a sense of accomplishment. The time of fearing vigorous exercise is over.

Tiger Energy and Emotions

"When I do the tiger energy exercise certain emotions and fears come up. Before when the fear came up the asthma would begin. Now when that fear comes up, instead of allowing the asthma to take control, I can get through it without the medication—by focusing on the hara.

"Strong emotion can trigger that muscle tightness and asthmatic reaction. The impulse I had was to use the inhaler as soon as that fear, panic, and awful sensation of tightening came up. The spray opens it right up but you no longer have the accessibility to what's going on. So by letting it come up, I'd maybe cry for ten seconds or so, but I had control over the feeling of asthma coming on. When I do the tiger exercise I'm bursting with energy in parts of my body. I start generating a lot of heat, the breathing just opens up, and the tightness goes. That's my big accomplishment. I'm not afraid to deal with terror or terrifying situations now. That's what I'd like you to say about me."

Other Ways to Connect to the Breath

Also helpful are low-impact aerobics classes where you can start out gently and get support and then move toward something more. Connecting your breath with your ability to move effectively is a way to empowerment and mastery of asthma. The martial arts–based activities as well as the Taoist and yoga exercises in this chapter lead us to greater mental, emotional, and physical health.

Modern dancing or ballroom dancing is also great exercise. Then graduate to square dancing. Anything that puts a smile on your face while you're doing it!

Important Reminders for Aerobic Activity

If you use medication be sure to premedicate before you leave home and take your bronchodilator with you. If you are working with your doctor to cut down on medication, be prudent; this may not be the time.

If you are not sure about your breathing, use your peak-flow meter (see

Resources) so you will be able to judge how you are at the time you want to exercise. This will help you decide about medication.

Dress appropriately. People with asthma should be covering up well indoors or out. You shouldn't be sweating and then getting chilled.

If you are going jogging out-of-doors, wear a scarf that can cover your mouth and nose. It will warm air if it's cold and keep out pollens in allergy season.

Warm up well before you start and do your yoga breathing.

Don't run at rush hour or where there is traffic. Inhaling exhaust fumes doesn't help. Jump rope in the house by the air conditioner during your allergy season.

Cool down after the workout and have an extra piece of clothing handy to put on to keep you warm.

Relax after your workout, let your awareness scan your body, and focus on the effects of whatever exercise you have completed.

CHAPTER 6

HORMONES AND ASTHMA

WOMEN'S HORMONES

Many women have commented that their asthma worsens when they get their periods or just before. This was first written about in 1931 although it has yet to be "proven."[1] Late-onset asthma has been noticed to occur often with the onset of menopause. And pregnant women report that their asthma has either improved or worsened during pregnancy. There seems to be an intriguing relationship between estrogen and progesterone hormone levels and asthma. I first noticed this when a workshop participant told how her asthma had returned when she was given synthetic estrogen and progesterone for menopausal symptoms.

Natural progesterone is sometimes thought of as a smooth muscle relaxer. It may have a bronchodilating effect because it is the smooth muscle encircling the airways that tightens during an asthma attack. But progesterone and estrogen must be maintained in a particular balance.

Then there is the problem of "xenoestrogens," which can mimic hormone functions in the body. We ingest, inhale, and absorb large amounts of xenoestrogens from pesticides, hydrocarbons from fuel emissions and other petroleum by-products, and PCBs (polychlorinated biphenyls), as well as synthetic estrogens from birth control pills and hormone-replacement therapy. Xenoestrogens mimic the chemical structure of our body's natural estrogens, and because they proliferate in our food, air, and water, women's hormones (and men's also) become imbalanced.[2]

Dr. Serafina Corsello, who is an expert on women's hormones, says that "toxic unopposed estrogen leads to many of our current gynecological problems. In this case there is too much estrogen in relation to the amount of progesterone. This is, in good part, responsible for the 'progesterone crisis' in which progesterone levels become too low in relation to estrogen." Dr. Corsello feels that "since progesterone is a natural bronchodilator, those with a proclivity to asthma will have more wheezing when progesterone levels fall."[3]

It is commonly known that more boys than girls start out with asthma in early childhood, but later women between the ages of twenty and fifty are three times more likely to be hospitalized for asthma than men. Estrogen rises sharply at ovulation in the middle of the menstrual cycle, then falls, and rises moderately again in the latter half of the cycle, falling off the last few days. Progesterone, however, rises sharply the latter part of the cycle and crashes suddenly at the end. Many women complain that their asthma gets worse when they begin to menstruate and the sudden lack of progesterone may explain why.

Dr. Corsello views it this way: "Progesterone plays the major role. We are in a progesterone crisis in Western culture, especially in America, where we eat junk. We ingest estrogen from feed with our meat, milk, cheese, and eggs, so we are besieged by estrogen all the time. To make things worse, by ingesting pesticides containing xenoestrogens, we are constantly exposing our kids and ourselves to toxic estrogen.

"Progesterone is a bronchodilator. I am talking about endogenous progesterone and natural progesterone. Fortunately, we now have natural progesterones that one can buy from compounding pharmacies. Natural progesterone relaxes the bronchial tree and the vessels and improves thyroid function. One has a far better balanced system if there are adequate amounts of progesterone. Adequate amounts of natural progesterone will diminish the estrogen, thereby reducing the chance of the unopposed estrogen crisis.

"Women get more asthma after menopause. They become more susceptible because in this phase one tends to have outbursts of estrogen production. Many of my patients who had allergies in childhood now have bronchial asthma. Progesterone also compensates for inadequate adrenal hormones. I call progesterone the 'masochistic mother hormone'; it becomes many other hormones we need—until it runs out of steam.

"During early menopause the body is in a state of hormonal disequilibrium. If all women took adequate amounts of progesterone throughout their life, including during menopause, that would diminish their chances of getting asthma. I'm not saying it will eliminate it, because it is multifactorial, but it would certainly help.

"I start with progesterone cream. If in two months symptoms do not

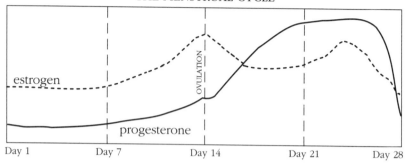

THE MENSTRUAL CYCLE

estrogen

OVILATION

progesterone

Day 1   Day 7   Day 14   Day 21   Day 28

change I add oral micronized progesterone. I am not talking about synthetic progestines. These interventions are medical in nature and need to be medically supervised."

Estrogen Hormone Replacement

Dr. Corsello's theory of "unopposed estrogen" being the culprit is supported by several recent studies. Israeli researchers at Ben-Gurion University followed fifteen postmenopausal women with mild to moderate asthma through two thirty-day periods in which they kept a dairy of their peak expiratory flow. The first thirty days was before estrogen hormone replacement and the second thirty days was during estrogen replacement therapy. They found that the women taking estrogen used the bronchodilators significantly more during the replacement therapy. Although there wasn't statistical significance between the spirometery measurements, the researchers felt that during estrogen replacement therapy there was a trend toward the worsening of the asthma.[4]

In another study researchers at Harvard Medical School, Harvard School of Public Health, and Brigham and Women's Hospital in Boston analyzing questionnaires from 121,700 women from the Nurses' Health Study (NHS) found that there was an increased risk of asthma among women who had used oral contraceptives, and that women receiving hormone therapy for ten or more years were at asthma risk. They concluded that "in some postmenopausal women, long-term use of high doses of estrogen may be associated with a moderately increased risk of asthma."[5]

So there is a relationship between hormone levels and asthma, and one hopes researchers will be paying more attention to it.

Dr. Corsello reminds us that the immune system, the adrenal system, and all the systems are interrelated. "The return to health is a very cumbersome and complex voyage. It doesn't happen overnight. The fact is that when the body falls apart, it's like a symphony when there's no harmony. You need a good director, all the instruments, and good players, and then you make music. It may take long but it doesn't have to be forever."

STEROIDS AND OUR ADRENAL GLANDS

The question of whether or not adrenal function plays a part in asthma has come up among researchers but has been dismissed. One study of the hypothalamic-pituitary-adrenal function of patients with "extrinsic" asthma found no abnormality in blood plasma levels of adrenocorticotropic hormone and cortisol.[6] According to Dr. A. Szentivanyi's 1968 theory, impaired beta-adrenergic receptors could cause asthma, because incorrectly balanced adrenergic receptors cause bronchial spasm.[7] Some researchers today feel that impaired beta-receptors may be from inflammation or from inhaler therapy.[8] No research, they say, has surfaced proving that poor adrenal function has anything to do with asthma.

"Two Little Glands"

In traditional Chinese medicine there is no respiratory system or endocrine system that corresponds to ours. But in the case of asthma, kidney weakness is often involved. Kidney weakness refers to a larger area that includes everything affected by the kidney meridian, including the adrenal glands.

The adrenals are two little glands that sit atop and in front of the kidneys on either side of the body in the area roughly corresponding to the lower back. The left kidney is usually larger and higher than the one on the right.[9]

The adrenal glands are each composed of two separate and distinct organs of glandular secretion, which together secrete more than forty hormonally active compounds.

The *adrenal medulla,* the inner portion, in instant response to nerve signals, secretes epinephrine, which Dr. Levin calls the "God-given prototype of beta-adrenergic drugs." Epinephrine, one of the most important adrenal hormones (but not a steroid), stimulates the adrenergic receptors of the sympathetic nervous system. In a healthy respiratory system there are more beta 2-

receptors, providing normal relaxation of bronchial smooth muscle. According to Szentivanyi's theory, people with asthma may have defective beta-receptors, a situation which would not allow a normal response of the bronchial smooth muscle. Your bronchodilating inhaler is a beta-adrenergic drug which evidently fills that gap.

The *adrenal cortex,* the outer portion of the adrenal glands, secretes cortisone, a glucocorticoid which is mostly inactive until it is converted to hydrocortisone (cortisol). Your steroid medications mimic the action of the cortisol. Oral steroids, particularly in large doses, will eventually suppress the action of your own adrenal cortex, which aggravates the problem.

By now you may also be wondering why we don't hear more about the adrenal glands in relation to asthma!

In traditional Chinese medicine the kidney energetic helps the lungs support the Qi. A weakened kidney meridian results in shallow breathing. And the adrenal glands are on this kidney meridian. An acupuncturist would determine if the kidney meridian was weak and work on releasing the blockage so that Qi or energy could flow through. An herbalist practicing traditional Chinese medicine would give herbs to strengthen the kidney-meridian function. These practices may not give instant relief such as your inhaler affords, and it could take up to several years to strengthen the kidney meridian. The proper diet, exercise, and rest will also affect the outcome. But one of the differences between prescription drugs and Chinese medicine is that the herbs and the acupuncture will work to rebalance the body, and allow it to heal itself.

Because the kidney works to filter toxins, such as chemicals, from the body, the constant use of the inhaler and other drugs will only further weaken your kidney function. This explains in part why asthma becomes a "chronic" condition.

Adrenals and Allergies

Adrenal problems may be epidemic in our society. Dr. John Tintera, an endocrinologist, wrote in 1959 that in his twenty years of working with thousands of patients, he hadn't met anyone whose allergies weren't due primarily to poorly functioning adrenal glands. He says they only found relief when the adrenals were again working properly, and that this included patients who suffered from asthma. Dr. Tintera says that the lymphocytes in the immune system cannot do their jobs without assistance from adrenal cortex hormones. "If the adrenal cortices are under-functioning, if they are semi-exhausted and unable to respond fully to stimulation, these essential hormones are either insufficient in amounts or they are chemically out of balance. Here, then is the basic cause of allergies and infections." Dr. Tintera says that some people are born with undersized or weak adrenals and that if the adrenals are not strong, every stress cuts into their reserve.[10]

WHAT STRESSES THE ADRENALS?

The word *stress*, as we now use it, was coined in the 1950s, when Hans Selye wrote his book *The Stress of Life*. Previously the word *stress* was used in industry and had to do with the endurance of metals.

In that famous and much quoted book, Selye lists a few of the stressors of adrenal function, such as diet, sound, light, vibration, electricity, magnetism, grief, constitution, temperature variations, immunity, hypoxia, hemorrhage, and exercise, including athletics.[11] Psychoanalyst Leon Hammer writes, "Chinese medicine agrees (with Selye) that stress is the principal issue in disease and that more than one stressor is usually necessary to produce symptoms and signs."[12]

Liberation from Steroids

Steroids, as so many of us know, are a major treatment for the inflammation of asthma. But steroids can cause unpleasant and deleterious side effects, and those dependent on this treatment wish to be free of them. *Steroids* is a broad term that includes cortisone and hydrocortisone (cortisol), naturally occurring steroids made by the adrenal gland. Steroids also include a host of pharmaceuticals such as prednisone, which is not found in the body except when used as a prescription.

Dr. Warren Levin has lectured to other doctors on the subject "Making Your Steroid-Dependent Patients Independent." He explains that all allergy represents—in addition to immune dysregulation—inadequate adrenal-cortical function. "It's something that clinical endocrinologists understood years ago but today is not evaluated accurately by the standard tests performed by today's laboratory-oriented endocrinologists.

"Our bodies run on an elegant control system," says Dr. Levin. "It's like a thermostat on the wall connected to the furnace in the basement and pipes to the radiator. And when it's fifty degrees outside and you say it's cold in here, I want it to be seventy, you turn the system on and turn the dial on the thermostat. The thermostat is a *sensing device* that says, 'It's cold in here,' and it's a *sending device* that sends a *signal* down to the basement to the furnace and says, 'Make some heat.' The furnace turns on and the heat comes up in the pipes. It warms the room and when the temperature reaches seventy

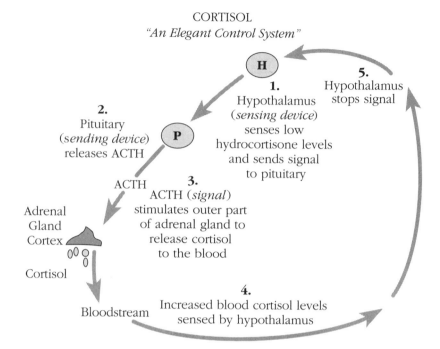

CORTISOL
"An Elegant Control System"

H

1.
Hypothalamus
(*sensing device*)
senses low
hydrocortisone levels
and sends signal
to pituitary

5.
Hypothalamus
stops signal

2.
Pituitary
(*sending device*)
releases ACTH

P

ACTH

3.
ACTH (*signal*)
stimulates outer part
of adrenal gland to
release cortisol
to the blood

Adrenal
Gland
Cortex

Cortisol

Bloodstream

4.
Increased blood cortisol levels
sensed by hypothalamus

degrees the sensing device says, 'That's enough,' and the furnace goes off, because the sending device stops sending a signal. And then the temperature starts to drop and at a sensitive point it goes on again. In a properly designed and engineered and functioning system you don't even notice because the temperature seems to be at seventy degrees all the time.

"The *sensing device* is a part of the brain called the hypothalamus. The hypothalamus constantly measures the amount of hydrocortisone, the representative hormone for all the steroids. And if the level of hydrocortisone drops below the current requirement it says to the pituitary 'Hey send a signal down and tell the adrenal gland that we need more steroids.' The pituitary gland is the *sending device* and it secretes ACTH (adrenocorticotropic hormone). ACTH is the *signal,* goes into the bloodstream, gets to the adrenal gland, the adrenal gland responds by secreting more steroids, puts it into the bloodstream, comes up to the hypothalamus and when there's enough, the hypothalamus says, 'Okay'.

"Because cortisone and hydrocortisone are stress-related hormones, the amount that we need varies from minute to minute and day to day, individual to individual, and stress to stress. All the stressors in our lives are mediated by the adrenal cortex, and that includes physical stressors, emotional stressors, chemical stressors, and everyday demands of living."

Adrenaline, though made in the adrenal gland, isn't a steroid. It's the emergency hormone for flight, fight, or fright. But its release leads to increased steroids, the major adrenal stress hormones. And steroids have all kinds of impacts on the body, including suppression of the immune system. When someone is having an acute allergic reaction, it can be suppressed with a large amount of synthetic steroids, more than the body is capable of making itself.

And here is the problem, says Dr. Levin. "When they started investigating these steroid hormones they used doses that far exceeded what the body is capable of making. When you're given prednisone or any of the other cortisone-type drugs in the enormous doses that are being used, the hypothalamus is fooled by the high level and stops pituitary release of ACTH. The adrenal is completely turned off. And when it isn't used, it shrivels up and atrophies. And when you stop the steroids it's incapable of giving a normal response. This is the most serious complication of adrenal steroids even in moderate doses over a long period of time."

LET THE ADRENAL GLAND REBUILD ITSELF

"On the other hand, small doses of natural cortisone or hydrocortisone—up to about one-half of a healthy daily output (i.e., five milligrams four times a day)—act like one or two space heaters in an overworked system—they reduce the demand but do not override the thermostat, so the adrenal continues to function and doesn't atrophy, but can heal. If you give small doses of adrenal hormones you can take some of the stress off of the gland and it can start to regain its health. It gets a chance to cool down and it may even function better when it starts up again."

SO WHAT'S THE SOLUTION?

"You need nutrients to make the adrenal steroids," explains Dr. Levin. "With artificial steroids you lose magnesium and you lose calcium. They also cause potassium loss and sodium retention. Anyone given high doses of cortisone should be given calcium and vitamin D and magnesium and potassium as supplements. That at least will reduce the impact of the damage.

"What I see over and over again is that in the hospital people are given steroids to control their asthma, and once it's under control they're tapered off and they feel fine. But little by little the steroids fade away and then the adrenal gland is not able to meet the demand again. And around six or eight weeks after a rapid tapering off of the steroids there is another flare-up. The problem is that people are not being given anything to stimulate the return of adrenal function in these cases.

"Vitamins and minerals and injections of ACTH should be used while going off steroids, because during that time your own adrenal glands are not being stimulated, and this gets them working again. Steroids are a great treatment for acute stuff but when you have to take them all the time it's a disaster. The better treatment is slower tapering, combined with stimulating ACTH, and nutrition.

"Allergies are the primary stressor in asthma. You can suppress allergic reactions with large amounts of cortisone, but that suppresses adrenal-cortical function, leading to increased allergies—a vicious cycle. A healthy adrenal response suppresses allergic reactions without a prescription!"[13]

WHAT ELSE CAN NOURISH THE ADRENALS?

- Nutritional deficiencies and imbalances must be corrected. Pantothenic acid, for instance, is a major antistress nutrient. It stimulates the adrenals to produce more hormones.[14] Vitamin B_3 (niacinamide), Vitamin C, Vitamin B_6, zinc, and magnesium are all important for adrenal function.
- Herbs can also strengthen the adrenals. Certain herbs called *adaptogens* have a balancing effect regardless of the condition. They will increase the ability of the body to withstand all kinds of stress, such as emotional and environmental stress, abrupt changes of weather and chemical pollution. Good adaptogens include Chinese herbs such as astragalus and codonopsis, which along with lycii berries and discoria can be cooked together in a soup.[15]
- Herbalist Susun Weed recommends dandelion and nettle to repair kidneys and rebuild adrenals.[16]
- Panax ginseng, one of the most famous Chinese medicinal plants, may also be useful and effective in preventing the atrophy of adrenal glands associated with longtime corticosteroid use, according to naturopath Michael Murray in *The Healing Power of Herbs.*[17] Ginseng has been shown to have an antistress effect which may come from its ability to act on adrenal function. It has been found that ginseng helps the pituitary gland to promote production of adrenocorticotropic hormone (ACTH).[18] This, as Dr. Levin just showed us, is needed to stimulate the adrenal glands to get going again. For people taking corticosteroids, Panax and Siberian ginseng may help restore adrenal function.[19]

- Stimulating drinks such as coffee, alcohol, and colas should be reduced and then eliminated.
- Proper rest and sleep are important.

WHAT WE CAN DO FOR ADRENAL EXHAUSTION

Many symptoms besides allergic reactions to foods accompany adrenal weakness. These include infections, chemical toxicities from heavy metals and organic chemicals, and sensitivity to chemical fumes.[20]

Avoid exposures to heavy metals and toxic fumes, both of which also affect the immune system. Fumes include combustion fumes, volatile organic compounds (VOCs), and organochlorines such as solvents, pesticides, dry-cleaning products, and wood preservatives. Avoid plastics and store food, for instance, in stainless-steel food containers.

Avoid phenol, formaldehyde, radon, and fluorescent light.

NATURAL LIGHT AND THE HORMONAL SYSTEM

Fluorescent light has a detrimental effect on adrenal function and the entire glandular system, particularly the pituitary gland.[21]

Daylight is the ideal light. John Ott, author of *Light, Radiation and You*, recommends lights which derive almost equal energy from all bands of the visible spectrum. Just as we can become malnourished from a diet lacking the proper balance of vitamins and minerals, Ott's studies indicate that we can also suffer malillumination from a lack of the full spectrum of wave lengths found in sunlight. According to Ott, even when we are exposed to daylight, we are often deprived of the benefits of the full spectrum because of windshields, windows, tinted glasses, contact lenses, smog, and even suntan lotions.[22]

What We Can Do for Proper Light

- We need light (not glare) in our eyes for at least a half hour daily for hormone balance. This should be without glasses, contact lenses, windows, or windshields. The shade is fine.
- We need to sleep in a dark room for correct melatonin release.
- We need the full spectrum of light for early winter morning doldrums and proper function of our hormonal system.
- If you can't get out of the house much or you work under fluorescent light, replace a tube or two with a full-spectrum Vita-Lite.

  John Ott says, "Light is a nutrient like food and the wrong kind can make us ill and the right kind can help keep us well."[23]

Rest, relaxation, and a good night's sleep are also needed for adrenal and immune repair. Taoist herbal practitioner Drew Di Vittorio advises eight or ten hours a day to replenish our energy at night. "When we sleep, between 11:00 P.M. and 3:00 A.M. the energetic points of our body open up and we accept energy from the universe, which replenishes us. It's one of the ways in which we are renewed. If we don't get rest we don't get better."

Learn to distinguish between nervous energy and real energy. When you start to overdo it, remember to let the tension go, relax, and start slow abdominal breathing.

For a Good Night's Sleep

- Don't eat after 8 P.M.
- Take a walk before bedtime.
- Warm feet in a hot foot bath.
- Make sure the room is dark. Staring at the bright light of the TV does not induce melatonin release necessary for sleep.
- Play some gentle, relaxing music while falling asleep.

What Are We Doing to Our Essence?

In Chinese medicine we saw that the Kidney Essence is the substantial basis of the body. To strengthen the kidney, one tries to support this Essence. As we have seen, some Western doctors also believe in strengthening and supporting the immune system rather than further weakening it with drugs. And adrenal function must be addressed because it will affect all the related systems of the body.

CHAPTER 7

ALLERGIES

THE IgE

S o did you know that I had asthma and I got better?" asked Dr. Warren Levin. A physician with "one wife, two kids, a German shepherd, two cats, and five kittens," Dr. Levin suffered from asthma for three years. "One evening I was reading in a reclining chair and one of the kittens crawled up and stretched herself out under my chin and went to sleep, and I took a nap and woke up with asthma. It certainly was a major change in my life; I had been active and vigorous and now couldn't do anything. I did not ever have to be hospitalized, but I took drugs for three years. Not any long-term steroids, but maybe one or two short courses. I got rid of the cats, and put in a central vacuum system."

Dr. Levin recalls that a patient he had been treating for depression read about hypoglycemia (a blood sugar imbalance) in a women's magazine and finally convinced him to look into the glucose tolerance test. After talking to several practitioners he found someone he admired for his scientific approach who introduced him to the work of Dr. John Tintera.

Dr. Levin's patient improved rapidly on a hypoglycemia diet, and so did his daughter, who had a similarly misdiagnosed blood sugar problem.

"When she did so well I started going to meetings about this kind of nutrition. I learned about food allergy. I went on a diet, took some vitamins, avoided the foods that I tested allergic for, and in six months I was well. I had never seen that before. Now I have had several episodes of asthma since, so that the word 'cure' has to be used advisedly, but each episode has been from an inadvertent and unknown exposure to cats who were nowhere to be seen."

The Allergy Connection

"All asthma is allergic," said the late Dr. Ralph Bookman in a 1988 interview in *Rodale's Allergy Relief Newsletter*. "If more physicians realized this, asthma would be treated much more efficiently in this country."[1] Dr. Bookman went on to say that asthmatics treated by good allergists are hospitalized less frequently than those who are not. This flies in the face of treatment of asthma by most pulmonologists.

Anything ingested or inhaled regularly may eventually cause an allergic reaction. Allergists, however, treat "classic" IgE-mediated allergies, allergies to common grasses, pollens, molds, and dander, which are only one part of the sensitivity problem.

THE IgE ANTIBODY

The IgE (immunoglobin E) allergy antibody was discovered in 1967. A 1980 NIH publication *Asthma and Allergies: An Optimistic Future* states that this discovery "brought the study of allergy into the mainstream of scientific research. Since that time, rapid progress has been made in unraveling the scientific basis of allergic disorders."[2] But in the 1980s the numbers of people contracting asthma rose drastically and the mortality rate soared. So the future wasn't so rosy after all.

WHAT HAPPENS IN AN IgE ALLERGIC REACTION?

In 1980, Dr. Alfred Zamm also wrote a book to explain allergies and to warn people about the danger of toxins in their homes. Here he describes a typical allergic mechanism at work:

What happens is that the body's defense system mistakenly recognizes an allergen as an enemy, as a foreign substance, as something that must be eliminated. The immune system starts churning out a special kind of antibody to neutralize or annihilate the invaders, just as though they were disease germs. Now the body is "sensitized," primed for the next invasion. (If it doesn't come, the antibodies diminish in number; that's why the longer one can stay away from an offending substance, the better.) Now the allergen particles reappear. Whenever an antigen meets its specific antibody, they lock together like two magnets. One effect is that the small blood vessels dilate; another is that some of the specialized mast cells release histamine that circulates and settles all over the body, and those tissues that are particularly sensitive react, swelling and stimulating surrounding nerves, causing itching, burning, redness, and all the uncomfortable symptoms associated with an allergic reaction. If the reacting organ is the skin, its blood vessels and cells—now swollen, distorted, broken down, and oozing their contents—appear as a rash. If it happens in the mucus lining of the nose, sinuses, or tracheobronchial tree, the glands produce surplus mucus, which the victim attempts to get rid of by coughing, sneezing, or nose blowing.[3]

When the mast cells release histamine it causes the inflammation of asthma. The leukotrienes, other chemical mediators isolated in 1985, are thought to be twenty to one thousand times more powerful than the histamines.[4] The release of leukotrienes increases mucus production and the narrowing of the airways. This early phase can happen fast and may peak in a half hour or go on for many hours. In this kind of reaction it is easy to connect the cause with the effect.

In the late phase or late response, certain white blood cells travel to the infected area to cause more inflammation. The late phase can occur hours later, or even the next day, making it more difficult to determine what was the trigger.

To What Are You Allergic?

When I ask people with asthma what triggered their asthma, the IgE-mediated allergies are usually the only sensitivities mentioned. IgE antibodies react to common allergens such as molds, pollens, grasses, mites, dust, dander, and certain foods. They are easily tested for and identified and are the ones that most doctors feel comfortable with. You may be sensitive to other substances but other antibodies are still poorly understood. Most food allergies are not IgE-mediated and attention is not paid to them in adults. Other substances to which you may be sensitive, such as chemical and automotive fumes, formaldehyde, perfumes, natural gas, and petrochemical products not mediated by this antibody, are also often not acknowledged by conventional allergists. Some people with asthma know that they are chemically sensitive, especially if they have connected the onset of their asthma with the sensitivity. Whether these are "true" allergies or not, the outcome is exactly the same.

A Major Cause

Dr. Levin also feels that the major cause of asthma is allergy. "I think that's one of the things many pulmonary specialists are ignoring to the detriment of their patients. I would put chemical sensitivities in the allergic category, but the official position of allergists in the United States is that the only way you know if someone is allergic is if they've got [elevated] IgE.

"In childhood, I think children outgrow asthma. People have pretty classical asthmatic bronchitis and they stop having it. Around puberty they just change. Now many times, later in life they'll get it back, but I think it's avoidable. The asthma is the last stage of what we call atopy. And it begins with a diaper rash in infancy, eczema, goes on to nasal congestion, allergic rhinitis, sinusitis, otitis, and then asthma, the IgE-mediated illness. And it also includes anaphylaxis, the most acute manifestation. Once whatever this ephemeral magical barrier is—the first acute episode of asthma in an adult, in most cases, irrevocably changes that person. I think that they become sensitive to things that they weren't sensitive to before."

IgE and Beyond

If your doctor administers a blood test that demonstrates a high level of IgE antibodies, you will be thought to be allergic. But environmental physicians know that you can have a low IgE and still have asthma.

They treat the whole spectrum of allergies, including chemical sensitivities, and try not to use more chemicals to treat what is already an imbalanced condition. Rather, as we saw earlier, they attempt to rebalance the body with what it lacks. An overgrowth of candida is sometimes associated with multiple chemical sensitivities. And low blood sugar or hypoglycemia is often found in people with allergies. Both of these conditions are often present in people with asthma and are worsened by the drugs treating the symptoms.

Does Ozone Exposure Make Allergies Worse?

Ozone, a potent destroyer of lung tissue, may increase permeability of the cells and make you more susceptible to pollens and grasses and other allergens.[5] So it could be possible that the chemical pollution comes first and the IgE reactions follow.

First we are going to look at some of the common IgE-mediated allergies and then at some chemicals and foods which may also be making you ill.

ALLERGY QUESTIONNAIRE

Variation by Time: Seasonal Incidence (Dates apply only to temperate climates; others may differ.)	Yes	?	No

Do Your Symptoms Get Worse:

1. In the spring—March to May? (Allergen could be tree pollens.) ___ — ___

2. In the early summer—May to August? (Perhaps grass pollen.) ___ — ___

3. In the autumn—mid-August to middle or end of September? (May be ragweed.) ___ — ___

4. From spring to first frost, with a peak from late July to frost? (Probably mold.) ___ — ___

5. In the winter—mid-September to spring? (May be house dust.) ___ — ___

(All allergy questionnaires are reprinted with permission of Alfred Zamm, M.D., and Robert Gannon from *Why Your House May Endanger Your Health,* Simon & Schuster.)

THE COMMON ALLERGENS

Pollens and Grasses

Pollens and grasses cause identical problems of sneezing, itchy eyes, runny nose, sinusitis, and for people with asthma, tightness of the chest and increased wheezing. In temperate climates tree pollen allergens produce symptoms which are worse from March to May. Grass pollen allergies worsen from May to August.

You may notice that you are worse out-of-doors, but when grass and tree pollens start blowing around they are going to find their way indoors as well. Air conditioners and air cleaners with HEPA (high-efficiency particulate arrestance) filters help in the bedroom. Try air filter panels if you want to open the windows (see chapter 10).

Ragweed

If your symptoms are worse mid-August to mid- or late September in the East your problem may be ragweed. However, in the Northeast and Central Plains, August through October is peak ragweed time. On the West Coast, seasons vary, from June to October in the California lowlands to July through September in the extreme Pacific Northwest.

If you are ragweed sensitive don't decorate with these: asters, bachelor buttons, calendulas, chrysanthemums, coriopsis, cosmos, dahlias, daisies, dandelions, goldenrods, marigolds, pyrethrums, sunflowers, and zinnias.

Tree Pollens

Tree pollen allergens can include mountain cedar, oak, sycamore, poplar, maple, birch, ash, and cottonwood.

Dust

House dust allergy often begins when the heating season starts and gets better in the spring. Sometimes people are worse when they get up in the morning but feel better as the day progresses.

House dust is really a combination of everything that is already in the house with whatever is tracked in. If house dust is the problem, air-conditioning may not help, and you will feel worse indoors. Children, who live much closer to the floor, are more likely to inhale these dusts in addition to the chemicals used to shampoo, mothproof, or stainproof the carpet. In winter, as bits of synthetic carpet fibers circulate through the heating system, they change their chemistry and may produce more than a hundred compounds adding chemical vapors to the air.[6]

Dust Mites

Some people are sensitive to dust mites, which, like molds, flourish in damp, warm conditions. The mighty dust mite is a microscopically small creature who feeds on the scales of human skin we constantly shed, which they find in carpets, mattresses, pillows, and upholstered furniture. The waste particles and tiny dead bodies of these mites (luckily for us, too small to be seen) may be a potent allergy trigger and are implicated as a prime suspect in asthma.

Mite Control

- For mite control in the bedroom, humidity should be kept below 60 percent relative humidity. A dehumidifier will help.

- Sheets and pillowcases should be washed in very hot water, and mattresses and box springs should be encased in zippered covers.
- Vinyl mattress covers may not be the answer, however, as many people cannot tolerate plastics. One hundred percent cotton barrier cloth mattress covers will protect the most sensitive person (see Resources).
- There are products available to control dust mites that can be sprayed on the suspect rug or mattress.
- Getting rid of the carpets helps get rid of dust and dust mites.

Use an air cleaner with an HEPA filter for all inhalant allergies.

MOLD   Yes   ?   No

Do your symptoms occur or get worse:

1. When you are exposed to a succession of days   ____ __ ____
   of damp weather?

2. When you rake dry leaves?   ____ __ ____

3. When you are near a lawn that's being   ____ __ ____
   mowed?

4. When you are in a damp basement?   ____ __ ____

5. When hay is being raked?   ____ __ ____

6. When you eat foods made by fermentation: ____ __ ____
   beer, wine, sharp cheeses, sauerkraut, pickles,
   vinegar, mushrooms?

7. Do you feel better when snow is on the   ____ __ ____
   ground? (Snow covers outside sources of mold:
   decayed vegetation, dry leaves, dry grass, and
   so on.)

8. Are you allergic to penicillin? (mold-based)   ____ __ ____
   If so, you are probably allergic to molds.

Molds like to grow in damp, dark, poorly ventilated places such as damp basements, bathrooms, kitchens, laundry rooms, and inside the refrigerator, as well as in the drip pan under the refrigerator. Molds grow at home, school, and places of work.

Anyone who consistently breathes mold spores can become allergic, and, unfortunately, the more you breathe the more allergic you will become. Molds grow indoors when there is sufficient damp. Leather, paper, plastic, wood, and cloth will all support mold growth if they have been subjected to high humidity (over 75 percent) or excessive dampness. Air ducts are especially vulnerable to harboring molds when the same ducts are shared by the air conditioner.

GETTING RID OF MOLDS AND MILDEW

- Zephiran is a disinfectant and mold inhibitor. Try mixing one ounce to a gallon of distilled water. You can use this to wipe down potentially moldy surfaces to keep mold from forming in the first place. Zephiran is available from most drugstores.
- Borax is an excellent fungicide and can be mixed with white vinegar and used to remove mildew around the refrigerator door and to clean bathroom tiles. Drip pans are havens for mold. Use this combination for cleaning the drip pan under the fridge regularly.
- Put a few drops of hydrogen peroxide in the air-conditioner drip pan every week when in use. Clean at the beginning and end of the season.
- Avoid stirring up mold spores. Use a triple-filter vac or install special filter paper in your existing vacuum cleaner.
- Repair water leaks.
- Vent clothes dryer to the outside.
- Rugs and rug pads should be aired out and dried or dry-cleaned within twenty-four hours of exposure to water.
- Try one or two teaspoons of tea tree oil in one cup of water in a plant spritzer to rid house of mold. Open closets and cupboards and close all windows. Saturate the room and leave for a couple of hours. On return, open windows and air for a few more hours before using the room. (Could be done overnight.) Lasts two months.[7]
- Use exhaust fans in bathroom and kitchen.
- Daylight, sunlight, and fresh air from open window can't be beat.
- Send for mold plates and find out where and what the mold is. (See Resources.)

You may be allergic to ANIMAL DANDER   Yes   ?   No

If your symptoms occur or get worse when:

1. You are exposed to mammals, such as cats,   ____ __ ____
   dogs, or horses?

2. You are exposed to animal hair (rabbit,   ____ __ ____
   mohair, wool in the form of blends, sweaters,
   gloves, liners, blankets), or rug padding, or
   furniture stuffing?

3. You are exposed to feathers (in pillows or   ____ __ ____
   down comforters), or birds (chickens, parrots,
   canaries), or to someone who has been
   working with fowl? (Some people sensitive to
   fowl dander also react to eating poultry or
   eggs.)

If you answered yes to any of these, animal dander is your problem.

THE PET CONNECTION

Pet dander is a classic allergen and the most heartbreaking, because no one wants to part from a beloved pet. In the pet kingdom there are many allergens, but cats far and away win the prize, perhaps because there are so many of them.

A Very Fine Dander

Some people with both asthma and cats swear that the cat is not giving them the problem. But when cats lick their fur, the saliva dries, and the resulting dander is extremely minute, making it easily inhaled into the lungs.

Here are some suggestions for those in co-dependent relationships with cats:

- If foster care is unacceptable the next best approach is to keep the cat out of the bedroom. It will not become neurotic as some have feared. And *you* need a danderless room to sleep in.
- An air cleaner with a good HEPA filter will remove 99 percent of particulates greater than 0.3 microns. This is a must because the fine cat dander may fly around when chairs are sat in or carpets are walked

on. Some machines are lightweight and can easily be carried into the bedroom, insuring a good night's sleep.

- Cat allergen is also sticky and clings to furniture surfaces as well as clothes and hair. Allergen levels can be reduced with a tannic acid solution. Test first for discoloration. Allergen concentrations will return to pretreatment levels if the cats are allowed back into the room.
- Even if tannic acid is used, damp mopping walls, ceilings, and hardwood floors is still in order.
- Start bathing the cat. Research conducted by Dr. H. James Wedner and his colleagues at the Washington University School of Medicine in St. Louis showed that repetitive washing of cats or kittens reduced the cat allergen protein to barely detectable levels in the bathwater. But cat washing takes time and commitment. Cats have to be washed for ten to fifteen minutes once a month for three to eight months. And all vertical and horizontal surfaces in the house still have to be cleaned thoroughly every few months. For the truly committed who want to cat-wash, the Division of Allergy and Immunology, Department of Medicine at Washington University offers a protocol. (See Appendix I.)
- The next recommendation will make some fur fly, but—learning to live without the cat will bring the greatest benefits with the least expenditure of time and money. You may even be thrilled by your new high level of functioning.

Overexposed

Today you don't even have to have a cat to be overexposed. Dr. Robert Lin, Chief of Allergy and Immunology at New York's St. Vincent's Hospital, says: "Fifty to seventy-five percent of people with asthma, with or without cats, are allergic to cats. Cat exposure is so ubiquitous in this society that even if you don't have a cat, you are exposed to enough cat allergens to become allergic. In schools, from friends and family, et cetera. The real test of cat allergy is if your asthma improved when you weren't exposed and got worse when you were. The only way to know for sure is to measure indoor dust levels for cat."

LATEX ALLERGIES

Allergy to latex is rarely considered when doctors talk about IgE-mediated allergy. But this allergy may not be as rare as one might suppose.

Latex, which comes from the milky sap of the rubber tree, has become a problem for hospital workers, perhaps because of the increased use of latex gloves. Reactions range from itchiness and rashes to breathing difficulties and anaphylactic shock.[8] A 1991 Canadian study found that latex allergies are on the rise as 7.4 percent of doctors and 5.6 percent of operating-room nurses reported allergies to latex.[9] Exposure to airborne latex, they found, produces symptoms of asthma.

Latex allergy is a Type I (immediate, IgE-mediated) allergy which can occur from contact with skin, mucous membrane, open wound, broken skin, or from injection or inhalation of the latex antigen. Inhalation occurs when latex gloves are discarded and the powder is released into the environment.

Doctors in Perugia, Italy, reported that people with no personal or family allergy history experienced symptoms of shortness of breath and wheezing from latex gloves.[10] They found that it took from one to sixteen years of use before onset of work-related respiratory problems and skin symptoms. Several of the study subjects reassigned to latex-free jobs still suffered chronic asthmatic symptoms one to seven years later.

Other sources of latex include adhesive on Band-Aids and other bandages, liquid bandage, rubber dams, tracheal tubes, adhesive tape, condoms, diaphragms, and surgical gloves.

For children who are latex sensitive, Mylar balloons could be used instead of rubber ones. Cotton socks should be worn with rubber shoes and cotton liners under latex gloves.[11]

If You Are Sensitive to Latex

- If you are having a medical or dental procedure, bring this sensitivity to the attention of the staff. Make sure it is in your records.
- Nonlatex gloves should be worn by any physician operating on you or by any health care provider with whom you have contact.
- Wear a Medic Alert bracelet that contains information of your latex allergy. The Canadian researchers suggest that you carry your own nonlatex gloves in case of an emergency.
- Bananas, avocados, kiwifruits, and chestnuts can cross-react with latex.[12] People with hay fever allergies and reactions to potatoes and tomatoes may also be susceptible to latex.[13]
- Carry an epinephrine autoinjection kit and know how to use it.
- If your child has asthma and has a latex allergy, the school officials and the school nurse should be informed.
- Check all manufacturers' product labels carefully before any purchase.
- Cotton liners, nonlatex gloves, and barrier creams can be used instead of latex gloves.

You can be tested and desensitized to common allergens either with allergy shots or drops that can be placed under the tongue. Drops are easy because they can be kept in the fridge and taken at home, saving many trips to the doctor's office. The scratch test on the skin; the RAST test, a blood test; and intradermal skin testing are the testing methods used by orthodox allergists.

A problem with all allergy serums is that some people are sensitive to the phenol used as a preservative while others become sensitive over time to both the phenol and the glycerine. Still, many people find marked improvement with allergy shots. Preservative-free serums are available from certain doctors.

SERIAL ENDPOINT DILUTION

Many environmental doctors feel that this is the best way to test although orthodox allergists have their doubts. In this method an antigen is tested and a dilution or endpoint (the concentration of antigen that gives no reaction at all) is identified. The endpoint varies from substance to substance. The shutoff dilution dose will rebalance the body's overactive antibody reaction. Shots or drops can then be given that eventually reduce allergenicity. Insurance carriers sometimes dispute payment for this testing, which they consider unproven.

NONINVASIVE TESTING

Although orthodox allergists use intradermal testing looking for a positive or negative skin reaction, and environmental doctors use it to find the endpoint dilution, testing the patient with asthma, who will have the greatest reaction, could be a problem. Either way, the greatest care should be taken. Some doctors feel that people with asthma should not be tested intradermally and desensitized until they have reduced their total load through avoidance of allergens, improved nutrition, and better digestion.

Aspirin-Induced Asthma

Aspirin-induced asthma is thought to be part of a triad which includes allergic rhinitis (runny nose), nasal polyps and/or sinusitis, and aspirin-induced bronchial asthma.[14] In aspirin-sensitive asthma there is usually a history of runny nose before the asthma developed. Then nasal polyps formed and then the asthma. Five to 10 percent of asthmatic adults experience severe or fatal reactions from aspirin.[15]

Leigh J. Lachman, M.D., an ear, nose, and throat specialist, says that the relationship of polyps with aspirin is not clear. "Allergy is the basic issue here—it doesn't help to get rid of the polyps."

People with aspirin-sensitive asthma have been told to use only Tylenol (acetaminophen). But some also react to acetaminophen. There are many over-the-counter medications on the market that contain aspirin. If you suspect an aspirin allergy, check with your doctor or pharmacist before purchasing any nonsteroidal anti-inflammatory drugs (NSAIDs).

FOOD ALLERGIES

In general, sensitization to allergens has traditionally been thought to happen between childhood and early adult life. Because many foods are not IgE-mediated, allergists often don't consider food an asthma trigger, particularly in adults. Most of the studies connecting food and asthma are done with children, who it is understood may be food allergic. Researchers at Baltimore's Johns Hopkins Children's Center recently found that many asthmatic children will fail to respond well to medication unless they avoid the foods to which they are allergic. Although food allergies had been connected with respiratory symptoms in the past, this was the first study to link them with changes in the airways through lung-function tests.[16]

But many alternative doctors feel that the number of older people with food reactions may be underacknowledged. Environmental doctors find that adults with asthma also improve by identifying all food allergies.

Food Reactions

There are two types of allergic reactions to foods:

Type I Allergies

These are reactions that occur immediately. Common foods causing Type I, IgE-mediated allergies are nuts, peanuts, fish, and shellfish. These are responsible for immediate onset reactions such as red skin patches, hives, swelling, and asthma. People having these reactions almost always test positive to skin tests and RAST tests.

Type II Allergies

Delayed onset or Type II reactions to foods such as milk, chocolate, legumes, citrus, and food coloring usually test negative for the IgE antibody. These delayed reactions may involve IgG, IgA, IgM, or IgD antibodies.

Other Types of Reactions

Some researchers have speculated that the delayed reactions of chemicals, drugs, and toxins in foods may be mediated by nonimmunological mechanisms.[17] These reactions are often called "sensitivities" rather than allergies.

LIFE-THREATENING ALLERGIES

Sometimes an allergy to a food such as peanuts can set off a life-threatening reaction. If a strong reaction has occurred, Dr. Jacqueline Krohn suggests complete avoidance of the food and caution when your food is prepared by someone else. She also suggests carrying epinephrine (Epi-Pin) at all times.[18] Sometimes foods such as peanuts are not easily detected. At a 1988 conference of the American Academy of Allergy and Immunology in Anaheim, California, researchers reviewed eight cases in which people who knew they had nut and shellfish allergies died of reactions to foods in which the ingredient was unidentifiable.[19]

AVOID LIFE-THREATENING FOOD REACTIONS

What better reason to adhere to a diet of freshly cooked whole foods?

Identify your allergens and stay away from foods with which you have had one bad experience.

MILD FOOD REACTIONS

On the brighter side, you may be allergic to a food in one state, but not in another. So before you give up a food that has caused only a mild reaction, steam it, roast it, or change the way you cook it. This may make it more tolerable to eat.

A FOOD CHALLENGE

Foods that are not mediated by the IgE mechanism are not well understood; some doctors think that most foods may be IgG mediated. Environmental and nutritional doctor Leo Galland, M.D., thinks that most foods may not be mediated through antibody mechanisms at all but through cellular mechanisms. Dr. Galland says that with a new asthma patient, after looking at molds and chemicals, he tries to ascertain food allergy from a dietary history; then he may do an intestinal permeability test, then an elimination diet and a challenge. The permeability test is done by giving a lactulose-mannitol drink taken fasting with no food, just water. The next day the patient takes the drink with a mixed meal of some regularly eaten foods, and he compares the results. If the second test shows an increase in permeability, it indicates an allergy to something that was eaten. The food challenge is done with a diet such as lamb and rice or a hypoallergenic product called Ultra-Clear, which is taken for five days, before regularly eaten foods are reintroduced, one by one.

POOR DIGESTION THE REAL CULPRIT

"The probability of the development of food allergy is much greater when digestion is suboptimal," says Dr. Martin Feldman. "Food allergies and environmental allergies are problems in asthma. Unfortunately, there is a lack of focus on foods as allergens in orthodox medicine. Every asthma patient needs to be a crusader to get their foods tested."

THE SPREADING PHENOMENON

And then there is the "spreading phenomenon." Food that we may never have had any trouble with before may now make our asthma worse. Dr. Levin says that in his own case, the foods that he had discovered he was allergic to that clearly gave him asthma, worsened the asthma while he was still asthmatic. So he avoided peanuts, pecans, grapefruit, and honeydew melon, and as he got well he continued to avoid them. But after some months of no attacks and perfectly normal lung function tests he started eating them without problems. Years later he had another episode of asthma when he stayed overnight in a house with a cat and was "absolutely flabbergasted," he said, "at how long that attack lasted. From a single exposure I wasn't well for weeks or maybe even a month. I took vitamins and I also used medication because I believed then and I believe now that the proper use of bronchodilators is important. By breaking that initial spasm, I believe you significantly reduce the complication rate. All during that time I had trouble with the same foods, the pecans and the peanuts, weeks after the exposure to the cats. And when it finally gradually died away I didn't have a problem with those foods anymore. I think that foods are a factor in at least 90 percent of the asthmatics that I see and it hasn't been entertained, let alone tested for."

MILK

Because milk is mucus-forming it may be the first item that people with asthma should avoid. Sensitivity to milk is not IgE-mediated and it can't be detected by ordinary skin tests.

Cow's milk was formulated by nature for cows, with more minerals, fatty acids, calcium, and protein than human milk.[20] These additions may not be in the best interest of the developing human baby. Although human milk contains less protein than cow's milk, it comes in a more digestible form, without the casein, which is one of many allergenic proteins found in cow's milk, and which creates problems in the human digestive system.

LACTOSE

Intolerance to lactose, a simple milk sugar, may be responsible for many cases of milk allergy. Lactose tolerability depends on lactase, an enzyme in the digestive system which breaks down the lactose. People of Asian, Native American, and African descent often have lactose problems. Caucasians' problems with lactose begin in the early teens.

AVOIDING COW'S MILK

- Milk creates mucus, which can add to asthma problems. Milk and milk products are best avoided.
- Goat's milk, however, is usually better tolerated.[21]
- Foods which may contain cow's milk include ice cream, cheeses, custards, biscuits, prepared mashed potatoes, junket, omelettes, pie crusts, chowders, waffles, and all kinds of processed foods—A good reason to stick to meals prepared from scratch.
- Food sources rich in calcium, and more easily absorbed than calcium in milk, are greens such as lamb's-quarters, collard greens, and turnip greens. One cup of collard greens contains 360 mg of calcium compared to goat's milk, which contains 320 mg per cup, more calcium than cow's milk.
- Other good sources of calcium include sea vegetables, sardines, almonds, kale, and broccoli.

FOOD ADDITIVES

Sometimes we are allergic to the pesticides, fungicides, preservatives such as sulfites and MSG, or food coloring on or in the food rather than the food itself. Try organic food and you may be able to give that carrot a second chance!

MSG

Monosodium glutamate–allergic people have mild to severe reactions from foods containing this flavor enhancer. MSG can be in wonton soup, sauces, bouillon cubes, and seasoning salts.[22] Vegetable protein and hydrolyzed vegetable protein contain MSG. Because it is found in many premixed commercial seasonings, restaurants often don't realize they are using MSG.

Sulfites

Common sulfite exposures can come from red wine, frozen potatoes, shrimp, and dried fruit. Sulfites are also ingredients in many medications, including some asthma medications. Check with your pharmacist about sulfites in over-the-counter medication.

Vitamin B_{12} can help diminish or prevent reactions to sulfites.[23]

MANAGING FOOD FOR POLLEN, GRASS, AND MOLD ALLERGIES

Our eating habits can contribute to our allergies, and what we are eating will affect to a great extent how we feel and how well we get through our worst allergy seasons. Of course, establishing good eating habits and maintaining them for life will make the greatest difference over the long haul. We'll learn more in the next chapter. For now we'll learn a few tricks to help us not react.

Ann, a forty-five-year-old writer, was very ill with asthma and sensitivities to just about everything for a number of years. She learned how to use food management as a tool for staying well in pollen and mold season.

"I noticed and was told by several less conservative doctors that foods can cross-react with certain pollens. If you find that your allergies are worse during the pollen and mold seasons, there are certain foods that will cross-react with those triggers. I put the list in my files and recently I got it out again. And for the first time I really paid attention to these foods and stayed away from them. The list contains a lot of the foods we eat all the time and it's very long, which is why I never bothered to do it before. But if you really pay attention and do it religiously you can avoid a lot of difficulty. For me, who gets so sick and feels so miserable at those times, it was really worth it. When ragweed season comes or anytime I'm feeling bad, I stop eating everything I'm used to eating. I also do this in mold season. It really helps."

Foods That Cross-react with

Grass Pollen
Cereal grains: grasses, wheat, barley, rye, rice, corn, and oats.

Birch Tree Pollen
Birch pollen allergy cross-reactions with apples can cause itchy mouth.[24] Other foods that cross-react with birch pollen include carrot, cherry, hazelnut, potato, pear, fennel, and walnut.

Ragweed

Chamomile, chocolate, tomatoes, green peppers, green peas, cane sugar, white potatoes, wheat, corn, eggplant, cantaloupe, paprika, milk, mint, watermelon, and rutin. Because sunflowers are in the ragweed family, you may also have a food problem with sunflower and safflower oils and sunflower seeds and nut butters.

Terpenes

Certain foods such as tomatoes, oranges, and saffron can cross-react with terpenes. If you are allergic to terpentine, perfume, fresh paint, and pine trees, you could have a worse reaction if you regularly eat these foods, according to French researchers.[25]

SELF-HELP FOR DISCOVERING FOOD ALLERGIES

Food Cravings

Sometimes we can identify the foods we are allergic to by looking at the foods we crave. We can also become allergic to common foods we eat every day over a long period of time. Sometimes we don't even realize how often we are ingesting corn, wheat, milk, or soy because they are hidden in so many other food items. There may not be any reaction because it is "masked." That is, eating the food we crave seems to make us feel better, so that we don't realize that we are allergic to it.

Allergic Symptoms

You may wheeze more or even have an asthma attack after you eat. Or you may have noticed certain other reactions when you eat a meal. Some people experience

- An itching at the back of the throat
- A blister on the tongue or lips or both
- A postnasal drip
- Itching or eczema on other parts of the body
- Hives
- An accelerated heartbeat
- Indigestion
- Rash on the face
- Exhaustion soon after eating
- Red ears
- A worsening of asthma symptoms

You may also recognize allergens as foods you eat every day. Foods commonly known to cause allergic reactions include:

eggs	fish
shellfish	nuts
citrus	corn
wheat	yeast
soy	peanuts
chocolate	milk

Check the items that you eat every day. Check the items you feel you can't do without. These are both good ways to identify possible trouble areas.

A Food/Symptom Diary

A food diary is a good way to keep track of food reactions. On the left side of the page write down what you eat that day and on the opposite page record any reactions, even if they happen hours later. Going back over the pages after several weeks will give you a picture of where your food problems lie. In the back of the diary have a minus page for reactive foods. Have a plus page for foods that you tolerate well. A food can cause a problem not only hours but one or two days after it is eaten.

Elimination Diet

This is a simple and cost-free way to uncover allergies. But don't test foods which you already know you react to. You want to avoid provoking serious symptoms.

Dr. Feldman says that the food being tested should be eliminated six days minimum and maybe ten to twelve days maximum. "If you eliminate for too few days you don't get good information because you may not have any reaction at all. But if you eliminate for too long and then reintroduce you may get a very severe reaction. So there is an ideal window in there of roughly six to eleven days." Look for symptoms or a change in condition. Write results in your food/symptom diary.

Five Day Rotation Diet

The rotation diet is also a simple, cost-free way to avoid high reactivity and to prevent becoming sensitized to things eaten regularly. In this diet you don't eat the same food again until the fifth day. The foods that you react to strongly should be completely eliminated for a while. Later they may be tolerated if only eaten occasionally. If you notice symptoms, cut that food out! Only foods that give a slight reaction should be rotated.

Ann, who showed us how certain foods cross-react with molds, grasses, and pollens, is also an expert at rotating foods.

"Another thing that really helped was taking seriously food elimination and rotating of foods. When my family and I went on vacation for a week, I took all my allergy cookbooks with me. I put all my amaranth and everything into little plastic bags and took it all along because we were renting a house and I could cook there. This kept me really allergy-free and happy. Wheat and corn are in everything, so I became much more allergic to them and although I might eat them at other times of the year, I have to rotate my foods and be really careful. I have every alternative grain known to humanity in glass jars in my freezer so that when I start to get really sick I can switch off. And then I start baking. Today I had buckwheat banana bread."

One Food Can Be Eaten within Twenty-four Hours

You can, however, eat the same food over a twenty-four-hour period. This is important so you won't be going crazy looking for new things to eat at every meal. When you cook dinner, pack up part of it in a stainless-steel container (put the plastic lid on when it cools) and save in the fridge to eat for lunch the next day. You will have your lunch all packed for work and you won't have to think about the new foods until dinner.

If you are severely ill with allergy or asthma you may have to be more focused and much more strict. As the asthma improves, the rotation can be relaxed.

Food Families

Some highly allergic people rotate not only the food but the food family. But you may have a reaction to only one or two foods in a food family. Doctors at the Mayo Clinic claim that only in members of the crustacean family (shrimp, crab, and lobster) is there a true cross-reaction. This probably varies from person to person. In a 1988 article in *Rodale's Allergy Relief,* Dr. Martin I. Sachs tells of a child who was very peanut allergic, yet had no reaction to peas.[26] Personally I've found it extremely useful to know that sunflower is in the ragweed family.

Pulse Testing

The pulse is tested at the same time every morning, such as at nine o'clock, five minutes before eating breakfast. You should be quiet and resting before you take this pulse. A resting pulse is usually between sixty and ninety beats per minute. The pulse must be taken for a full minute and retested fifteen to thirty minutes after eating each food, one at a time, by itself. A sensitivity may be indicated by a rise of twenty. The data has to be kept for at least five days to get a stable value. A fast heartbeat may be experienced when there is a strong allergic reaction with a food that is more easily tested.

Sublingual Food Testing with Kinesiology

In this noninvasive test the food substance is placed in the mouth under the tongue. The tester will first test the strength of a muscle (such as that of an outstretched arm). If the food substance is energizing to the body the muscle will hold its strength. If it is deenergizing or is negative to the body's energy, the muscle used for testing will weaken and the arm will not be able to resist being lowered by the tester. Each food should be tested on its own. This should be done by a skilled practitioner such as an osteopathic or chiropractic physician.

Provocative Neutralization Test

This technique was discovered in 1957 by Carleton H. Lee while he was looking for a better way to diagnose and treat food allergy. The allergen is injected under the skin and from the size of the wheal, or reaction that may be seen on inspection ten minutes later, the tester can decide how high or low the neutralizing dose should be. This is similar to serial endpoint dilution.

Cytotoxic Testing

Cytotoxic testing is the most controversial test for allergies because it has a reputation for inaccuracy. However, many doctors feel it is valuable.[27] One advantage is that many food allergens can be tested fairly inexpensively with one blood sample. This can give you a quick overview of what to watch out for. A patient's blood sample is sent to a laboratory and cells and parts of the blood, one drop at a time, are mixed with food extracts (the allergen) under a microscope and the reactions or nonreactions of the blood to these foods are measured. The technician rates the white blood cells' response to an allergen as marked, moderate, or slight. The PRIME test is the latest technologically advanced version of cytotoxic testing.

Elisa/Act Test

With one drop of blood over three hundred items can be tested for hyper-sensitivity of immune response. In addition to TYPE II, III, and IV food reactions, certain pesticides, chemicals, and toxic minerals can also be tested.

HYPOGLYCEMIA

People with asthma also often have blood sugar imbalances. Hypoglycemia, or blood sugar imbalance can also be allergy-related. Symptoms such as sudden exhaustion, panic attacks, and mood swings are often related to foods, especially those containing sugar. If you are hypoglycemic you may crave sweets which temporarily make you feel better but cause a tremendous let-down soon after. With this condition the body isn't metabolizing sugar correctly. The flood into the bloodstream of excess sugar puts a strain on the pancreas and the adrenal and other glands of the endocrine system that are responsible for regulating blood sugar levels.

You may not think that you eat much sugar, not knowing that sugar exists in many hidden forms in foods. Orange juice, for instance, is 13 percent sugar.[28] Alcohol, caffeine, tobacco, and salt can all contribute to hypoglycemia as well as nutritional deficiencies, food allergies, and emotional stress. Many doctors advise a high-protein, low-carbohydrate diet to stabilize blood sugar. However, naturopath Paavo Airola in *Hypoglycemia: A Better Approach* advises that for optimum health, the protein should come from sources other than animal products. Airola points out that proteins are made up of twenty-two amino acids, eight of which, essential amino acids, we need to take in every day. And all eight of these essential amino acids are contained in foods such as soybeans, pumpkin and sunflower seeds, almonds, avocados, potatoes, and green leafy vegetables.[29] In countries where meat is scarce, foods combined properly, such as corn tortillas and beans in Central and South America, become a complete protein.[30]

Dr. Airola suggests a diet of grains, seeds and nuts, vegetables, certain fruits, and fermented sour milks as the best route for recovery from hypoglycemia.

A CASE HISTORY: FOOD ALLERGIES, CANDIDA, AND HYPOGLYCEMIA

Donald's case is a saga of undiagnosed food allergies, candida, and hypoglycemia—often found together in adults with asthma. Donald, a forty-two-year-old businessman from New Jersey, developed asthma at the age of three. Although it subsided in his early twenties, it came back "pretty strong" when he was thirty-five. "When I was a kid I was allergic to ragweed and grass and was given prednisone and antibiotics. Later I went to an allergist and got shots, but from July to the end of September nothing would work and I was given antihistamine. From the age of thirty-five to forty I basically couldn't breathe and I had general malaise along with hypoglycemia."

Donald tells how this last five-year episode coincided with his and his wife's getting a cat and manifested in the form of food allergies. He was given a drug, Reglan, for digestive problems and Zantac for gastroesophageal reflux. A pulmonologist treated the asthma with Theo-Dur and a Ventolin spray. "I don't like to think about that, because between the Ventolin and the Reglan I developed sleeping problems. The Reglan also caused mood swings. I don't know what the Theo-Dur did. I didn't know about adverse reactions because the doctors don't tell you about that. Because of the sleeping problem, the doctor who gave me the Zantac started me on Adivan, a sleeping pill. My general practitioner was also giving me one and it was really screwing me up.

"I began having a lot of problems from the reactions to all the pills. I would have insomnia for long periods of time, which led to depression from lack of sleep. The sleeping pills became addictive and I had to keep taking more and more of them. It was difficult coming off of them. The only thing that worked was a mild antidepressant called Imiprimine, which allowed me to stop. Besides making me sleepy, it was supposed to regulate my moods.

"Throughout all this I was still having asthma problems. I was using the spray several times a day, not knowing that the food I was eating was causing the asthma. I would have an asthma attack and clear it up with Ventolin.

"In order to be on the antidepressant Imiprimine you have to check in with a psychiatrist every six months. I called her and told her that even with the drug I still had these tremendous mood swings. She told me about the five-hour glucose tolerance test, but said it was such a pain that I should just write down what I thought I may be reacting to. When I later had this test and found I was very hypoglycemic, I became very resentful of regular doctors. I told my pulmonologist that I try to stay away from dairy products, for example, and he said, 'Don't worry, just take your medicine.'"

Donald found an alternative doctor through a magazine article about allergies and realized that he had experienced everything that was discussed in the article. "Luckily, he only lived an hour away. He did a battery of allergy tests including a cytotoxic test for food allergies. I was found to also be allergic to yeast, molds, and to my cat. He said that people may be more allergic to some cats than to others, which explained why when we tried to get another cat it didn't work out and we had to settle for just the one."

As a result of the food testing Donald was put on a strict diet, rotating foods that are not problems and those to which he is only slightly allergic. Today he doesn't have to rotate foods but stays away from dairy products, fermented foods, and especially sugar because of the hypoglycemia. He was also found to have candida, for which he took Nystatin for a year. The doctor prescribed vitamins, acidophilus, and allergy drops under the tongue.

GETTING OFF MEDICATION

"I went to the hospital about once a year before I started seeing this doctor. I would have asthma attacks in which I couldn't breathe at all. Besides the Ventolin and theophylline, when nothing else was working they would put me on prednisone and it made me crazy. I was also given antibiotics.

"The new doctor scaled down the medications relatively easily. After about a month of treatments and the diet, I started feeling better and seeing a lot of improvement. My wife and I also made many environmental changes, got rid of our rugs and now run an air purifier all the time. I still take the allergy drops. I think the last time I used the inhaler was when I stayed at a very moldy place where everyone had colds."

CHEMICAL ALLERGENS

How many doctors have inquired about your exposure to cigarette smoke, carpets, or to chemicals at your job or workplace? Most people with asthma have not considered or been tested for occupational allergens or chemicals.

Chemicals and Asthma

"I would say that asthmatics and allergists who treat them underestimate the importance of indoor pollution as a provocative factor in asthma," says Dr. Leo Galland. "That's why they just test for IgE allergies, because they are thinking about conventional allergies. But it's hard to know whether chemicals are the primary factor which causes asthma, or are aggravating the asthma as secondary factors. Natural gas, formaldehyde, those are things that will generally make asthmatics worse but they may not be the reason why the person is asthmatic. That's a very individual matter."

Multiple Chemical Sensitivity (MCS) syndrome seems to be running rampant these days as our homes, food, air, and water are inundated with chemicals. I've heard a number of accounts of onset of asthma from exposures to man-made products: nurses contracting asthma during construction work in hospitals; architects at construction sites; teachers overexposed to formaldehyde in new schools; a middle-aged man and woman (who never met) contracting asthma during two-week stays in newly renovated luxury hotels. Most recently, a psychotherapist told how she and a formerly healthy and very surprised young psychiatry resident both contracted asthma after a move to a new wing in a hospital. Exposure to formaldehyde or petrochemicals (from fresh paint) is often the cause, and this can result in a lifelong sensitivity problem. Mobile homes and trailers have left many elderly people with health problems that include asthma. And often their conditions have orthodox doctors stymied.

"Had to retire it got so bad," said Jim, a seventy-eight-year-old Harrisburg man who had worked for an energy company. "I don't know what I inhaled at work, but I didn't get sick until 1977, when my wife and I took our vacation in Virginia. The place we usually stayed was full so we were put up for one night in a brand-new trailer. That was a Thursday night and by Monday I couldn't breathe. I was tested for Legionnaires' disease, saw a lot of lung specialists, and was in the hospital a couple of times. They loaded me with antibiotics, inhalers, and breathing machines. For a long time I was on Keflex at $1.50 a pill. Several doctors diagnosed asthma, others weren't sure. Before I got to an environmental doctor I was on a breathing machine four times a day and was about to have my knees operated on for arthritis. For five years I slept sitting up in a lounge chair and was tired all the time."

Jim was treated for his yeast problems from the many years of antibiotics, and given a special diet, vitamins, and allergy shots. "Most people want something to happen instantly; they don't want to go to any trouble. I credit this doctor for keeping me alive. Those other guys—they do the best they can but they're just 'practicing' medicine, they never learn it! They can't believe how much better I am. You'd think they'd want to know about this and share it but they don't. Actually it makes 'em a little mad!"

Vapors

The relationship between strong odors and asthma was documented three hundred years ago by John Floyer. Today, according to the "American

VAPORS

	Yes	?	No

Start noticing—do you get worse when you are
exposed to:

1. Tobacco smoke?

2. Insect sprays or powders, including lawn
   products?

3. Mothproofing chemicals?

4. Perfumes, lotions, shampoos?

5. Paint fumes?

6. Resinous wood (Christmas trees, knotty-pine
   walls, cedar closets, pine-scented products,
   turpentine)?

7. Gas fumes (cooking stove, gas dryer, gas hot-
   water heater)?

8. Auto or bus fumes?

9. Smoke (fireplaces, furnaces, candles)?

10. Solvents (gasoline, kerosene, nail-polish
    remover, alcohol, varnish, lacquer, cleaning
    fluids—including visits to the cleaners)?

11. Polishes (furniture, floor, metal, shoe, nail)?

12. Lubricating greases or oils?

13. Room disinfectants and deodorants?

14. Petroleum residues (roof or road tar, or
    creosote from railroad ties or telephone
    poles), fresh newspaper ink, new leather and
    its polishes or dyes, weed killers?

15. Rubber products (gloves, mattresses, rug
    pads, rubber-based paints)?

Asthma Report II," 95 percent of people with asthma attributed their odor-related asthma attack to pesticides from fumigations and roach sprays. Next came household cleaners, especially those containing ammonia. Seventy-five percent attributed the attack to fresh paint, perfumes, and colognes; 50 percent to gasoline fumes or car exhaust; and 33 percent to cooking smells. (And those are only the people who have been able to make the connection!)

CIGARETTE SMOKE

Secondhand or sidestream cigarette smoke is one of the most often encountered forms of chemical pollution. It contains over thirty-five toxic chemicals, including formaldehyde, carbon monoxide, acetone, toluene, hydrogen cyanide, and nitrogen oxides. As we have seen, women who smoke are more than twice as likely to give birth to babies who develop asthma. In my asthma workshops about 75 to 85 percent of the participants grew up in houses with a smoker. Luckily, today you may not have to linger in public places full of cigarette smoke. And I'm not even going to ask if you smoke yourself!

HEALTHY HOME AND WORKPLACE

Every man-made synthetic material offgassing into the home can be a problem for people with asthma, but many have no awareness that synthetics are making things worse. In some of the upcoming chapters we will learn more about home and workplace problems. There are also many wonderful books on this subject. (See Bibliography.)

DEVELOPING AWARENESS

You may have difficulty determining if the vapors from man-made products are bothering you. When I was ill with chest tightness, wheezing, choking with phlegm, and taking a lot of medication, it was difficult to make the connection between what I was inhaling and the symptoms being produced. Except for overexposure to fresh paint fumes, it was really hard to smell anything at all. Add prednisone to the mix, which is actually depressing immune response, and you might not ever figure out what the source of the problem is. It was only when the asthma symptoms began to clear and the medication was reduced or done away with that my sense of smell returned with a vengeance. At that point, none of the "inhalant" allergens bothered me anymore except for cat; foods that previously made me wheeze now triggered other reactions, and many, many chemical vapors that I hadn't paid attention to before now gave me headaches, sore throats, exhaustion, and brain-fog.

It's important to understand that there is a distinction to be made between allergens such as pollens, pets, and foods, which are really harmless to most people, and chemicals to which some people develop sensitivities, but are really toxic to everyone—whether they know it or not!

When All Is Said and Done

Overwhelmed by allergies and testing? Remember that the best approach is to work on your digestion and reduce your total load. Strengthen and detoxify the body through the proper nutrients, good eating habits, and avoidance of chemicals and allergens. In the next chapter we learn more about food, eliminating the negative and accentuating the positive for rebuilding good health.

CHAPTER 8

YOUR NEW EATING ADVENTURE

A NEW LIFESTYLE

W hat we choose to eat is the one area of our lives over which we can have control. But unfortunately, how we eat is the area that seems to be out of control much of the time. We will of course continue to eat three meals a day, so it's important that we learn to use food as a tool for wellness.

When we think of a diet we usually think of a short-term eating regimen that deprives us of the things we love the best. For a little while. Just until we whittle off some extra pounds. Then we go back to eating anything we want until we decide to do it all over again. Diets don't work because they don't last. People count calories and fat content rather than nutrients. They don't examine ways to permanently change their eating habits.

How About a Brand-new Lifestyle?

The word *diet* comes from the Greek *diata*. It meant a lifestyle, a "scheme of living, a pattern for life."[1] And a new lifestyle is what we are after. One of the reasons we became ill was because the body was lacking in needed nutrients. Then the illness itself created more deficiencies that now must be addressed. So what we need to do is learn a new way of eating that will help enhance our immune systems, detoxify and rebalance our bodies, and support our overworked adrenal glands. A new way of eating in which every bite gives nourishment to encourage the body to repair itself. Let's stop worrying about fat and start thinking about the nutritional value of food. The idea here is to enhance our resistance rather than stress it further with junk food and known allergens. We don't need foods that work against us by adding even more toxins to our already overburdened body.

Along the way you may notice that your asthma symptoms are decreasing and other aches and pains may have ceased; you have more energy than usual and those extra pounds disappeared without counting calories! At this point you will probably notice that you use your inhaler less, and you should be able to start working with your doctor to decrease other medications.

Why Pay Attention to What You Eat?

We learned in an earlier chapter that in traditional Chinese medicine our basic constitution depends on the Prenatal Essence we inherited at birth. From the food that we eat, however, we derive our Postnatal Essence. Food is digested and transformed and eventually helps produce Qi, life force or energy. A more specific kind of energy, Kidney Essence, is partly inherited and partly replenished by this Postnatal Essence which we get from the food that we eat.

Understand the importance of Kidney Essence: The growth of your body depends on it—your bones, your teeth, the regulation of your hormones, your fertility, and your sexual energy. It also creates Kidney Qi; it builds marrow which nourishes the brain and it keeps the immune system strong.

THE ALLERGY CONNECTION

"I've eaten ———— all my life and it's never bothered me."

You may have had asthma all your life and never connected what you ate with how you felt. Or you may have started suffering from asthma as an adult and felt that food had nothing to do with it. Many of the foods that you handled perfectly well in your pre-asthma existence may now be making your condition worse. Once you get sick there is a spreading effect, and many things that were tolerated when you were strong are not tolerated when you are sick. As you recover you will be able to better tolerate many more foods.

Now is a good time to ask yourself, "How well do I want to feel?" Maybe you'd like to feel your best! Let's see how you are going to get there.

THE FOOD DIARY

When you read the allergy chapter of this book you started keeping a food symptom diary. And you are using this diary to keep track of and plan what you will eat every day, so that you can do a five-day rotation of foods.

The Minus Page

In your food diary you should also have a minus page in which you have listed the foods to which you are allergic and the foods that you crave so that you can eliminate them, and perhaps later rotate them back into your meal plan.

The Plus Page

All of the foods that are discussed here as possibilities for creative cookery can be listed on your plus page to give you meal ideas. Of course, everyone's allergies are different, so if you have identified a food as an allergen, keep it on your minus page and eliminate it from the recipe. If you open your heart (and your stomach) to some of those vegetables you have been avoiding all your life, and to new foods like sea vegetables, your plus page will soon fill up with delicious possibilities.

Understand that food restrictions are more stringent at the beginning or healing phase of the diet. So the strictest dos and don'ts should apply especially to the first few months. When you get stronger and breathing improves, the maintenance phase will allow you to modify this a bit, until you don't experience setbacks from the foods you are adding in again. As you strengthen yourself through better digestion, better diet, replaced nutrients, more sleep, and regular exercise, you may be able to tolerate foods, once in a while, that you couldn't tolerate at all when you started out. Hopefully by that time you will be enjoying your better health so much that you will want to make a nutrient-rich, junk-free diet part of your permanent lifestyle.

A Plan for Better Breathing

There are certain items that many of us used to consider essential, but they are the items that many doctors and nutritionists now tell us must be eliminated. Anyone experiencing a health problem needs to address these first. If you can, try to slowly cut down. If you're not addicted try a week without, just to see how it feels. Better breathing may compensate for that sense of loss.

Sugar (and alcohol), caffeine, white flour, milk products, and red meat are on the list. Pick the one that's easiest to do without. Develop awareness of how you feel. We begin with sugar because that often makes a noticeable difference for asthma. But eliminating any of these is bound to help.

SUGAR

Begin by eliminating sugar—if sugar has never been "your thing," you could cut it out completely now. If you have a serious addictive sugar habit, better cut back slowly. When you succeed it will definitely be worth it.

This includes all white and brown sugar in desserts, colas, cookies, and processed foods. Look carefully at labels—sugar is added to many products you may not suspect, such as mustard, ketchup, vinegar, salad dressings, and hundreds of other products. Sugar masquerades as fructose, sucrose, sorbitol, glucose, glycogen, lactose, maltose, mannitol, corn syrup, monosaccharides, and polysaccharides. Maple syrup can also cause phlegm.

Sweet fruits like dried fruit, apples, bananas, raisins, and oranges can also be eliminated for now. Then apples and raisins can be used cautiously in the cooked recipes. Unless you live in the tropics, bananas may not be the ticket. Your improved breathing will surely make up for any feelings of deprivation!

Why Cut Down on Sweets and Sugar?

- Because sweets are absorbed too quickly into the bloodstream, raising blood sugar to dangerous levels.
- Because sugar depletes the body of nutrients including B vitamins and minerals such as chromium and magnesium (which asthmatics are already short of).
- Because sugar depletes the adrenals.
- Because sugar encourages candida!
- Because sugar, according to Chinese medicinal cooking, has a cold energy which is contracting, and may shut down the digestive fire.

And no alcohol! Some people who wonder why they don't improve feel that "a couple of drinks won't hurt."

Two reasons for getting rid of alcohol:

- Alcohol contains sugar, which plays havoc with your blood sugar levels. No wonder we feel "hungover" the next day.
- Alcohol washes all those nutrients, vitamins, and minerals right out of the body.

On the plus side—for sweets try

- Blueberries, cherries, blackberries, kumquats, tangerines, pineapple, papaya, pears, apricots, peaches, and plums.

- Sweet vegetables such as squashes, yams, and pumpkins.
- In a sugar emergency, look in health food stores for local honey, or rice syrups.

CAFFEINE MUST GO

This includes all coffee, decaf (which contains about 10 percent or more caffeine), nonherbal tea, colas, and chocolate. Chocolate also sometimes causes the pain of arthritis. (You are not eating this anyway because of the sugar, right?) Aspirin and Excedrin are included in this list.

Why No Caffeine?

Because caffeine stimulates, but weakens the adrenals. Some people report that cola makes their asthma feel better. But that little lift is only temporary. You may have heard that famous advice for stopping an asthma attack with a strong cup of coffee. The coffee or cola *will* temporarily allow you to breathe better because it will stimulate the adrenals. In an extreme situation in which you've forgotten your medication, a cup of black coffee may just save the day. But in the long run it will only succeed in further exhausting you. We're aiming for truly better functioning. I know you don't want to depend on steroids forever.

If you are caffeine dependent, start eliminating it slowly.

On the plus side try

- Occasional weak kukicha and bancha teas from the health food store. These teas may have a tiny amount of caffeine, but also other things that support immune function.
- Breathe Deep tea (Yogi teas) achieves a mild bronchodilating effect with a combination of herbs that include eucalyptus and licorice.
- Rotate herbal teas and avoid herbs that give you problems. If you are allergic to ragweed, for instance, you may want to avoid chamomile.
- Pau D'Arco, also known as Taheebo or Ipe Roxo, helps with the yeast problem. It is made from the bark of a Brazilian tree on which molds don't grow.
- Red clover, burdock, and plain hot water with lemon are teas that are great blood cleansers.
- Dandelion tea is good after dinner to help cleanse the liver.
- Fennel tea is good for mucus.

Say Good-bye to Dairy Products

Especially milk products. But also yogurt, all cheese, especially blue or moldy cheese, and ice cream. If you must, butter is better than margarine. And ghee (clarified butter) is best of all, considered very tonifying in Ayurvedic medicine. You can buy this in specialty and health food stores. If you are devoted to yogurt, Ecrivan yogurt and YoGoat don't have additives but contain acidophilus cultures, the best reason to eat yogurt.

Why No Dairy?

It clogs the system and creates mucus.

Soy milk and rice dream may be all right occasionally for oatmeal or rice cereal, or used in baking, but they are not substitutes for the calcium in milk. Some people have soy allergies, others are allergic to the safflower oil in rice dream. Soy milk can also create mucus. Try oat milk instead of soy. However, soy, rice, and oat milk are *not* suitable substitutes for milk, especially for babies, children, and pregnant women, who all have special calcium requirements.

You can get your calcium from lamb's-quarters (they're greens, not lambs), cooked turnip greens, cooked collard greens, sea vegetables, almonds, almond milk, sunflower seeds, watercress, amaranth, quinoa—all of which, ounce for ounce, contain more calcium than milk. Goat milk is rich in calcium and may work well for you. If you are pregnant, check with your doctor about calcium supplementation and any diet changes. Pregnancy may not be the time to begin a new food program.

Give Up Red Meat, Pork, and Shellfish

Pork and shellfish are major allergens because they encourage the mast cells to release histamine. You can still have a little fish several times a week. Because the fish industry so far is completely unregulated, stick to the white unfatty fishes that may not have absorbed as many toxic chemicals.

Studies have shown that red meat encourages the mast cells to release leukotrienes, which are even more potent than the histamines.

With all the fat, hormones, and antibiotics in meat these days, giving it up will probably save you from a host of other problems. However, some people need red meat. If you do, be sure to buy organic.

Eliminate White Flour

Or go further and eliminate all flour products. As one doctor said, "Pretend the flour mill was never invented." Why? It clogs the system with mucus, and has no nutritional value.

EGGS

Eggs are a major allergen. Give them up for a while—it's not forever. Many people eat just the whites of eggs because the yolk is reputed to be very high in cholesterol. However, the yolk is where all the nutrition is. If you are concentrating your eating on whole grains, vegetables, and legumes, you will not have to worry about cholesterol! If you eat eggs they should be organic.

NIGHTSHADES

The nightshade family includes tomatoes, potatoes, peppers, and eggplants. People with arthritis are usually told to eliminate these to reduce inflammation. They also can cause allergic reactions. So be moderate if you eat nightshades. And if you are allergic to them, watch out for vitamin C tablets or capsules that may be made from a red or green pepper source.

THE OPTIMUM WAY

no shellfish	reduce nightshades
no pork	no yeast
no meat	no white flour
no dairy	nothing cold from the fridge
no sugar	nothing dry, smoked, or burned

Stay away from processed foods, preservatives, additives, and store-bought food with long lists of chemicals and other unpronounceable items listed under ingredients.

If you must use an egg, eliminate the white, or make sure it is thoroughly cooked, for less allergic reactions.

What is being suggested here is the optimum way to improve. If you can eliminate the negative for a while you will be better off. This is the healing phase of your eating regimen. Remember, not all these precautions are forever. But don't get so discouraged that you make no changes. Anywhere you start here is going to be an improvement.

Sandy, a single mother with two daughters, has had asthma most of her life: "Since I came to your cooking class I've cut out milk, ice cream, cheese, junk food, and cut down on wheat bread and meat, although I still eat them. I find I'm not as congested. I'd say that the diet plays a very important role. I also got a water filter because I think clean water is important.

"I had asthma as a child and it got worse in my late twenties after the birth of my children. I've been on this medication for fifteen years. Many different kinds. The doctor told me to use Theo-Dur every day—three times a day. But in May I just made up my mind not to use it and go cold turkey. [Usually not a good idea!]

"This is the best that I've felt in my whole life."

What's left to eat? Plenty! Let's take a look at some of the interesting ways around which we can organize our eating. And let's approach this with a spirit of adventure.

The Macrobiotic Diet

In the past macrobiotics was sometimes thought of as a "brown rice" diet. Actually the diet is based mostly on grains, legumes, certain vegetables, some fermented foods, a small amount of fish and seafood, and sea vegetables. Today there are organizations that suggest similar diets, but often these new food group diets leave out the fermented foods, which are there to promote better digestion (for those with no candida and/or mold allergies) and the sea vegetables, which are powerful sources of vitamins and trace minerals.

Although I wasn't "cured" on a macrobiotic diet, I did improve, and undoubtedly three years of changed eating habits had a positive effect on the outcome. The tofu, tempeh, and seitan in the diet are items that I would not eat today were I ill and weak with asthma. Anyone with a yeast problem will want to avoid the ferments, and the wheat-allergic will want to avoid seitan. Although tofu is a fine source of protein, it is also very cooling, and overconsumption can weaken your kidney energy. When I travel or have strayed too far from the basic principles, I am always comforted to know that I can return to a modified version for a few weeks to regain balance.

A typical American diet is very acid-forming, which is why antacids are such a big seller in this country. It is also why a macrobiotic diet is excellent for those who typically eat a cheeseburger, french fries, and ice cream kind of diet. Macrobiotics keeps you more neutral, in the center. Too many years of strict macrobiotics, however, may create other problems.

Vegetables

In macrobiotics you choose from three groups of vegetables: those that grow beneath the ground, those that grow on the ground, and those that grow above the ground. This provides a balance.

Root vegetables include carrot, parsnip, onion, radish, turnip, daikon, lotus root, and burdock.

Ground vegetables include cauliflower, broccoli, all kinds of winter squash, pumpkin, brussels sprout, and cabbage.

Leafy vegetables include bok choy, collard greens, daikon greens, kale, mustard greens, parsley, scallions, turnip greens, watercress, and leeks.

Other vegetables used occasionally in macrobiotics include peas, string beans, sprouts, romaine lettuce, escarole, endive, cucumber, shiitake mushrooms, and summer squash.

Grains

Short-grain brown rice for winter, long-grain brown rice for summer; my favorite is a medium-grain rice called Golden Rose. Then there are millet and barley. These three grains may be the best for those of us with asthma. Barley, especially Hato Mugi barley, helps drain mucus from the body. Sweet brown rice mixed with brown rice is useful in winter for more energy. Buckwheat groats (kasha) can be used occasionally.

Rolled oats, rice cakes, cornmeal, couscous, and soba and udon noodles are also used.

Legumes

Aduki beans, lentils, lima beans, black beans, chickpeas.

Sea Vegetables

Kombu, nori, hijiki, wakame, arame, kelp, and others. Sea vegetables are rich in vitamins and contain all the important trace minerals and amino acids that are necessary for good health. They alkalize blood that is too acid and dissolve fat and mucus. According to Steven R. Schecter, N.D., in his book *Fighting Radiation and Chemical Pollutants with Foods, Herbs, and Vitamins,* alginic acid found in darker sea vegetables transforms toxic metals in the intestines into harmless salts that can be easily assimilated.[2] The sea vegetables can effortlessly become a part of your life and change it for the better.

Let's take a closer look at these gifts from the sea.

Kombu (the kelp or laminaria family)

Kombu is cooling and moistening. It soothes the lungs and can help relieve phlegm. It can help you breathe deeper and helps gets rid of candida.[3] It can also protect against degenerative disease.[4] You can wash kombu in cold water and throw it into a pot of soup or soak for five minutes and cut into small pieces to arrange on the bottom of the pot when cooking legumes. It makes beans more digestible. Kombu is extremely nutritious and was one of my mainstays for relieving phlegm and shortness of breath.

Hijiki

Hijiki is the seaweed richest in calcium. It helps to detoxify the body and it's also rich in protein. It helps support hormone function and balance blood sugar.[5] Hijiki is rich tasting, dark, and coarse and is good cooked with small slices of onion and carrot. It is also used in salads.

Wakame

Wakame is high in protein, calcium, iron, and magnesium. Good for miso and other soups. It is also good cooked with vegetables.

Dulse, Irish Moss, and Kelp

These are high in potassium. Dulse is rich in protein, iron, vitamin A, iodine, and phosphorus. Great for soups.

Arame

Arame is the finest and fastest cooking of the sea vegetables. It's high in complex carbohydrates. After being well washed it can be sautéed with vegetables or cooked in miso soup.

Nori (porphyra family)

Nori is the most digestible of the sea vegetables and is the best one for protein. Nori is the mainstay for making rice and vegetable sushi and snacks. It can also be toasted and broken, to be eaten alone or sprinkled on grains or veggies.

Other unusual and useful foods that I discovered in macrobiotic cooking include:

Umiboshi plums—a little stimulate the appetite and digestion and aid in maintaining an alkaline blood quality. Antibiotic.

Lotus root—especially good for the sinuses and lungs. Helps relieve coughing and drains mucus.

Daikon root—helps dissolve stagnant fat and mucus deposits. Freshly grated raw daikon is good for digestion of oily foods.

Burdock root—strengthening, it cleans the kidneys of wastes and acids and is also a blood cleaner.

Kuzu—cooling. Like arrowroot, it comes from a root and can be used as a thickener for sauces and stews.

Teas

Teas can be used medicinally:

- Burdock tea is good for overall vitality.
- Kombu tea helps remineralize the body.
- Shiitake mushroom tea acts as a mild relaxant to relieve tense muscles and nerves. It also helps dissolve animal fats.

CHINESE MEDICINAL COOKING

When I got beyond crying in my kitchen and burning my macrobiotic food I felt I was ready to move on and signed up for a special cooking class. I arrived late—the instructor was already chopping and saying, "Scallions have a warming quality that expels cold and an ascending nature." This really spoke to me and opened up the whole wonderful new world of Chinese medicinal cooking.

Whereas macrobiotics is a generalized system formulated in recent years, Chinese medicinal cooking developed over thousands of years and is more specific and complex. According to this theory there are no "healthy" or "unhealthy" foods. Rather, food is chosen for certain energies and how they relate to the condition of the particular person. In Chinese medicinal cooking all of these vegetables and foods and herbs are chosen for their energy, temperature, and relationship to what is called the "Five Elements." In China today, of course, most people do not eat like this. Nor will you find this food in your favorite Chinese restaurant. However, the knowledge is far from lost. Every time I visit Chinatown and pause before a display of herbs and vegetables I know nothing about, a passerby with some knowledge of English invariably appears and says, "That (vegetable) is good for arthritis," or "Those herbs are perfectly balanced," or "Cook these for three hours with chicken bones for more energy."

Understanding something about Chinese medicinal cooking can make a great difference in your day-to-day feeling of wellness. So let's try to be open to this totally new way of looking at food.

Henry Lu, author of *The Chinese System of Food Cures,* points out how we in the West consider food for its nutritional content: its vitamins and minerals, carbohydrates, calories, and proteins. The Chinese diet, on the other hand, looks at the five flavors of foods, the five energies of foods, the movements of foods, and common and organic actions of foods.[6] Each of the Five Elements is related to paired organ systems of the body:

Wood: liver/gallbladder
Fire: heart/small intestine
Earth: spleen/stomach
Metal: lungs/large intestine
Water: kidney/bladder

FIVE TASTES OR FLAVORS

In Taoist Five-Element Theory, those elements and organ systems also correspond to a particular taste. The taste will lead the food to nourish the particular organ. Each meal should contain all five tastes. You could create several meals with all five tastes using the suggestions below:

Sour (liver/gallbladder): collards, chicken, raw fruit
Bitter (heart/small intestine): broccoli, cauliflower, celery
Sweet (spleen/stomach): squash, rice, carrots, string beans
Spicy (lung/large intestine): parsley, garlic, onions
Salty (kidney/bladder): sea vegetables, saltwater fish, egg

YIN AND YANG

As you can see, the organs are paired. Each pair contains a yin and yang organ. For instance, the lung is a yin organ paired with a yang organ, the large intestine.

Foods, as well as organs, are thought of as yin and yang: Cool and cold are yin (contractive); warm and hot are yang (expansive).

FOOD ENERGIES

Foods may be thought of as cold, hot, warm, cool, or neutral. We are not talking about the temperature of the food here, but the energetic quality of the food. Foods thought to be either cool or cold will have a contracting energy; warm or hot foods will have an expansive energy. Foods will be combined to balance energies—fish, for instance, which is cool, can be balanced with carrot, or ginger, which is warming. This provides for good food metabolism and digestion.

In addition, people are spoken of as having a cold or hot condition. Very simplified, if your condition is cold (such as being chilled) you would eat warming foods (such as chicken broth). To some extent we do that instinctively in all cultures. But in Chinese medicinal cooking, every food and condition is assigned one of these properties.

DOCTRINE OF SIGNATURES

The doctrine of signatures was part of early folklore about plants in China. Also, in the Middle Ages in the Western world, it was thought that God had left clues in a plant, flower, or root that would tell us for which organ of the body or disease it was intended. In traditional Chinese medicine a specific plant relates to a certain organ based on its shape and color. Therefore, vegetables good for the lungs would include cauliflower flowerets, lotus root, and white fungus, which all are white and look like lungs. Mustard greens are also thought to have a shape which makes them specific for the lungs.

COLOR

Colors are also assigned to each organ and each element. Eating a food of the right color, according to the doctrine of signatures, is supposed to guide that food to benefit the corresponding organ. That is not so far-fetched as it might seem—modern physics sees color as electromagnetic energy of different wavelengths.[7] Since we experience color on both physical and unconscious levels, couldn't that energy affect the functioning of the body?

In the Five-Element Theory, the colors correspond to organs of the body and related foods like this:

Liver: Green (green vegetables, leafy vegetables, mung beans, blue-green algae)

Heart: Red (aduki beans, red lentils, Chinese dates, beets, apples)

Spleen/stomach: Yellow (yellow peas, soybeans, yellow round millet, yellow squash)

Lungs: White (lotus root, daikon, cauliflower, lima beans, white beans, white fungus)

Kidneys: Black or blue (black beans, dark lentils)

David, the college student who had been to China, was told that to strengthen the kidneys or lungs you should eat food the color of the lungs. "The idea was that food the color of my lungs would be good for me—and anything that was grayish white would be beneficial. White fungus and pear soup are supposed to be good for your lungs. It was a cold soup and sweet—we would have it for dessert. At a doctor's house where I had dinner, they tried to make things that would be beneficial and I was given lotus root on several occasions."

GENERAL ADVICE BEFORE YOU START COOKING

Oils

Unrefined cold-pressed olive oil and sesame oil are the only oils used for cooking because they can safely be heated to high temperatures. Monounsaturated fats such as olive oil and sesame oil are also less likely to turn rancid than other oils. They reduce only harmful LDL cholesterol and leave protective HDL cholesterol in the body. Olive oil is commonly used in Mediterranean countries, where heart disease is less common than in the United States.

Other monounsaturated oils such as canola, apricot kernel, and almond can be used on salads.

Cooking Pots

Pots should be stainless steel, glass, lead-free Corning Ware, or Chinese clay pots, such as those available in Chinese herbal stores. Before using your clay pot: Soak it completely overnight in water. Dry it. Half fill it with water and slowly heat it on a low flame before the first use. This will seal your pot.

Organic food should be used, or grow your own. Otherwise:

Pesticides on food should be reduced:

- Wash thoroughly in purified water.
- Soak with a few drops of citricidal in the water; scrub and rinse thoroughly.

Bacteria should be avoided:

- Vegetables, fruit, and poultry can be soaked in water containing a few drops of food-grade hydrogen peroxide.

- Use a water-and-vinegar soak for salads.
- Spring or purified water should be used for cooking soups and stews.

Promote Good Digestion

- Most food should be cooked and eaten warm until your digestion is in order.
- Chew your food thoroughly.
- If you are ill and just embarking on a new way of eating, keep it simple. Steamed or cooked vegetables, a small amount of grain, and a well-cooked protein, plus a sea vegetable is best at first.

Unusual Ingredients

Macrobiotic items and vegetables you may not have heard of previously are available at health food stores in the macro section or in the fresh vegetable bins. Asian food stores also carry many of these vegetables.

Chinese Herbs

They can be ordered from the Resources at the end of the book. Herbs are dried, come in boxes or bags, are inexpensive, and can be kept for a year or two. Store in tight dark containers behind closed doors. Red Chinese dates are best stored in the freezer. Dishes containing these herbs should be cooked in clay, glass, or Corning Ware pots. The clay pots sold in Chinese herbal stores are inexpensive and easy to clean.

THE RECIPES

Many of the recipes that follow have been organized around the principles of macrobiotics and/or Chinese medicinal cooking, and the ingredients are used mostly for their energetic qualities.

Some recipes will be for strengthening, some will be for specific asthma conditions, and some will help get rid of colds. As you work with these recipes, you will develop more skills for dealing with your asthma specifically and your overall health in general.

CALMING CARROTS AND KOMBU TEA (excellent for breathlessness)

4" kombu (cools, relieves cough)
4 2" pieces of daikon (breaks up mucus)
2 whole carrots, cut in large chunks (strengthening)

• Wash salt from kombu.
• Put all ingredients in a heavy pot. Cover with 4 cups of water and simmer for 1½ hours.
• Drink the liquid. Eat the carrots.

It works fine to drink some of the liquid after only 20 minutes.

DISPEL GREEN MUCUS TEA (very strengthening)   *4 servings*

6" kombu
2 carrots
1 onion
2 Chinese dates

• Wash kombu.
• Cut vegetables in half.
• Put ingredients in pot with 6 cups of water.
• Boil 1 hour and drink liquid.

DISPEL STUCK MUCUS TEA   *4 servings*

12" kombu
 6" wakame
4 cups water (cooked to 1½ cups)
1 tbs grated fresh daikon (at the end)

If daikon doesn't work use ½ tsp fresh ginger.

   This should enable you to cough up dry, stuck mucus. (This tastes as bad as it sounds, but it really works! And the ingredients are good for your lungs.)

DISPEL STICKY PHLEGM TEA

Boil almonds in spring water and drink the liquid.

CALMING CHRYSANTHEMUM TEA   *3 servings*

1 tsp kuzu (pueraria—relaxes spasms and tightness)
A medium handful Chinese dried chrysanthemum (calming)

- Dilute kuzu by adding a teaspoonful to a little cold water.
- When it's fairly liquid, add a little tea at a time.
- When it's very liquid, put the diluted kuzu back into pot with tea and simmer slightly, stirring constantly for a couple of minutes, until the powdered, white kuzu has become clear. (This drink releases heat from the exterior of the body.)

CALMING HEAVY BREATHING DRINK   *1 or 2 servings*

4" kombu, washed
2 cups water

- Simmer ½ hour and reduce to 1 cup.
- Grate in a couple of drops of lotus root.

You can drink this twice a day if you feel dry and thirsty.

COOLS HOT PHLEGM, STRENGTHENS SPLEEN TEA   *2 servings*

6" kombu (breaks up phlegm, soothes lungs)
2 jojube dates (energize, dry up mucus, and moisten tissues)
1 onion (warming, strengthening)
⅔ tsp kuzu (sweet, clears heat)

- Wash kombu.
- Cut up onion.
- Add kombu, dates, and onion to 4 cups of water. Reduce to 2 cups.
- Add kuzu to a small amount of cold water and stir until dissolved. Then add a few spoonfuls of hot tea, one by one.
- Stir well, add to pot of tea, and simmer, stirring for a few minutes.

TEA FOR KIDNEY (for winter; warming)

1 oz. cinnamon bark (warms kidney fire)
1 oz. licorice root (good for digestion, harmonizes)
½ oz. lycii berries (helps blood)
½ oz. Chinese ginseng root (warming, good for winter)

- Boil with three quarts of water for one hour. Discard herbs and drink.

COOLING FOR SUMMER TEA

Mint-and-chrysanthemum tea is good for cooling.

BURDOCK, LOTUS ROOT TEA (cooling)

4" burdock root, washed and chopped (blood cleaner)
2" kombu (breaks up phlegm, softens hardened masses)
5 pieces of lotus root, chopped (clears heat, tonifies yin)
6 cups water

- Boil together for 1½ hours. Strain, reserving liquid. Burdock and lotus root can be eaten. Sweeten with barley malt, if desired.

SHORTNESS OF BREATH TEA

- Boil a few cloves in a pot of water.
- Drink this tea in the fall for better breathing.

Cooking Grains

BROWN RICE

4 servings

1 cup medium brown rice rinsed thoroughly
1¾ cups filtered or spring water
Pinch of salt

- Combine and simmer on medium burner in covered stainless-steel saucepan until excess water is absorbed.
- Put flame deflector under pot, reduce heat, and cook until rice has completely absorbed water, about 40–45 minutes.

For more energy in cold weather
- Combine ¼ cup of sweet brown rice with ¾ cup of small-grain brown rice.

For draining mucus:
- Combine ¼ cup Hato Mugi barley (also called Job's Tears) with ¾ cup of small-grain brown rice.

Sometimes Chinese recipes call for white rice, which can be more digestible and better when you feel weak. Brown rice, of course, has more nutrients, but not if you are not absorbing them.

In general brown rice is neutral, barley (for draining mucus), and millet are cooling. These are the most highly recommended grains. However, there are others to use for variety as well as their energetic qualities. Amaranth and Job's Tears cool; oats, quinoa, spelt, and sweet rice warm. Buckwheat groats (kasha) is neutral. In my mother's house, however, kasha was always a cold winter dish.

Kasha   4 servings

1 cup buckwheat groats
1 diced onion
1 tsp olive oil
Pinch of salt
2 cups water, boiled
Chopped parsley

* Sauté onions in a little oil until soft.
* Add the buckwheat groats and continue to stir until groats are a little toasted and covered with oil.
* Add the salt and boiled water. Cover, reduce flame, and simmer very slowly until water is gone. Open and stir after 20 minutes.
* Taste for doneness. Add liquid and cook longer if necessary.
* Garnish with chopped parsley.

Kasha for Breakfast

Cook leftovers in another cup of water and serve hot. Buckwheat strengthens the intestines and is alkalizing. Not good for fever, red tongue, or sore throat.

Cold Winter Energy Breakfast

¾ cup short-grained brown rice
¼ cup sweet rice
¼ cup Hato Mugi barley
A few small pieces of dried orange peel
Cinnamon
Grated apricot or almond kernels

- Cook brown and sweet rice, barley, and orange peel in 1¾ to 2 cups of water until soft.
- Sprinkle with cinnamon and grated apricot pits. (Optional—cut up apricot pits or almonds and cook with rice.)
- Use the remainder of the rice for dinner or use for a cooked pear dessert.

QUINOA

Gluten-free quinoa (keen-wa) was the grain of the Incas for five thousand years until the Spanish conquerors stopped its cultivation in Peru. However, quinoa is still being grown in South America and is a good source of protein, calcium, iron, and fiber.

½ cup quinoa (this will expand quite a bit)
1 cup water

- Cook for 15 minutes and serve for breakfast.
- Use leftovers to make quinoa soup with carrots, onions, celery, and shredded cabbage.

AMARANTH

Look also for amaranth, which grew in Mexico, and was also used by the Incas until they were forbidden to grow it. The seeds survived over centuries in the jungles, and amaranth is still used in Africa and Latin America, where its high protein, calcium, and lysine content help prevent malnutrition. Amaranth is cooling, dries dampness, and is good for the lungs. It is often combined with other grains in cooking and baking.

MILLET WITH CARROTS, CELERY, AND FRESH HERBS
(cooling grain dish)   *4 servings*

1   cup millet, well washed (less mucus-forming grain, cool energy)
1   bay leaf (heating, expectorant)
¼   tsp sea salt
2   cups filtered water
¾   cup carrot, small dice (neutral, strengthens spleen)
¾   cup celery, small dice (cooling, calms the liver)
1–2   tsp extra virgin olive oil
2   tsp fresh basil, minced (warm, relieves cold headaches)
1   tbs fresh thyme, minced (heating, reduces mucus)
1   tbs fresh oregano, minced (heating, promotes digestion)
Dash of vinegar

- In a 2-quart heavy pot with a tight lid, bring millet, bay leaf, sea salt, and water to boil, covered. Do not stir or lift the lid off. Turn down to a simmer and cook for 20 minutes, until all the water is absorbed.
- While the millet is cooking, sauté the carrot and celery in the olive oil for 4–5 minutes, until the vegetables are just tender. Add the herbs and vinegar. Toss and cook for 1 minute longer.
- Adjust seasoning.
- After the millet has cooked, remove the pot from the heat and let it sit covered for 5–10 minutes. Remove the bay leaf and fork into a large bowl. Toss with the vegetables and serve hot. (If you are hot and dry, omit the herbs.)

Soups

SWEET VEGETABLE SOUP
This soup is rich in carotenes and vitamin A, soothing for the lungs, and good for digestion.

6" kombu seaweed
Any winter squash plus two other vegetables from the following: acorn squash, buttercup squash, butternut squash, Hubbard squash, Hokkaido pumpkin, pumpkin, carrots, fresh or dried lotus root, onions, daikon, cauliflower, or green cabbage

- Soak kombu for 5 minutes and place in bottom of pot.
- Cut vegetables in chunks and add to pot.
- Add 4–5 cups of spring water and bring to a slow boil.
- Reduce heat and simmer for 20 minutes.
- Drink two cups of the warm liquid daily and eat vegetables with a grain for lunch or dinner. (Cook with barley to drain mucus.)

Before you make the following recipes, you should know that beans should not be eaten regularly by anyone who is thin, weak, or dry.

BASIC LENTIL SOUP

6" kombu
1   medium onion
2   stalks celery
2   carrots

1   cup lentils
5   cups spring water

- Soak kombu until soft, cut into squares and arrange on the bottom of a heavy pot.
- Cut the onion into quarters, and cut the celery and carrots into medium-size chunks. Add the vegetables to the pot.
- Wash the lentils and pick through. Add the lentils to the pot.
- Add water, bring slowly to a boil, and simmer from 45–60 minutes.
- Add a drop of tamari or liquid aminos for flavor.
- Garnish with parsley.

Lentils stimulate the adrenals, increase vitality. Kombu disperses mucus, soothes the lungs, and makes the lentils more digestible.

ASTRAGALUS CHICKEN SOUP   *6 to 8 servings*
(Strengthens kidney and spleen)

1   cup chickpeas, soaked overnight and drained (mildly sweet, warming, harmonizing)
½   oz. astragalus tied in string (strengthens immune system; sweet, warm)
2   quarts chicken stock made from a whole organic chicken with the cooked breast meat sliced and reserved (warming)
½   cup brown rice
1   onion (helps expel phlegm)
2   cloves garlic, minced (warming)
2   tbs extra virgin olive oil
1   tsp ground cinnamon (warming)
½   tsp ground cumin (warming)
Black pepper (warms the stomach, relieves cold)

- In a covered 3-quart pot, cook the chickpeas and astragalus in the stock for 20 minutes.
- Add rice and continue to cook for 1 hour.
- In a small skillet, sauté the onion and garlic in the oil until soft, about 15 minutes.
- Stir in the spices and cook for 1 minute longer.
- Add the spice mixture and reserved chicken to the beans, remove the astragalus, adjust seasonings, and serve.

ADUKI BEAN, WATER CHESTNUT, WHITE FUNGUS SOUP   *4 servings*
(Eliminate fungus for mold allergies.)

¼ cup aduki bean (tonify kidney/adrenals, detoxify)
1   4" piece kombu (balances beans, cooling)
1   carrot (alkaline, good for lungs)
3   pieces white fungus or tree ear (lubricates lungs, eliminates damp)
4   water chestnuts (transforms sputum, not for weak condition)
4   olives (good for lungs, tonifies Qi)
1   bunch watercress (cooling and pungent)
A little salt

• Combine ingredients with 6 cups of water and cook slowly for 1½ hours.

Stews and Congees

Congees are a kind of well-cooked porridge made with grains such as rice or barley with many times the water. Because they are easy to digest they are excellent for those who are ill. You can create your own congees choosing ingredients for their energetic qualities.

STRENGTHENING, SAVORY CONGEE

1   large turnip, peeled and cut into ½-inch cubes (clears heat, dissolves phlegm)
2   carrots, peeled and cut into ½-inch cubes (calming, good for lungs)
1   clove garlic, minced (warming)
1   onion, chopped
2   pieces of black fungi, chopped (sweet, neutral, tonifies Qi)
¼ cup sweet rice
4   cups water
Dash sea salt

• In a heavy saucepan, sauté onion and garlic over medium heat for 5–10 minutes.
• Add carrot and turnip; sauté for an additional 5 minutes.
• Add sweet rice, fungi, and water to vegetables. Cover the pot.
• Bring to a boil, reduce heat, and simmer for 1 hour.
• Season to taste with sea salt.

3   oz. white fungus (You can eliminate the fungus and make this with yam.)
1   cup white rice
16 cups water
Scallions, cut into diagonals
Sweetener (barley malt or rice syrup)

- Place white fungus in bowl or pot and cover with water. Let sit until well softened, up to several hours. Wash carefully and cut up the larger pieces. Reserve water for congee.
- Place rice and white fungus in large pot.
- Measure water and add enough to total 16 cups. Pour into rice pot and begin cooking. Once the water boils reduce the heat to maintain a slow bubbling. Cook an hour or longer.
- Slice the scallions and add the whites during the cooking.
- Sweeten to taste with the barley malt syrup, and use the greens of the onion for garnishing.
- Cook 1–1½ hours.

Vegetable Dishes

STRING BEANS WITH ROASTED WALNUTS AND LYCII BERRIES
(for the kidney)

¾ cup walnuts (strengthen the kidneys)
Sesame oil
1   lb. string beans (strengthens spleen, tonifies kidneys)
1   oz. ginger root, freshly grated (warming, good for digestion)
Soy sauce
½ cup lycii berries (tonify blood, replenish Jing essence)

- Roast the walnuts in a couple tablespoons of sesame oil in a skillet over moderate heat.
- Wash and trim the string beans. If large, cut into lengthwise strips.
- Heat ¼ cup of sesame oil in skillet or wok and sauté the green beans a couple minutes. Remove and drain. Pour off excess oil.
- Sauté ginger briefly; add string beans and walnuts.

- Season with soy sauce.
- Pour boiling water over the lycii berries and let them plump briefly. Then drain and use to garnish the dish.

MUSTARD GREENS WITH LOTUS ROOT

1 lotus root segment (moistens)
3 garlic cloves
1 bunch mustard greens (or kale if mustard greens are too strong)
kuzu

- Slice the lotus root into thin rounds. Mince the garlic. Chop the mustard greens.
- Cook the lotus root slices in 2 cups of water, covered, for 20–25 minutes until nicely softened.
- Add the garlic and cook briefly.
- Then add the mustard greens and cook down for 5–8 minutes until tender.
- Season to taste. Thicken with kuzu.

These vegetable dishes can be served as main dishes:

ROOT VEGETABLES WITH CHINESE HERBS AND ALMONDS

2   oz. astragalus (for stamina, dispels dampness)
2   oz. glehnia (moistens lungs)
2   oz. polygonatum (relieves dryness, thirst, and cough)
1   oz. pseudostellaria (strengthens lungs)
1   oz. lily bulb (eliminates phlegm, good for cough)
2   daikon (dissolve fat and mucus)
4   small turnips (detoxifying, removes damp and phlegm)
2–3 sweet potatoes (cools, promotes Qi energy)
2   cups almond (good for lungs)
Salt (moistens)
White pepper (helps move phlegm)
Parsley, minced for garnish

- Cook herbs in 10–12 cups water for 45–60 minutes (or pressure cook for 20 minutes).
- Remove the herbs from the stock and let cool.
- Discard the astragalus. Cut the other herbs into smaller bite-size pieces.

- While the herbs are cooking, cut up the root vegetables into cubes about fork size.
- Roast the almonds in a 350° oven about 8 minutes. Grind coarsely in a Cuisinart or coffee mill. Mix about half the almonds in with the stock.
- Place herbs and stock in the bottom of baking dish, and put the root vegetables on top. Sprinkle with salt and white pepper.
- Sprinkle the remaining almonds on top. Bake covered at 375° for about an hour. May also bake uncovered for the last 10–15 minutes.
- Check the seasoning. Garnish with minced parsley.

FAST VEGETABLE MELANGE   *4 servings*

1   bunch of broccoli flowerets and stems peeled and cut in matchsticks
2   carrots cut in pieces on diagonal
1   cup buttercup squash, peeled & cut in small pieces
2   scallions cut in one-inch pieces on diagonal

- Steam together, and cover with sauce made from a bit of mashed carrot and scallion. Sprinkle with sesame seeds. Serve with brown rice.

SQUASH STUFFED WITH WILD RICE   *2 servings*

1   squash (halved and seeded)
½   onion
1   piece burdock (cut fine and shaved)
Olive oil
½   cup wild rice
Handful of sunflower seeds

- Chop onion and burdock finely and lightly sauté together in olive oil.
- Roast sunflower seeds and stir into mixture.
- Add wild rice, mix, and cook together with other ingredients for ½ hour (keep moist with water).
- Stuff squash, cover with tin foil, and bake until done.

Other Main Dishes

WATERCRESS FISH STEW   *4 servings*

1   onion, chopped
2   carrots, peeled and medium diced

1 celery stalk, medium diced
2 slices fresh ginger, minced
1 Chinese date, chopped
1 cup water
8 oz. white fish, cut into ½-inch chunks
½ bunch watercress

- In a large heavy pot, sauté the onion until transparent (about 10 minutes).
- Add carrots, celery, chopped date, ginger, and water.
- Bring to a boil and reduce heat.
- Simmer partially covered for 15–20 minutes, or until vegetables are soft.
- Add fish and watercress, and cook just until the fish is done (about 5 minutes).

CHICKEN TOMATO DISH

1 piece chicken, or breast with skin removed (sweet and warming)
6" wakame (resolves phlegm, moistens dryness)
Watercress
1 tsp barley miso
¼ cup millet (cooling)
5 cups water
1 large tomato, peeled, seeded, and chopped (detoxifies liver)

- Wash salt from wakame and cook in large pot with water, millet, chicken, and tomato until chicken and millet are done.
- Add watercress last 10 minutes.
- Dilute miso in a little of the hot soup.
- Add to pot and simmer on low flame a few minutes.
- (Millet, tomato, and wakame cool down the warmth of the chicken.)

ASTRAGALUS, CODONOPSIS STEW   *2 servings*

6" kombu
1 oz. astragalus
1 oz. codonopsis
5 red Chinese dates (optional)
2 sticks celery
1 carrot
1 large yam
1 small slice ginger

1 large dry shiitake mushroom
½ cup brown rice

- Cook astragalus and codonopsis and pitted dates in 10 cups of water for several hours.
- While herbs are cooking, wash vegetables and cut into chunks.
- Wash salt from kombu.
- Soak shiitake mushroom in hot water and slice. Preserve water for stew.
- When herb stock is ready, discard herbs (leave the dates) and add shiitake, soaking water, kombu, and vegetables. (If using a clay pot, let stock cool first.)
- Add ½ cup of brown rice.
- Cook until done. (You may have to add water, so watch carefully.)

CARROT SEAWEED SALAD (side dish)   *4 servings*

6 organic carrots
2 oz. organic raisins
1 oz. hijiki seaweed
½ cup red cabbage
½ cup white cabbage
Umoboshi vinegar
Balsamic vinegar (lemon juice could substitute for vinegar)
Apple juice

- Peel and cut into matchsticks 6 table carrots and set aside.
- Wash and strain hijiki seaweed. Julienne and blanch ½ cup of white cabbage and ½ cup of red cabbage. Poach hijiki in equal parts of vinegar, apple juice, and water.
- Let all cooked ingredients cool. Toss ingredients with sesame dressing. Serve alone or on a bed of mesclun.

Sesame Vinaigrette

1 tbs lemon juice
1 oz. red vinegar
2 oz. mirin (sweet rice wine vinegar)
1 oz. tamari
½ tbs sesame oil
1 tbs olive oil
1 tbs chopped cilantro

Mix all ingredients with a whisk or food processor. Dressing does not emulsify.

Desserts

FRESH AND DRIED PEAR DESERT

⅛ oz. dried tangerine peel (chen pi) (good for indigestion, removes stuffiness in chest; drying, not for dry cough)
¼ lb. dried pears
Peel of an organic orange
1 oz. fresh ginger
3 fresh pears (good for coughs, moisturizes)
1–2 oz. apricot pits (expectorant, helps to clear phlegm)

• Cover tangerine peel with water and cook for 30 minutes to soften. Cook the pears separately in 6 cups of water. When the peel has softened, add the water to the pears. Thinly slice the tangerine peel, and add it to the pears.
• Peel the orange with a vegetable peeler and slice the peel into thin strips. Add to the pears.
• Peel the ginger root, cut it into thin strips, and add to the pears.
• Quarter and core the fresh pears, cut them once more lengthwise, and when the dried pears are well softened, add the fresh pears and continue stewing until the fresh pears soften.
• Grind the apricot pits (in spice mill or coffee grinder).
• Serve the pears garnished with the ground apricot pits.

SWEET CONGEE WITH RAISINS AND FRESH RASPBERRIES   *6 to 8 servings*

2 cups white rice
8 cups water
1 tsp sea salt
1 tsp cinnamon (warming)
¼ tsp nutmeg (warming)
¼ tsp cardamom (warming, strengthens digestion)
1 cup raisins
1 large Chinese date, chopped (good for lungs)

2 pints raspberries (tone the liver and kidneys)
2 tbs rose water

- Sort and wash rice. Place rice, water, and salt in a medium-size heavy pot, cover, and bring to a boil. Reduce heat and simmer for 30–40 minutes or until the rice is soft and the water somewhat thickened.
- Remove rice from heat. Stir in spices, raisins, and chopped date. Spread the rice mixture into a greased 9 × 13 × 2 inch baking pan. Bake in a 350° oven for 30–40 minutes or until the mixture thickens.
- Wash the berries and mix them with the rose water. Garnish the pudding with the berries.

SWEET KUMQUAT TREAT   (good for the lungs)

- Wash and soak overnight a couple dozen kumquats.
- Rinse and cook slowly with half apple juice and half water to cover until the fruit becomes dark and candylike. May take 4 or 5 hours but it's worth it. Eat one a day.

CHINESE HERBS LISTED IN THE RECIPES

Chinese name is in parenthesis in pinyin. Herbs can be ordered from Chinese herb stores (see Resources).

almond seeds (*xing ren*)
astragalus root (*huang qi*)*
black fungus (*hei mu erh*)
Chinese red dates (*hong zao*)
chrysanthamum flower (*ju hua*)*
codonopsis root (*dang shen*)
glehnia (*bei sha shen*)
honeysuckle flower (*jin yin hua*)*

jujube fruit (*da zao*)
lily bulb (*bai he*)
lotus seeds (*lian zi*)
lycii berries (*gou qi zi*)
polygonatum (*yu zhu*)
pseudostellaria root (*tai zi shen*)
pueraria root or kuzu (*ge gen*)
tangerine peel (*chen pi*)

---

*These are too stringy to eat and should be removed before serving. They can be tied in cheesecloth before cooking. All the other herbs can be sliced and eaten.

WHAT SHOULD I EAT WHEN?

A macrobiotic diet needs to be fine-tuned by a macrobiotic counselor who knows your particular condition. When I was wheezing and called in a panic, mine advised me to "eat widely." Meaning: not the same things every day. Sensible advice. But when I called my Chinese medicinal cooking teacher one night when I was breathing heavily and had a frightening cough, he said, "You'll feel fine tomorrow. Just cut up two carrots . . ." And he proceeded with instructions for cooking and drinking the liquid of the calming carrots and kombu tea. He was right. The mucus began to subside and the heavy breathing stopped. I use this as an example of the energetic nature of food and why I find this cooking so interesting. Of course if it hadn't worked, I would have gotten myself to a doctor or hospital.

The best way to assess your condition energetically is to get a diagnosis from a practitioner of Chinese medicine. If that isn't possible, you can read and study more about it. (Books are in Bibliography.) Experiment with food and herbs carefully, and keep track of the results in your food/symptom diary. Be moderate. Eat widely. If you find something that works, use it over a twenty-four-hour period but don't start eating it every day! Use it when you need it. And avoid those foods which are allergens or are excluded from your diet for other reasons. This is a very simplified version of Chinese food energetics; nevertheless, the lists below should take some of the hit or miss out of eating.

FOR COPIOUS WHITE PHLEGM AND PRODUCTIVE COUGH

+ *Eat pungent herbs and foods*	− *Do not eat phlegmy foods*
garlic	sugar
fresh ginger	dairy
cayenne	soy
nutmeg	honey
turmeric	peanut
coriander	sweet rice
cinnamon	
rosemary	
sea vegetables	
papaya	
mustard greens	
daikon	
fennel	
pumpkin	

continued

+ Eat pungent herbs and foods	− Do not eat phlegmy foods

string beans
tuna
barley
papaya
strawberries

Recipes

* SWEET VEGETABLE SOUP
* ASTRAGALUS CHICKEN SOUP
* STRING BEANS, WALNUTS, AND LYCII BERRIES
* SWEET CONGEE WITH RAISINS AND FRESH RASPBERRIES
* MUSTARD GREENS WITH LOTUS ROOT AND GARLIC
* DISPEL PHLEGM DISH
  COOK PUMPKIN WITH GINGER
  COOK TUNA WITH BARLEY

FOR COLD, WHITE STUCK PHLEGM

+ Add more pungent warming food	− Do not eat cooling foods
garlic	tofu
onion	millet
ginger	fish
chili peppers	asparagus
hot peppers	potato
turnips	salt

Recipe

* FRESH GINGER AND GARLIC TEA

FOR YELLOW OR GREEN PHLEGM (HOT) (AND/OR A BAD SORE THROAT)

+ Use cooling herbs and foods	− Do not eat hot and spicy
sage	garlic
marjoram	ginger
skullcap	walnuts
chamomile	mustard greens
asparagus	again no sugar
celery	
cauliflower	
bok choy	
white fungus	

continued

sea vegetables
carp
millet
barley
kasha
kuzu
persimmon
peach
pear
papaya
plantain
watercress
turnip

Recipes

* COOL HOT PHLEGM, STRENGTHEN SPLEEN TEA
* FRESH AND DRIED PEAR DESSERT
* MILLET WITH CARROTS AND CELERY (LEAVE OUT THE HERBS)

FOR HOT, YELLOW OR GREEN, STUCK PHLEGM

+ *Use pungent, cooling food and herbs*	− *Do not eat hot foods*
cabbage	(see above)
daikon	
radish	
white pepper	

Recipes

* DISPEL GREEN MUCUS TEA
* STUCK MUCUS TEA

FOR SLIGHT SORE THROAT, NIGHT SWEATS, AND THIRST

sea vegetables
chicken broth with yam (don't eat
   the chicken)
baked apple
pears cooked with walnut
yams
pumpkin
sweet potato

Recipes

* SAVORY CONGEE (with excess mucus)
* BURDOCK LOTUS ROOT TEA
* CALMING CARROTS AND KOMBU TEA

FOR DIFFICULTY BREATHING

* ORANGE PEEL AND CRUSHED ALMOND TEA
* CLOVE TEA
* CALMING CARROTS AND KOMBU TEA
* CALMING CHRYSANTHEMUM TEA
* CALMING HEAVY BREATHING TEA

FOR LUNG/KIDNEY/ADRENAL-RELATED PROBLEMS

(shortness of breath, chilliness, weakness and fatigue, breathlessness on exertion, edema, lower back pain, depression, or feel worse at night)

+ *Use strengthening-kidney food and herbs*

Recipes

* CODONOPSIS, ASTRAGALUS, YAM STEW
* BASIC BROWN RICE
* BASIC LENTIL SOUP
* MILLET CHICKEN SOUP
* ASTRAGALUS CHICKEN SOUP
* STRENGTHENING SAVORY CONGEE
* CHICKEN DISH
* STRING BEANS WITH WALNUTS AND LYCII BERRIES
* ADUKI BEANS AND TOFU (only once in a while)
* BASIC CONGEE WITH PAPAYA OR PEACH

(dry lungs, tightness in chest, thirst, irritability, emotional strain causing asthma)

+ *Eat cooling and moistening foods*	− *Do not eat hot or drying foods*

asparagus
bamboo shoots
grapefruit
lemon
millet
peppermint
potato
salt
tofu
watermelon

Recipes

* Burdock lotus root tea
* Pear congees
* Fish stew

To Disperse Old Mucus and Moisten the Lungs

Try kombu, fenugreek tea, marshmallow root.

AVOIDING AND RECOVERING FROM COLDS

There are teas and herbal formulas for getting rid of colds, but the most important thing to do for a cold is to avoid getting one.

- Watch out for sudden drops in temperature. Thermal stress is real. Sudden changes in temperature imbalance the body.
- Dress warm. Don't pay attention to what everyone else is wearing. With asthma, you need to keep your throat and chest warm.
- Carry a scarf for windy or cold days. Don't be caught without something to wrap around your neck.
- Wear an extra cotton layer under your regular clothes on chilly days.
- Wash your hands often. You don't have to be Lady Macbeth, but hand-washing before you leave work, when you come home from the mall, and before eating really helps.
- Rinse your nostrils with salt water, regularly.

- Exercise enhances resistance, but don't overdo it.
- Get plenty of rest. Do your deep breathing and relaxation exercises. When your body tells you it's time to slow down, pay attention.
- When you get a cold, you must concentrate on getting rid of that before addressing other conditions.
- Drink warm liquids; eat mostly soups and soft cooked food such as congees.

At the first signs of a cold:

FIRST SIGN OF COLD TEA   (for cold condition, white tongue)

1 entire fresh ginger root (hot and spicy)
3 scallions (warm and spicy)
2 cinnamon twigs (warming and spicy)
Some citrus peel (warm and sweet)
Honey (only if there is a cough) (neutral and sweet)
Pot of boiling water

- Slice up the ginger root and scallions.
- Put the cinnamon, some citrus peel, and then a little bit of honey into the pot of boiling water.
- If this tea does not make you sweat, add more ginger and scallions. Then get in bed.

- YIN CHIAO CHIEH TU PIEN—an herbal Chinese patent medicine. An anti-inflammatory for the first signs of a cold. Six tablets every three hours for the first day are usually recommended. Only to be taken for the first day.
- CHICKEN BROTH
- ECHINACEA AND GOLDENSEAL. At first sign of cold, take only first day, then taper off. (Available as tinctures and capsules)
- ASTRAGALUS. Enhances the immune response and can be taken over a long period of time. (Available as tinctures and capsules)
  Increase liquids.
  Soak feet in hot water for ten minutes before bedtime.

FIRST SIGN OF COLD SOUP   *6 servings*
Promotes perspiration, relaxes muscles. Good for first day of a cold but not for sore throat. If you don't want to sweat, leave out the chrysanthemum and rosemary.

1   onion, diced
4   cloves of garlic, minced
1   tsp oil
2   carrots, sliced
3   ribs celery, sliced
1   small bulb of fennel, sliced
4–6 cups of stock
½   oz. dry chrysanthemum flower and
¼   oz. fresh rosemary tied together in cheesecloth bag
1   tbs kuzu dissolved in ¼ cup cold water
1   bunch of scallions, chopped

• In a large pot sauté the onion and garlic in the oil for 5 minutes.
• Add the carrot, celery, and fennel and cook for 5 minutes longer.
• Add the stock and cook until vegetables are soft, about 20 minutes.
• Steep the herbs in the broth for 5 minutes and remove.
• Thicken soup with kuzu, garnish with scallions, and serve hot.

If cold becomes well established:

OLD COLD, SORE THROAT TEA   (Hot, dry condition, yellow tongue) For
hot condition (also for headaches):

Chrysanthemum, cool, diaphretic cooling
Honeysuckle, purges heat and inflammation from the body
Honey (for cough), neutral

Combine equal parts of dried flowers and steep in boiled water.
Add honey only for a cough.

ZINC LOZENGES with vitamin C, beta-carotene, and bioflavonoids
ZHONG GAN LING—Chinese herbal patent for more established cold
or flu
CHICKEN BROTH
BURDOCK AND RED CLOVER TEAS
FOR BAD WHEEZING FROM COLD, fill sink or a basin with hot (not
too hot) water. Rest and soak arms in water to above the elbows for ten
minutes.
KEEP WARM AND REST.

RECOVERY FROM COLDS STEW   (For lingering colds, coughs, and headache. Replenishes Qi and Moisture, eliminates Wind and Phlegm.)

1   oz. pueraria root (helps eliminate phlegm)—(kuzu comes from this)
1   oz. polygonatum rhizone (good for dry throat and thirst)
½   oz. orange peel (helps to eliminate phlegm)
1   oz. lotus seeds (stops sweating, strengthens, helps to retain moisture)
12 red dates
8   cups vegetable or chicken stock
5   scallions, sliced
3   carrots, cubed
2   celery sticks, diced
⅓   cup white rice

- Slice the pueraria, polygonatum, and orange peel into small pieces.
- Simmer these along with the lotus seeds, red dates, and ginger in the stock for 1½ hours.
- Add the vegetables and cook an additional half hour.

DISPEL PHLEGM DISH
Cook these together:

½   oz. orange or tangerine peel (1 oz. fresh)
½   oz. apricot or almond seeds
1   fresh pear (diced)
1   cup daikon radish
2" ginger

Cook this with leftover sweet rice for a rice pudding dessert, adding a little cinnamon.

CHAPTER 9

VITAMINS AND HERBS

DON'T FORGET YOUR VITAMINS

U ntil recently, current medical wisdom has been that vitamins are not necessary if one is eating a "balanced" diet. Four to six servings of vegetables and fruit are now recommended. There is no doubt that food is the best place to get your nutrients, but, according to newspaper reports and sightings in supermarkets, lunch counters, and hospital cafeterias, Americans are eating more junk food than ever. Some feel they are eating healthfully if the food is "fat free." And some count calories instead of looking at nutrition. But precious few eat anywhere near the recommended four to six servings of fruit and vegetables, and even if they do, if it is not organically grown, the nutrition value will be lower.

Some people take vitamin pills because they don't have time to eat. Dr. Warren Levin says that vitamins, minerals, and amino acids can work only if they are superimposed on a really good diet. We really can't substitute pills for food. "We should be striving to get our basic requirements from food, but what they call the recommended daily allowances are ridiculously low. You still need them as a base, but they are designed to prevent deficiency disease as opposed to promote optimum health."[1]

Dr. Robert Atkins, who sells his own brand of vitamins, believes that the body is capable of healing itself if presented with the proper substances. Nutrients enable, drugs block. However, he feels that his patients benefited as much from withdrawal from conventional medications as from the vitamins that he gave them.[2]

But if the body is ill and out of balance, what is needed to recover may be too great to be met by even the most nutritious food. A 1981 workshop sponsored by the Department of Food and Nutrition and its Nutrition Advisory Group of the American Medical Association found that immune system dysfunction can come from single-nutrient deficiencies.[3] This is why most alternative or complementary doctors test their patients for nutritional deficiencies and use supplementation as one mode of restoring the body's balance. The best way to find out what you are lacking and establish a program of nutrients suited for you is through a nutritionally oriented practitioner, someone who works toward health with food, vitamins, and/or herbs.

Let's Learn Our ABC's

Vitamins, minerals, and amino acids synergistically work in the body to restore balance. Testing the effects of one vitamin at a time isn't going to tell you much, although that is the way they are tested. Likewise, ingesting one without the others that may be necessary for the vitamin to get to the right place and be utilized properly may create serious imbalances.

Let's take a look at some of these vitamins, minerals, and amino acids. Let's see how they affect immune function and look at ways in which they can work specifically in helping asthma.

ANTIOXIDANTS

Vitamins C and E, beta-carotene, selenium, and zinc are antioxidants, important because they "scavenge" free radicals. Free radicals are molecules which can damage tissue, leading to many degenerative processes. Antioxidants prevent this damage. Free radicals can be created as a result of pollution, chemicals, infections, and other stressors. Let's look at the major antioxidants that go after free radicals.

Vitamin A and Beta-carotene

Illness depletes stores of vitamin A and those of us with allergies and asthma need it for lung tissue repair. Vitamin A can also become depleted by chemical pollution and other stressors. However, vitamin A is one of the few vitamins that can be stored in the body, because it is fat-soluble, not water-soluble like most vitamins. Because vitamin A is not excreted, too much can have a toxic effect. Pregnant women are especially at risk from large doses. Blood levels should be checked if you take a lot of vitamin A.

Where to find vitamin A: butter, egg yolk, green peas, lima beans, soybeans.

Beta-carotene is a precursor of vitamin A and has always been considered a safe and effective way of letting your body make its own. Vitamin A is essential for health; it helps protect the mucous membranes, speeds tissue repair, and boosts immunity by helping T cells produce antibodies.[4] It fortifies the cells of the lining of the respiratory tract and helps against infiltration by viruses and bacteria. Much of the research on vitamin A has been cancer research in which it has been found that vitamin A increases T-helper cells. Vitamin A needs zinc, vitamin E, vitamin C, and vitamin B complex to work really effectively.

THE BETA-CAROTENE STUDIES

The public may have become wary of beta-carotene based on the results of a study of Finnish smokers.[5] That study and a second study of smokers and asbestos-exposed subjects found that cancer rose in the supplemented groups.[6] However, in the May 1996 *Townsend Letter for Doctors & Patients,* nutritionist Jeffrey Bland, Ph.D., reports that in a third study, the Physician's Health Study, of a low disease risk group "beta-carotene was found to have no effect on either morbidity or mortality, even in the 11% of the group who smoked."[7] The negative studies, it should be remembered, were evaluating cancer risk with high-risk groups.

Bland concludes: "The story which emerges when all the studies are reviewed is that beta-carotene is *not* toxic, but rather needs to be part of the full complement of balanced antioxidant nutrients which are delivered as a group in food or supplements. It is well known that vitamin E, vitamin C, selenium and carotenoids work together to protect one another against oxidative damage."[8] Because there are 499 other carotenoids in food, that is a good place to go for all the carotenes.

Where to find beta-carotene: Cod liver oil is rich in beta-carotene. Spirulina, a wild blue-green algae, wheat/barley grass, and chlorella are dried sources. Other rich sources in descending order include: dandelion greens, kale, parsley, carrot, sweet potato, yams, turnip greens, beet greens, watercress, collard greens, winter squash, egg yolk, endive, green onions, persimmons, apricots, broccoli, whitefish, romaine, papayas, apricots, mangoes, nectarines, pumpkin, peaches, cherries, asparagus, and kumquats.

THE B-COMPLEX

Deficiencies of B-group vitamins such as B_6 (pyridoxine), pantothenic acid, and folic acid have produced important compromising immunologic effects.[9] We shall see that certain B vitamins are highly recommended for asthma.

The B vitamins work best as a team although some people report problems with taking all of the B vitamins.

B_6 (Pyridoxine)

Vitamin B_6 is essential to life because it is necessary for protein synthesis, red blood cell production, and many aspects of nervous system and immune function. B_6 works best with magnesium. When B_6 is deficient there may be lymphoid tissue atrophy and decreased hormone activity.[10]

B_6 sometimes gets a bad rap because it can be toxic in very high doses. However, in people with asthma, B_6 levels may fall short. The Department of Agriculture studied the possible use of B_6 for sickle-cell anemia and accidentally discovered that asthmatics were low in B_6. They found that as little as 50 mg twice daily could decrease the number of asthma attacks.[11] Some researchers suggest that the deficiency may occur only in those who have used theophylline. Studies have shown that when theophylline is used for asthma, there is evidence of a B_6 deficiency. In a 1988 study, University of Pretoria researchers concluded that theophylline can affect liver metabolism of vitamin B_6.[12] In another study, all fifteen participants felt the frequency and severity of their asthma attacks or wheezing decreased dramatically while taking the supplement, even though B_6 status was not normalized by supplementation.[13]

Where we can find vitamin B_6: in brown rice, wheat, soybeans, rye, lentils, sunflower seeds, salmon, walnuts, beans. Vitamin B_6 and folic acid, another important B, are concentrated in green vegetables.

B_{12}

Vegetarians need extra vitamin B_{12} and anyone taking folic acid should be taking B_{12}.[14] Vitamin B_{12} can prevent or diminish reactions to sulfites[15] and activate the body's detoxification pathways,[16] making it an important nutrient for those with asthma. B_{12} supplements are best absorbed under the tongue.

Where to find vitamin B_{12}: sardines, flounder, hake, salmon, eggs, haddock.

Ascorbic Acid (Vitamin C)

There are hundreds of studies testifying to vitamin C's immune-stimulating effect.

In an 1985 article in *Medical Hypotheses,* Dr. Robert Cathcart discusses his positive experience in treating over eleven thousand patients suffering various illnesses with large doses of vitamin C. He finds it especially beneficial for infectious disease. In toxic conditions the body is using up its vitamin C stores to scavenge free radicals, so not enough is left for "vitamin C–dependent housekeeping functions."[17] Dr. Cathcart feels that large doses are mostly safe and often in order.

Several recent studies have shown that blood levels of vitamin C in those with asthma were reduced as compared to control groups.[18] A study in Nigeria showed that the number and severity of attacks was reduced with high doses of ascorbic acid.[19] Ascorbic acid is also shown to have a beneficial effect on asthma and in preventing airway hyperactivity in people with upper airway infections.[20] In light of vitamin C's many positive effects, moderately high doses appear to be important to people with asthma.

Where to find vitamin C: Rose hips, guava, and papaya have the highest amounts. Also cabbage, peppers, parsley, watercress, broccoli, oranges, and tomatoes.

VITAMIN E

Vitamin E is an important antioxidant, valuable for strengthening blood capillaries and getting oxygen to all the organs of the body. One reason Vitamin E is essential is because it helps the lymphocytes, which produce antibodies for protection. For optimal immune function, vitamin E needs to be taken in quantities higher than the Minimum Daily Requirement (MDR).[21] Vitamin E protects against common pollutants and chemicals. Some researchers found a "positive association" in combining vitamins C and E in adult asthma supplementation.[22]

VITAMIN E AND OZONE

Researchers have found that rats with reduced vitamin E fared poorly (edema and mortality) when exposed to ozone.[23] So vitamin E may have an important ozone-protective effect.

Where to find Vitamin E: wheat germ oil, raw wheat germ, sunflower seeds, sesame oil, soy oil, almonds, olive oil, sunflower and safflower oil, and cabbage.

MINERALS

Selenium

We have already seen how selenium can protect us against mercury toxicity. Because too much selenium can be devastating to the body, it wasn't until the 1950s that researchers found that small amounts were essential for good health.[24] Now it is thought that proper amounts of selenium can prevent many types of cancers. And selenium, contained in the enzyme glutathione peroxidase, can help reduce the leukotrienes that are responsible for much of the misery of asthma.[25] In decreasing the production of leukotrienes, major mediators of hypersensitivity and inflammation, supplementary selenium could be invaluable for managing asthma and other inflammatory disorders.[26]

Alcohol consumption and exposure to metals such as cadmium, copper, and lead (which can leach from water pipes) can lower levels of selenium. In a double-blind study of twenty-four patients, six asthma patients taking selenium improved, compared to one patient in the placebo group.[27] British researchers at Southampton General Hospital found that asthmatic patients showed a reduced selenium status in plasma and whole blood consistent "with a significantly increased risk of having this disease" compared to normal healthy subjects. Patients with asthma and eczema tended toward lower selenium levels than those with only asthma. They note that the prevalence of asthma and asthma mortality is greater in New Zealand, where there is a lower dietary intake of selenium than is found in the United Kingdom.[28]

Selenium may also help inhibit candida. A deficiency in mice was shown to impair the ability of neutrophils to kill *Candida albicans* in invitro tests.[29] Selenium works well taken with vitamin E.[30]

Where to find selenium: corn, tuna, eggs, asparagus, broccoli, rice, wheat, beans, peas, onions, chicken, beets, barley, tomatoes, soybeans, and sea vegetables.

Magnesium

Magnesium is a major mineral for benefiting asthma as well as many other serious conditions because it is antispasmodic. When there is not enough magnesium, calcium and sodium flood the cells, causing constriction of muscles.[31] Back in 1940, a Philadelphia researcher noted that 50 percent of patients having acute asthma attacks had low magnesium levels.[32]

In a 1985 study, pulmonary function improved when serum magnesium levels were highest.[33] At the Department of Emergency Medicine at the Medical College of Pennsylvania, in 1989, after beta-agonist therapy failed to show significant improvement in the peak expiratory flow rate of thirty-eight asthmatics, those receiving magnesium did significantly better than those given placebos.[34]

Where to find magnesium: sea salt, kelp, blackstrap molasses, sunflower seeds, almonds, soybeans, and sea vegetables.

Zinc

Zinc, another valuable mineral and anti-inflammatory, can prevent cells from releasing up to 40 percent of histamine and leukotrienes.[35] Zinc is available as picolinate, gluconate, and chelated zinc. The elderly are often zinc deficient.[36]

In a book about amino acids, *The Healing Nutrients Within,* the authors suggest that vegetarians may be zinc and vitamin B_6 deficient. Grains, legumes, and beans added to the diet by vegetarians may eliminate minerals from the digestive system. This can be avoided by the addition of sprouted grains, beans, and seeds.[37]

Where to find zinc: oysters, wheat germ, pumpkin seeds, squash seeds, sesame seeds, blackstrap molasses, soybeans, sunflower seeds, egg yolk.

Fish Oils—Omega-3 Fatty Acids

In the late nineteenth century, cod liver oil was recommended for the treatment of asthma and it was thought to affect the improvement of a patient's health. Now fish oils have been found to be effective. However, aspirin-sensitive asthmatics don't do well on fish-oil supplements.[38]

Fish oils contain two important omega-3 fatty acids, EPA and DHA. The omega-3 fatty acids not only decrease inflammation, but protect the heart by decreasing cholesterol and triglycerides. In one study, researchers found an "anti-inflammatory potential of a fish-oil enriched diet." There was also a significant improvement of the later asthmatic response to inhaled allergens.[39]

Where to find omega-3 fatty acids: in oily fish such as salmon, mackerel, sardines, and anchovies.

Amino Acids

Amino acids are the building blocks of protein. There are eight essential amino acids, and other amino acids, including cysteine, a sulfur amino acid which we are discussing here: N-acetylcysteine (NAC), (a derivative of L-cysteine).

At the Princeton Brain Bio Center, researchers say that L-cysteine (500 mg morning and evening) has helped certain patients with asthma "totally eliminate their need for inhalers and medications."[40] Other researchers have reported L-cysteine to be effective in breaking up mucus in the lungs and bronchial passages. (Do not confuse with L-cystine.)

A Swedish study compared the effects of oral acetylcysteine with a placebo in 203 patients with chronic bronchitis over the course of six months. They found that 40 percent of the cysteine users had no "exacerbations" compared with 19 percent of the placebo group.[41]

N-acetylcysteine has antioxidant properties and is used to break down heavy mucus. It's a precursor of glutathione, an amino acid important in scavenging free radicals and in boosting the body's ability to detoxify. Studies have also shown that it can protect the liver from heavy metal poisoning.[42] Cysteine is a high quality source of sulfur which is good for allergic reactions.

Where to find sulfur: kale, brussels sprouts and cauliflower, raspberries, the onion family, and watercress.

HERBAL HEALING

Herbs and green and growing things have been used for healing and strengthening since the beginning of time. The Bible, Revelations 22:2 says, ". . . and the leaves of the tree were for the healing of the nations." The earliest written records list plants that were used as medicines. In China, Shen Nung, founder of the Shen Nung Dynasty in 3494 B.C., researched the properties of herbs and their relation to human beings; his "herbal," based on centuries of earlier folk uses of plants, lists 365 medical preparations.[43] For thousands of years Taoists have kept written records of their experiments with herbs and the formulation of herbal combinations.[44]

Hippocrates, born about 460 B.C., was a Greek physician who is considered to be the father of modern medicine. His writings list nearly four hundred medicinal plants. Throughout the Middle Ages, herbal gardens and plant medicine developed in monasteries; botanic gardens were developed by universities during the Renaissance; and physic gardens were established throughout Europe beginning in the sixteenth and seventeenth centuries. London's Chelsea Physic Garden was founded in 1673 and in 1993 opened the "Garden of World Medicine" displaying medicinal plants used by the Native North Americans, Aboriginals, and Maoris, as well as South American tribal, Ayurvedic, and Chinese medicinal plants. Today Glaxo looks to the plants in this garden for possible new drugs.[45]

In Colonial America people depended on their gardens to supply medicinal plants. Hundreds of millions of people today, in developing countries, depend on plants for their traditional medicine.

Many pharmaceuticals are based on the actions of plants. But today plants are fast disappearing because of deforestation and the destruction of the rain forest. Drug companies are scouring parts of the world looking for beneficial plants. They are talking to native peoples and "witch" doctors for information before these peoples and their plants completely disappear. With "civilization" galloping at the current rate, the knowledge, the forests, and lands where the plants can still be found could be lost in our generation. Alliances have been formed of scientists, traditional healers, entrepreneurs, governments, and pharmaceutical companies working together to preserve these resources.[46] It sounds good, but let's look closer.

Experts are working to find the part of the plant that has the active ingredient, isolate this ingredient, standardize it, and synthesize it in the lab. Why? One reason is that you can't patent a plant. You have to change it in some way, add a molecule, to make it your own. Another reason is that medicine is practiced by targeting symptoms. But when a drug is made from the active ingredient, the other equally important parts of the plant are gone. We know nothing about how all the parts are balanced to work together, perhaps to protect us.

Originally in China, herbs were used for their nutritional and energy aspects, to promote life—not to address symptoms. In traditional Chinese medicine, an herb is rarely used alone. Rather, a Chinese herbalist would prescribe a combination of at least four or five herbs to balance and strengthen the body, rather than to simply address symptoms. Herbs included would counteract side effects and harmonize other herbs in the formula. Herbs can help the body reset its own healing mechanisms, but they will work best with a comprehensive approach to health.

EPHEDRA (MA HUANG)

Ephedrine, found in many medications, is the active constituent of the herb *ephedra sineca* (ma huang), used by the Chinese for thousands of years to relieve fever, calm coughing, and dilate the bronchioles to relieve asthma. But it can also elevate the blood pressure, increase heartbeat, and affect the central nervous system.[47] Andrew Weil, M.D., says that his asthma patients do much better when they learn to make Chinese ephedra tea, which is slower acting, but without the unpleasant side effects of ephedrine.[48] A small amount of ephedrine can sometimes have a toxic effect.[49] In China, ma huang was sometimes prescribed with other herbs such as licorice, apricot, and gypsum for pulmonary problems.[50] Ma huang is a drying herb, should be used carefully, and shouldn't be used regularly by anyone in a weak condition.[51]

Chinese ephedra should not be confused with the American desert version, *ephedra nevadensis,* which is a more potent nervous stimulant.[52]

ASTRAGALUS

Astragalus is a popular tonic herb and a mainstay of Chinese medicine. Because it is a very safe herb, it is used often in Chinese medicinal cooking. It tonifies the lung, strengthens the limbs, and promotes adrenal function regulating sugar metabolism, especially if combined with licorice root.[53] Cancer and AIDS researchers are currently investigating the many beneficial qualities of astragalus which help enhance immune function.

Astragalus is used for shortness of breath and for frequent colds, but not for hot conditions such as sore throat.[54] Astragulus root can be purchased at Asian herb stores and used in cooking soups and stews.

GINKGO BILOBA

The ginkgo tree is the oldest living species; it has been in existence for over 200 million years. It is extremely resistant to disease, pollution, and insects, making it the perfect street tree for large cities. Although the herb ginkgo may be best known for its memory-enhancing effects, in China it has been used to treat the symptoms of asthma and cough.[55]

The extract of *Ginkgo biloba* and the ginkgolides have a powerful inhibiting action on the platelet-activating factor, which helps prevent inflammation. It has antiallergenic properties and affects smooth muscle contraction, making it an important herb for symptoms of asthma.[56] It is also very safe to use.[57]

SKULLCAP OR SCUTELLARIA

Scutellariae radix has been used in China for centuries for the treatment of many conditions. It is a cooling herb with anti-inflammatory and antiallergenic properties.[58] Chinese skullcap helps with allergic inflammatory reactions, perhaps because it contains numerous bioflavonoids which work somewhat like cromolyn sodium to inhibit formation of leukotrienes.[59] Researchers in Osaka, Japan, found that ogon, the dried roots of *Scutellariae baicalensis,* showed a relatively marked antibacterial activity.[60]

ANGELICA POLYMORPHA

Angelica has shown significant antiallergy effects for persons sensitive to pollens, dust, dander, and other IgE-mediated allergies.[61] It is used by Chinese and Japanese herbalists to prevent and relieve allergic symptoms by inhibiting the production of IgE antibodies. It also helps to relax smooth muscle.

CHINESE LICORICE ROOT (*GLYCYRRHIZA GLABRA*)

Licorice is very important in Chinese herbology as it harmonizes all other herbs and helps them go where they are needed. It is a detoxifier and energy builder, and has an antibacterial effect. Its anti-inflammatory action works similarly to natural adrenal steroids.[62] At the same time it can decrease some of the undesirable side effects associated with cortisone in other parts of the body.[63] If licorice is used over a long period of time it's important to increase potassium-rich foods. It should not be used by those with high blood pressure or hypertension.

PATENT CHINESE HERBALS

It is best to take herbs by working with a qualified herbalist who will put together a combination to suit your particular condition. However, there are patent herbal formulas that are mild and are available in pill form from Chinese pharmacies. See Resources for mail-order information.

Chinese Patent Herbal Combinations for Asthma

Chi Kuan Yen Wan. Contains eriobotrya (loquat) leaf and codonopsis root among its thirteen ingredients. Good in hot conditions for a dry cough and sticky phlegm with labored breathing. Not to be used for "colds." Twenty tiny pills, twice a day is recommended.

Ping Chuan Wan or Ping Chuan Pill. Contains ten herbs including codonopsis root and licorice root. Good for chronic asthma with white lung phlegm due to weak kidney condition. It will help the cough by resolving the phlegm. Not to be used with heat signs such as yellow or green phlegm, headache, or fever. Ten (tiny) pills, three times a day are recommended.

CHINESE HERBS FOR ASTHMA USED IN JAPAN

Perhaps one of the reasons for better asthma management and low asthma mortality rate in Japan is the use of Chinese herbal therapy. The Japanese use Saiboku-to, a formula that includes ten Chinese herbs. Bupleurum is one of the major herbs in Saiboku-to, a formula that also contains scutellaria, licorice root, and Panax ginseng in lesser amounts. Saiboku-to has been reported to inhibit histamine release from mast cells and suppress Type I and Type IV allergic reactions in animal studies. These results have not been consistent in asthma patients but it is used because it is free from side effects.[64] The action of Saiboku-to may also work by hormonal stimulation of the adrenal cortex.[65]

Magnolia officinalis, which comes from the outermost layer of the bark of the magnolia tree, seems to be the ingredient in which researchers are most interested. Magnolol (the part being tested) has gentle antibiotic and anti-toxic properties.[66]

HERBS FROM HAWAII

Mamane (*Sophora chrysophylla*) was one of fifty-eight native Hawaiian herbs for asthma selected to be investigated for therapeutic purposes. This herb and others closely related have been used for hundreds of years as a tea in China and India, as well as in the United States. *Sophora chrysophylla* and *Sophoras* alkaloids have been shown to have bronchodilating, anti-inflammatory, and anti-allergenic effects.[67]

ECHINACEA ANGUSTIFOLIA AND *PURPUREA*

Echinacea is an herb used by Native Americans over one hundred years ago. In recent years its immune-stimulating and antiviral properties have been more appreciated in Europe, especially in Germany, where it was researched and developed. The polysaccharides in echinacea stimulate T-lymphocytes and interferon production. Echinacea's immune-stimulating effects make it popular for treatment of colds. People with weakened immune systems are said to benefit the most.[68] Because it's very heating, herbalist Letha Hadady recommends only using echinacea the first day or two of a cold.[69] Use should be monitored because high doses or long-term use may cause problems.[70]

Echinacea, as well as the Chinese herbs listed here, can be purchased in capsules or liquid extracts.

AYURVEDIC HERBS

Ayurveda is a complete science of medicine that comes from ancient medical traditions of India. There are many books that attempt to explain Ayurveda and its herbal science. Although you can buy Ayurvedic herbs in health food stores today, remember that a diagnosis should be based on knowing your particular body type according to this system, which takes into account every aspect of your being. As with any vitamin or herbal remedy, those that address symptoms should only be used as an adjunct to a comprehensive program to strengthen the body.

Tylophora asthmatica. Used in Ayurvedic medicine for asthma and other respiratory illnesses because of its antiallergenic qualities. Its alkaloids may contribute to its antihistamine and antispasmodic effects.[71]

Boswellin. Addresses the leukotrienes. Comes in chewable pill form at health food stores. It is an anti-inflammatory.

Ashwagandha. An energy tonic with bitter, sweet, and heating properties. Not to be used with severe congestion.

SPIRULINA (BLUE-GREEN ALGAE)

Spirulina is not an herb but a blue-green algae which is found in high salt alkaline lakes in various parts of the world, including Mexico and Kenya. The Aztecs made bricks of spirulina harvested from Lake Texcoco and ate it the way we might eat cheese today.[72]

Spirulina is thought to be the best source of digestible protein in the vegetable kingdom. Essential amino acids comprise 47 percent of the protein in spirulina. It is also a good source of B vitamins, beta-carotene, and gamma linolenic acid.[73]

Japanese researchers at Kagawa Nutrition University found that feeding mice *Spirulina platensis* which has a "high protein content and good amino acid composition" enhanced antibody production. Because it may enhance immune function through the modulation of macrophage function, it could be valuable for reducing allergic reactions.[74]

CHAPTER 10

CREATING A HOME THAT'S TRIGGER-FREE

TRIGGERS AND FLARES

Much has been written about different kinds of asthma: intrinsic, extrinsic, and "mixed." But categories haven't been useful in helping us recover. Most of us have been told that the condition is chronic, that we should learn to manage our "flares" through proper use of medication while avoiding asthma "triggers." Those who develop "occupational" asthma are told to stay home or change jobs. However, doctors are the first to admit that they know little about the way that asthma works. We've seen that usually only symptoms are treated, while little attempt is made to find out why it is getting worse. I feel that the word "trigger" trivializes what may be of utmost importance. And has anyone had an asthma attack that feels like a "flare"?

Our Chemical Exposures

When asthma sufferers are questioned as to the cause of their illness, molds, pollens, dust, and dander are almost always cited. All of these are allergens that can be measured with an IgE antibody test. Because there are no biochemical markers, most doctors are not trained to take into consideration the thousands of other irritants we are exposed to daily. You may have been cautioned about dust mites in your mattress, but have you been warned of petrochemicals in your living room?

In 1945 Du Pont coined the slogan "Better Living Through Chemistry," and since then billions of tons of chemicals have been manufactured yearly in the United States, thousands of new ones every year. If you were born after World War II you are part of the first generation to be exposed to this chemical onslaught. Because our bodies haven't been able to keep up with and adapt to this assault, we develop toxic overload.

All of the irritants that we deal with in this chapter could possibly "trigger" an asthma attack. But reducing your toxic load is as compelling a reason as avoiding an asthma attack, to get them out of your life. Let's face it, many of these "triggers" are toxins that are not good for anyone. Maybe we should consider ourselves fortunate that our bodies tell us to practice avoidance and change our lifestyle. For when our toxic load is reduced, real recovery can begin.

Is "Occupational" Asthma Really Occupational?

You've undoubtedly read about occupational asthma. Or you may have been told that asthma can be triggered by an offending agent in the workplace, sometimes after years of chronic exposure.

In the manufacture of detergents, for instance, workers can develop asthma from the constant inhalation of enzymes. Farmers, fumigators, and manufacturers develop asthma from ongoing exposure to pesticides and insecticides. Nurses, pathologists, lab workers, rubber processors, textile workers, and people in dozens of other professions are at risk from formaldehyde.

You might not be thinking about the dangers of formaldehyde if you are working in the fashion industry. One woman developed asthma from working with fabric she later discovered is heat treated with formaldehyde resin to make it stronger. It took twenty years of exposure to constant cutting and handling of the material releasing its vapors before she became ill. Once asthma developed, she quickly became reactive to everything, including foods, other chemicals, and outdoor air pollution.

At Home with Pesticides and Formaldehyde

As you will soon see, you don't have to have a risky occupation to be constantly exposed to agents causing "occupational" asthma. Formaldehyde and pesticide residues are only two of the "occupational" triggers to which we are all exposed at home, sometimes to a shocking degree.

Pesticide production has actually tripled in the last three decades. Billions of pounds of pesticides are sold in the United States each year, with much of it ending up on the food that we eat. It is used in fertilizer and sprayed on growing crops. And when the produce reaches the supermarket it is sprayed again with fungicides so it will last longer. The lawn-care industry produces thousands of tons of chemicals a year to keep the suburbs green and weed-free. Is the lawn-care truck going from house to house on your block? Does an exterminator call once a month? Chlorpyrifos (Dursban), an insecticide, Diazinon, and products containing pyrethrum may be particularly bad for the respiratory system.

THE FORMALDEHYDE STORY

Nine billion pounds of formaldehyde are produced in the United States every year.[1] Although millions of people are exposed to the vapors in the workplace, many more were exposed in their very own houses by urea-formaldehyde foam. Also known as UFFI, it was blown into the walls for insulation of 150,000 homes a year before 1982, when the public was made aware of its dangers.

You may remember formaldehyde as an embalming fluid from high school biology lab, but you probably did not know that it is used routinely for disinfecting, deodorizing, and flameproofing common products and as a preservative. Although there may be legal limits set on how much formaldehyde can outgas in the workplace in an eight-hour day, no one is monitoring the effect of it outgassing from hundreds of products in your home twenty-four hours a day. These products include kitchen cabinets and furniture made of particleboard, plywood, and plastics, as well as paint, adhesives, newsprint and other paper products, carpets, drapes, shampoos, soaps, facial tissue, nail polish, hairspray, deodorants, grocery bags, permanent-press clothes, and *cigarette smoke*. One young man in my workshop recounted how his asthma improved considerably when he inherited ten large handkerchiefs from his father and stopped using tissue to blow his nose!

Irritation of the eyes, the respiratory system, and the mucous membranes can result from acute exposure to formaldehyde. Low levels can be a potent sensitizer and may induce asthma in asthmatic persons.[2]

CLEANING UP THE LIVING SPACE

Chemicals are a major stress to the immune system. Our task is to see where this stress is in our lives, learn to make changes, and allow our immune system to recover.

BECOME AN ASTHMA SLEUTH

When you get up in the morning, shower, shave your legs or face, brush your teeth, put on makeup or aftershave, and dress in freshly washed clothes, you may feel clean and fresh and ready to start the day. You probably don't think of yourself as being loaded down with chemicals. But let's take a closer look. You may have already noticed having allergic reactions to products that seem to have nothing to do with your breathing. But whatever is causing the itchy skin, eczema, tearing eyes, or exhaustion is probably making your asthma worse.

Your favorite shampoo may contain perfumes and chemicals or para-aminobenzoic acid (PABA), to which many people are allergic. Hairsprays are plastics which can be inhaled. Some of these even contain shellac and polyethylene glycol. When you wash, mousse, and spray your hair all of these chemicals are with you all night on the pillow!

You may wash your face with care but the scented soap can linger with you all day long. And after the washing, men use shaving cream and after-shave lotions which may contain ethanol and ammonia. Women use cleansers, masks, lotions, moisturizers, perfumes, and cosmetics of every kind. These may contain phenol, formaldehyde, fragrance, and PABA as well as other irritants and allergens.

Many people wear clothes made of synthetic materials or cotton with no-iron, no-press treatments containing formaldehyde. These interfere with good breathing. Detergents and fabric softeners contain petrochemicals, perfumes, and enzymes which cause respiratory problems.

Dry-cleaning chemicals such as percloroethylene can give you asthma or heart arrhythmia, or can attack the central nervous system.

As you can see, there's a lot of room for improvement!

WHAT WE CAN DO

One workshop participant writes, "What helped me 1000 times more than anything else: I removed everything scented from my house, along with all cleaning substances other than Bon Ami, lemon, vinegar, and baking soda."

Let's get rid of our scented products. People are extremely devoted to certain items. I've noticed a great reluctance about changing laundry products or giving up a favorite perfume that might not have been a problem in preasthma days. Remember: Breathing well is your first priority.

Have a pencil handy as you go through this chapter so you can check off the items that you feel can be most easily changed. I'll bet you can already think of some things that need substitutions. Your local health food store or mail-order houses (see Resources) may be the best places to find simple nonscented products.

Soap. Olive oil soap is well tolerated. Avoid washing hands with scented soap. The smell could ruin your whole day.

Shampoos. Look carefully at herbal formulas, which may contain allergens.

Moisturizers. These may contain perfumes, menthol, and camphor. Health food stores sell nonscented herbal brands.

Hair conditioners, setting lotions, and rinses. These should come from natural sources. Smell first to make sure there is no scent. Do not use hairsprays of any kind and avoid any product which is sprayed into the air, even if it isn't an aerosol.

Toothpaste. Yours may be causing more of a problem than you know, especially if you've been using the same one for years. Avoid fluoride. Baking soda makes the best toothpaste and can double as a deodorant. If it causes a rash underarm, mix with cornstarch.

Cosmetics. Lipsticks, rouge, and face powder can also contain talc, perfumes, and heavy metals, which may be absorbed. When you buy these from natural sources, still watch for allergic reactions. Itching, scaling, redness, or eye problems indicate an ingredient that may also affect your asthma.

Shaving. Shaving lotion, your own or your spouse's, can be extremely irritating. Again, health food stores have brands without ethanol, perfumes, and ammonia. Or use a hot towel before shaving.

Fabrics. Wear clothes made of cotton without permanent press or no-iron finishes. Wash without detergents or fabric softeners. You can't imagine until you try it the difference that scent-free sheets and clothing can make on your breathing. To remove detergent residue or finish on brand-new clothes use one-half to one pint of vinegar to a washer full of water; soak clothes for twelve hours, agitating occasionally. Launder using one-quarter cup of baking soda and rinse well.

LAUNDRY

Laundry soap. Perfume-free soap flakes, ½ cup washing soda, and ½ cup borax.

Fabric softener. Add ¼ cup baking soda to wash water.

Bleach. Nonchlorine bleach or ½ cup borax.

Grease spots. Cover with baking soda for several hours, brush before washing.

Chemicals in fabric softeners include:

Alphaterpineol. Irritating to the mucous membranes.

Benzyl acetate. Vapors irritating to respiratory passages.

Benzyl alcohol. Irritating to the upper respiratory tract.

Chloroform and camphor. Should not be inhaled.

Ethyl acetate. Irritating to the respiratory tract.

Pentane. Avoid breathing vapors, which can cause nervous-system depression.

Moving through the House

With our cities choking with pollution from factories, incinerators, and auto exhaust fumes, it may seem strange to be worrying about the living room. However, most people spend 85 percent of their time indoors at home or at work, and believe it or not, the air inside your home can be up to one hundred times as polluted as the air outside. Sometimes people move to a cleaner, less-congested part of the country and take all of their problems with them.

So now that we are clean and scent-free, let's go through the house and locate problem areas. Cleaning up our living environment may mean more than a thorough dusting.

The two main ingredients for breathable indoor air are the open window and the air cleaner.

Open windows for at least ten minutes morning and evening even in cold weather. This will help to get rid of the buildup of vapors outgassing from cooking, combustion, cabinets, and rugs. Often windows are never opened out of fear of traffic fumes or pollen. Pick a time when the pollen count is low and the traffic has died down. Attach an air-conditioning filter from the hardware store to an adjustable screen and put it in the open window. This should filter out the worst pollutants and give you a change of air. Just make sure that there are no openings between the window and the screen.

Air cleaners are a necessity for people with asthma. Make sure yours has an HEPA filter plus a charcoal filter which is changed regularly according to the manufacturer's instructions. Some sensitive people are allergic to the glues, so you may need an all-stainless-steel model. The air cleaner will take particulates such as dust, pollens, and dander out of the air and can help with cooking, formaldehyde, and other odors.

Air fresheners of any kind should be disposed of. Flower scents are simply chemicals that mask harsher odors. For freshening air try zeolite (which can be purchased in bags) or open a box of baking soda. Or open a window.

CLEANING MATERIALS

Liquid soap. From health food store.

All-purpose cleaner. 1 tsp. liquid soap, 2 tsp. borax, and some lemon juice in 1 qt. water in spray bottle.

Scouring powder. Bon Ami or baking soda with vinegar.

Air freshener. Open boxes of baking soda.

Tile cleaner. Vinegar and borax.

Dishwasher. Equal parts borax and washing soda.

Windows and mirrors. 3 tbs. vinegar to 1 qt. water, spray.

Furniture polish. Oil and lemon juice.

Cleaning copper and brass. Rub with ½ a lemon.

Aluminum. Lemon juice and warm water.

Silver and stainless steel. Baking soda and water.

Ovens. Steel wool, washing soda, and water.

Drain cleaner. Equal parts baking soda and vinegar; after a few minutes, rinse with boiling water.

THE KITCHEN

Start your house survey in the kitchen by sniffing in the cabinets under the sink. Cleaning products may be making you feel worse than you realize.

Products. Products containing chlorine and pine are extremely irritating to respiratory conditions and should not be used. Others with strong odors have got to go. This includes detergents, ammonia, solvents, waxes, polishers, and chlorinated cleansers. Despite propaganda to the contrary, housework can be done with a few simple ingredients—white vinegar, baking soda, borax, lemon, vegetable oil, and water. Get rid of that deodorizer in the garbage pail now!

Water Filters. This is a necessity for toxin-free living. Reverse osmosis with a carbon filter is best but expensive. Have your water tested first to find out what you need to remove. A good water filter will remove giardia (a common parasite), solvents, heavy metals, and chlorine. Request test results from the company before buying. Whole house filters are available.

Kitchen Cabinets. Cabinets made of particleboard or plywood usually have unfinished back and side surfaces which should be coated with a formaldehyde sealer to keep vapors from outgassing. Solid wood is best for new floors or cabinets. In an emergency, aluminum foil can be used as a vapor barrier.

Appliances. When purchasing new appliances look for porcelain, stainless-steel, or used items that have finished outgassing.

Stoves. Gas is a major irritant for some asthmatics. Have your stove checked for leaks. However, many people are even more sensitive to electric stoves. I find the heated coils extremely irritating, especially when food or liquid has spilled and burns. And electric stoves have strong electromagnetic fields which can be detrimental to health. Keep your electric stove clean, limit your cooking time, and try to stay at a safe distance. If you are considering having the gas stove removed, you can be tested for gas sensitivity first, to make sure that gas is really a problem. Kitchen stoves should have a hood and exhaust fan to draw odors out of the house. Avoid self-cleaning ovens. If you must use a microwave have it checked for leaks and don't linger close by. Corning Ware, glass, or stainless-steel pots and pans are best for cooking.

Flooring. Solid wood subfloors, tile, and natural linoleum are best for the kitchen floor, but make sure that the glues and grouts used are formulated for chemically sensitive people. Natural linoleum may contain resins and a jute backing so test a piece by your pillow for a few nights before you cover the kitchen floor. Remember, everyone's sensitivities are different.

Pest Control. Do not use commercial chemical products, or natural ones containing pyrethrum or diatomaceous earth. Pyrethrum is made from chrysanthemums (which are part of the ragweed family) and is sometimes used in flea collars and other insecticides labeled nontoxic to humans and pets. Products containing diatomaceous earth can be extremely irritating to the lungs.

PEST CONTROL

Moths. Brush clothes thoroughly. Make cheesecloth bags of equal parts dried rosemary and mint. Good for one season only.

Ants. Boric acid in cracks. Plant mint or onions outside house.

Roaches. Boric acid in cracks.

Mice and rats. Seal holes in walls and around pipes with fine steel wool. Mix 1 part plaster of paris with 1 part flour and some cocoa powder and use for rodent control.

Termites. *Do not apply termiticides.* Call Bio-Integral Resource Center in Berkeley, California, for advice. (See Resources.)

Flea control. Sprinkle lavender oil over rock salt, let salt absorb the oil, and distribute this under furniture as a flea repellent. Vacuum thoroughly.

LIVING AND DINING ROOMS

Upholstered Furniture. Your furniture may have been impregnated with chemical stainproofing and mothproofing.

Joyce, a fifty-year-old Toledo woman, developed asthma and exhaustion after the arrival of a new living-room set. She spent a lot of time on the couch, which only worsened her condition. Eventually she traced the problem to the couch's synthetic material treated with stainproofing. But formaldehyde-treated wood or glues in new furniture may cause some of the same symptoms. Sometimes conditions worsen after the purchase of new nonupholstered furniture because of vapors that outgas into the air for years.

Joyce got rid of the couches, bought wicker furniture, and had a cushion made from foam untreated with formaldehyde. Finally she had a seamstress make curtains from untreated cotton material purchased from a mail-order house.

Used Furniture. If you can't find new furniture without formaldehyde glues or tolerable foam cushions, used furniture may be the best bet. But avoid thrift shops which fumigate everything with pesticides. And be particularly wary of movers who may spray your perfectly tolerable furniture or who regularly fumigate their trucks.

Carpets. At Joyce's house, when the carpeting was pulled up and she started reacting to the subfloors, her husband bought a sealer varnish from an allergy mail-order house and sealed the wood. Then she purchased new room-size cotton rugs and left them outside in the sun for a few days before putting them on the floor. Feeling better takes a lot of initiative!

If you must have carpets, watch out for synthetic carpets, stain- and moth-proof treatments, and carpet shampoos. You can obtain nonscented, nontoxic shampoos from an allergy company. Some people tile when they get rid of carpets. If you go that route, make sure the grout and glues are less-toxic products. The wrong glue can worsen your asthma as much as the wrong carpet.

Vacuuming. Should be done with a water canister or triple-filter vac so that very fine dusts are not blown back into the room. If a new model isn't possible, you can order just the filter material and cut it to fit your current cleaner.

Dust Mites. These may also be a problem if you test allergic to them. There are several sprays on the market with which to treat upholstered furniture and rugs. Keep the humidity low.

Dusting. Thoroughly dust walls, ceilings, and floors. Walls and furniture can be dusted with a damp rag or a combination of mineral or olive oil and lemon juice. Wear a dust mask while cleaning! Throw pillows can be fluffed in the dryer with no heat to remove dusts. Dust lightbulbs, fixtures, and radiators. Radiators heat up dust and change it to something more toxic.

Forced-Air Heating. Another common problem for people with asthma is pollutants emanating from forced-air heating units. A contractor can be called in to examine the hard-to-reach insides of heating and air-conditioning units. These can be contaminated with highly allergenic molds.

Forced-air heating units can be equipped with special HEPA filters which are far superior to the ones that come with the unit. The room vents should be cleaned regularly and special filter material inserted to trap dusts and mold spores. In old-fashioned systems where heat rises, these won't work. Several layers of cheesecloth inside the grate should help. Ductwork should be maintained properly. Find a professional service that will vacuum the ducts once a year. This is a must!

Have chimneys cleaned once a year and watch out for combustion fumes from oil or gas burners. Some people don't feel better until they switch to electric baseboard heat. Just be sure to remove the covers of the units for frequent vacuuming.

Air-Conditioning. Air conditioners should be maintained by giving the vents a regular cleaning with a hydrogen peroxide solution or vinegar. Wash and change filters often during the season and examine the unit closely for molds. Trouble often begins in a clogged drip pan and spreads to the ducts.

Clean drip pans every month and inhibit molds by leaving a hydrogen per-oxide solution or diluted vinegar in the pan.

Fireplaces and Wood-burning Stoves. Even with the best of flues, fire-places and woodstoves create an air problem that makes breathing extremely difficult. A high-efficiency air cleaner with a HEPA filter, makes a dramatic change in air quality appreciated even by those without asthma.

Anything burning is going to be a problem for asthmatics. That includes barbecues and kitchen grills, in the home or in a restaurant. Burning wax is a respiratory irritant, so don't use candles. Incense is also an allergen. If you have ever suddenly experienced chest tightness and your throat closing up while dining out (as I have) it could be from a grill or the result of a fat fire in the kitchen. Go outside immediately for fresh air and from there assess your next move.

Window Treatments. Curtains are dust catchers, but cotton washed reg-ularly could be okay. Cotton window shades are simpler. Avoid slats, which collect dust.

PLANTS AS AIR CLEANERS

Philodendrons. The whole family—for formaldehyde fumes from new carpets and fumes from benzene.

Aloe vera. For reducing formaldehyde in low concentrations in a tight space.

Spider plants. For benzene and carbon monoxide.

English ivy. Benzene.

Remember to cover soil with an inch of aquarium gravel to keep down molds. Fumes are absorbed through the root system, so you'll need lots of pots.

Plants. Houseplants make a great window treatment, are good to look at, and provide oxygen. The best ones for us include spider plants and philo-dendrons, which actually help take chemicals such as benzene and formal-dehyde out of the air. A layer of aquarium gravel over the surface of the soil should help keep down molds. And always transplant outside the house. Don't use houseplants in the bedroom.

Printed Material. Don't let newspapers, magazines, and professional journals pile up in corners of the room. Vapors from the inks and chemicals in paper can build up, adding to the mix in the air.

THE BEDROOM OASIS

Your bedroom should be an oasis free of allergens from the outside world. Although we can't control all the pollutants in our lives, the bedroom should be a retreat in which you can recover from exposures to outside pollution. Sleeping time should be recovery time. If you are taking all the other proper precautions and still wake up wheezing, the bedroom needs to be examined more carefully.

Air Conditioners. They help with heat and humidity and keep pollen and pollutants from entering. But they must be well maintained as outlined previously.

Air Cleaner. This is a must. A portable one with an HEPA filter can be brought into the bedroom to keep the room dust- and pollen-free for a good night's sleep.

Bed. The bed should be of solid wood or metal, or be old enough to have finished outgassing. Make sure neither the bed nor the mattress has been sprayed with pesticides. All mattresses are flameproofed but you can buy an untreated cotton one from Janice Corporation with a letter from a doctor. Or you could cover yours with silver foil and pad it with layers of cotton blankets. A miteproof mattress cover should be made of all-cotton barrier cloth. (See Resources.) Cotton flannel sheets, pillows, cotton thermal blankets, and quilts will keep you cozy in winter. Polyester sheets make breathing more difficult.

Closets. They should be free of cedar, mothballs, or moth repellants. Try to buy clothes of natural fabrics that can be washed. If you must have clothes cleaned, ask cleaners to make sure they are completely dry when they are returned. Air them out-of-doors if possible, don't store them in plastic bags, and keep them out of the bedroom closet. Closets should be free of sachets or deodorizers and the doors should be kept closed.

Carpets. Synthetic carpets are a bane to the bedroom. Some chemicals found in their manufacture include formaldehyde, tetrachloroethylene, toluene, xylene, benzene, and styrene, all of which are highly toxic. They are often backed with jute, rubber, or urethane foam, which may outgas when new or when exposed to heat, sunlight, and high humidity. Many people become ill when the bedroom is carpeted. A small cotton rug that can be washed is best. Do not use rubber or hemp pads under rugs. If you're stuck with carpeting that is outgassing and can't rip it out, you could treat it with a formaldehyde sealer. (See Resources.)

Curtains. Curtains and blinds can be dust catchers. Cotton window shades that can be wiped down are better. Don't use plastics in the bedroom.

Windows. If you can, open windows when you go to sleep, even in cold weather. If it is really too chilly, open them for five minutes to air the room and close before retiring. In pollen season it's better to keep them closed and run the air conditioner. (See page 207.)

Electrical Appliances. Keep clocks and radios at a distance from the bed to avoid sleeping near strong electromagnetic fields. Don't use electric blankets except to warm the bed. Be sure to unplug completely before going to sleep.

Hot Air Vents. Keep them clean and insert filter material or seal them closed and use an electric radiator.

Pets. "That darn cat" (and dogs and gerbils) should be kept out of the bed and out of the room!

Renovations. Many people become ill after renovating their bedrooms, although some haven't made the connection between the materials and the wheezing. Common pitfalls include papering with vinyl wallpaper, wallpaper paste containing fungicides, pressboard furniture, new polyester quilts, drapes, and synthetic carpeting. After renovation everything is new and outgassing.

In this case some people get relief by renting an ozone machine, leaving the house, having the machine turned on, and running it for twenty-four hours. The house must be empty when the machine is on and should be aired out for another day or two before people return. The use of ozone is controversial but some find it effective. Another option is turning the heat up high to hasten the outgassing for twenty-four hours and then airing the house. Again, you don't want to be there until the fumes are gone.

THE BATHROOM

Products. Start sniffing under the sink. Although your scented soap and toilet tissue didn't give you asthma, the combinations of scented bathroom products do stress breathing more than you may know. Rid yourself of any perfumed soaps, lotions, and moisturizers. Ditto for tub, tile, and toilet cleaners made with pine scent, Clorox, or ammonia. The health food store has a variety of all-purpose cleaners like Uni-Clean, which can clean practically anything without odor.

The air freshener in the toilet bowl has to go. Scented tissues and toilet tissue should be replaced with the unscented variety. But beware of earth-friendly products that have been bleached with Clorox! Any products in bottles you can't part with, wrap with silver foil for occasional use.

Shower. We absorb more chlorine in the shower than by drinking several glasses of water. The chlorine inhaled in a hot shower is also very irritating to the lungs. A shower filter is a real boon to people with asthma and helps start the day with a lot less stress. Avoid commercial tile sprays. When product warning labels say "Use with proper ventilatation," you know this isn't for you. There is no way to ventilate a bathroom well enough to spray tiles with such an irritating substance. (See Box 2 for a safe solution.)

Mold. After the shower remember to open the window to help get rid of moisture. Bathrooms can be sprayed with Air Therapy for molds, but don't inhale. Spray and leave the room.

Shower Curtain. Cotton is better than plastic because of the aggressive odor emanating from plastic shower curtains. This can be helped somewhat by putting it in the sun for a day until odor dissipates.

GARAGES AND CELLARS

If your garage is attached to the house, make sure your bedroom is not over it. Seal off the garage from the house and make sure the garage is aired thoroughly periodically. Products stored in the cellar or in an attached garage will affect the air in your house. Dispose as hazardous waste all old cans of solvents, paints, varnishes, shellac, and automotive products. Those being currently used should be stored away from the house in a metal cabinet. Combustion fumes from the cellar can enter the house from the oil burner or gas heater. From the hardware store buy rubber strips called "sweeps" and seal up the space at the bottom of the bedroom door.

TAKE A DEEP BREATH

We really do have the power to feel a lot better. Don't be overwhelmed. The goal here is to take control of our own wellness little by little. Isn't it wonderful that we don't have to wait for someone to invent a new pill?

If you have been watching your diet for allergens, eating whole foods, and taking your vitamins or herbs and you still don't feel well, this environmental cleanup may be just what you need to get you where you want to be. You can start right now by getting rid of the items you have marked and proceed slowly to make additional changes. The more changes, the less stress on your breathing. Use the boxes as a guide for easy to make products. Safer commercial products are available at health food stores and through mail order houses. Inhale deeply and let the breath out slowly. Bet you are doing better already!

CHAPTER 11

THE SCHOOL, THE OFFICE, AND THE STUDIO

SAFER SCHOOLS

A hundred years ago Ellen Swallow Richards, a chemist and educator, wrote, "In the 20th century it will be a criminal offense for a college to lure students to its halls under the pretense of education, and then slowly poison them by bad air and poor food."[1] Little did she know what a hundred years would bring, not only to colleges, but to schools and students at all levels.

According to Irene Wilkenfeld, a Louisiana-based environmental school consultant, 9 percent of the student population is asthmatic and asthma is the cause of most absences of school-age children.[2] Asthma is increasing faster in children than among adults, up 55 percent in the last twelve years. Now more than 3.7 million children and adolescents in the United States have asthma.[3]

After Lead and Asbestos, the Deluge

The serious and much-publicized problems of lead paint and asbestos in schoolrooms are being cleaned up, sometimes only after parents organize and make a terrific racket. Regulatory agencies finally made the public aware of the dangers of these materials in older schools. But their job is far from finished. The load of toxic chemicals and poor ventilation in which children and teachers live every school day is just beginning to be addressed.

According to a study completed for Yale's Lung Research Center, a person's pollutant load is determined mainly by indoor exposures, and children in the United States spend 60 to 80 percent of their time indoors.[4] Children are more susceptible to toxins than adults because of their size and body weight. All of the teachers I have interviewed are acutely aware of the increased numbers of allergic and asthmatic students in their classrooms.

And teachers are becoming ill themselves; some are no longer able to work, and some are involved in long-term litigation. Pesticides and solvents seem to be the main culprits, although toxic carpets have also been a problem. If your child has asthma, a toxic school situation is going to exacerbate the problem. And research suggests that high exposure to allergens early in life may trigger a latent genetic susceptibility to asthma.[5] Let's take a look at what is causing most of the trouble.

A CLOSER LOOK

Pesticides. School lawns and playing fields are routinely sprayed, as are cafeterias and kitchens. Pesticides have also been detected in classrooms and elevators. A 1988 Public Citizen's report entitled *Contaminated Classrooms* tells how pesticide use in most schools studied was out of control, and dangerous chemicals were applied with complete disregard for health.[6]

Solvents. Highly toxic organic solvents are often used in schools. Solvents are particularly irritating to anyone with asthma. Solvent-containing art materials include turpentine, paint thinner, silk-screen inks and their solvents, lacquers and thinners, shellacs, permanent markers, spray fixatives for pastel and charcoal, cleaning solvents, aerosol spray cans, and solvent-based glues and adhesives. Art processes involving solvents include pen and ink, intaglio, lithography, oil and alkyd painting, relief printing, silk-screen printing, and woodworking. Even "water-based" silk-screen paints may contain up to 20 percent solvents, often in the form of glycol ethers.

Janitorial supplies. These irritants include floor cleaners and waxes, window cleaners, bathroom deodorizers, disinfectants, and furniture polish. Today however, janitors are supposed to receive formal training in the use of chemicals under the OSHA hazard communication rule. The late Dr. Theron Randolph once wrote that fresh air, sunshine, hot water, and unscented soap are still the best disinfecting agents.[7]

Carpeting. Schools with funds are beginning to actually carpet classrooms. In addition to the dozens of chemicals outgassing from new carpets, and the glues used in installation, carpets harbor dirt, dust, molds, and bacteria. Children also bring in dander from pets at home so that children who are petless are still at risk for asthma attacks from the dander that may linger in school. Carpets don't belong in the schoolroom.

Arts and Crafts. Children can also develop asthma from exposure to pottery kiln gases, solvents, and photoemulsions.[8]

OTHER PROBLEM AREAS

Faulty ventilation: Heating, ventilation, and air-conditioning (HVAC). The amount of fresh air entering the school should be adequate to dilute contaminants. Many schools have systems in which all areas are sharing the same ductwork. Wilkenfeld calls the HVAC the "heart and lungs" of the building. These ducts, when not well maintained, are circulating molds and bacteria which create serious problems. Molds themselves may emit volatile organic compounds which researchers have found are identical to those originating from solvent-based building materials and cleaning supplies.[9]

Vapors from fixatives, solvents, janitorial supplies, and photo chemicals may be recirculated to other rooms or other floors through the central ventilation system if it does not supply enough fresh air. Formaldehyde used to preserve specimens from biology rooms could circulate to other rooms if they all share the same system. Poorly ventilated and poorly maintained ductwork may be the biggest problem for asthmatics. And this will be a greater problem if there are windows that don't open.

Copy machines and other irritants. School offices and libraries often have copy machines that emit ozone and trichloroethylene. One librarian reports that the photocopier is often near the librarian's desk, where inks, glues, and adhesive sprays are also found. There may be mimeograph machines that use methyl alcohol or other solvents that make teachers and children ill.

Electromagnetic fields are another underinvestigated school problem, especially where a number of computers are in use and rooms are lighted by fluorescent light. Although Scandinavian countries take the threat of elevated electromagnetic fields seriously, in the United States no laws pertaining to EMFs will be passed for now. Meanwhile, schools should practice prudent avoidance. There should be at least several feet of space—front, back, and side—between each child using a computer. And plastic-cased computers and other electronics can heat and outgas, making children ill.

Then there are scented personal products, fabric softeners and detergent from children's clothes, dusty chalk, outgassing furniture, and exhaust fumes wafting in from the parking lot. And if children go home to an environment full of the same odors and vapors they are dealing with all day at school, parents and school personnel should not be surprised that more and more children are wheezing.

WHAT TO DO IF YOUR CHILD HAS ASTHMA

School consultant Irene Wilkenfeld says that some of the case histories in her environmental company's "Safe Schools" files are "so poignant that it's heartbreaking." To avoid school hazards for your asthmatic child, especially if you are moving to a new district, she recommends finding out if any indoor air quality testing has been done and asking to see the report. "Inquire specifically as to the carbon dioxide levels taken over the course of a typical day. It should be on the indoor air quality report and it's a good surrogate marker for other indoor air quality problems. If these levels are elevated, probably not enough outside air is being introduced, so other pollutants are also elevated. It tells you that the ventilation system is not as efficient as it should be. A fair number is 750 ppm of carbon dioxide. The test should not be performed in the early morning in an unoccupied space. But if the air tests below that in the middle of the afternoon in an occupied space, the air probably isn't too bad although there could still be other problems. Sometimes parents tell me that carbon dioxide in the classroom tested in the two and three thousand ppm range and sometimes even higher."

BE SURE TO ASK QUESTIONS!

- Are pesticides routinely sprayed?
- What kind of chemicals are being used? Does the school look for safe alternatives?
- Are there carpets in the classrooms?
- Are renovations going on? Have there been renovations in the last year? These could have an adverse effect on an asthmatic child. Are pollutants being drawn into the school from renovation work or other sources of pollution outside the building?
- Are ventilation ducts adequately maintained?
- Are there windows that open? This is a must. If renovations must be done and windows are not opened, you can't get rid of the volatile organic compounds (VOCs).
- Can you smell disinfectant? Are safe or less-toxic janitorial supplies being used? Take a walk through the building and look for any unusual, mildewy, or moldy odors. Do you notice harsh cleaning chemicals? Formaldehyde? These are red flags. Odor in a part of the building where

it shouldn't be—such as cooking odors in the gymnasium—tell you that the ventilation system is wanting.

Arts, Crafts and Theater Safety recommends these substitutions of art materials for children under twelve:

Dusts and Powders

Use talc-free, premixed clay (Amaco white clay) instead of clay in dry form. Sponge and wet-mop well after use.
Use water-based paints instead of ceramic glazes. Waterproof dried clay with acrylic-based mediums.
Use black-and-white newspaper and white paste instead of premixed papier-mâché.
Use liquid paints instead of powdered colors.
Use crayons and oil pastels instead of pastels and chalks.

Solvents

Use water-based silk-screen inks, block printing, or stencil inks with safe pigments instead of solvent-based inks.
Use water-based paints with spatter techniques instead of aerosol sprays.
Use glue sticks and school paste instead of rubber cement, epoxy, and airplane glue. White glue may contain vinyl acetate monomers.
Use water-based markers instead of permanent felt-tip markers, which may contain toulene or other toxins. Avoid scented markers. Children should not be tempted to taste or smell a marking pen.

Toxic Metals

Avoid pigments containing cadmium, chrome, arsenic, lead, and manganese.

What Parents Can Do

- Communication. "The first thing that I would recommend," says Irene Wilkenfeld, "is open communication. You need to approach the principal and find out if there is an environmental manager or an indoor air quality task force at the school. Talk to the school nurse. Make it very clear what the child's health status is and what the child's special health needs are. If they say your child is only one of 750 and we can't cater to him/her—that's absolutely not the place for your child." However you may not have another option. In that case you will want to try to work with the classroom teacher to implement, as well as possible, the suggestions made in this chapter, which will benefit everyone's health.

- Parents should work with the physical plant to make certain that the HVAC system is well maintained. If problems persist, have the school contact an industrial hygienist or ventilation engineer.
- Make sure pesticides are used only when necessary according to the recommendations of Integrated Pest Management.
- Renovations should be done during the summer break and completed in advance of the first day of school. The building should be aired thoroughly before children return.
- Good housekeeping should be encouraged. Ask teachers to avoid using harsh cleaning products or any spray product in the classroom. Cleanup can be accomplished with safe soap; windows can be cleaned with water and vinegar.
- Have the PTA sponsor a special chemical-awareness meeting so that parents and teachers can exchange information.
- Make sure that there is an environmental-awareness table included at all health fairs.
- Check the school's arts-and-crafts room. Is there an unvented kiln, toxic felt-tip markers, clay dust, moldy clay, solvents, shellacs, varnishes, wood dust, or projects involving grout and plaster of paris? Plaster should be mixed by teachers in ways that keep the dust down. Read labels carefully, remembering that all the ingredients in a product do not have to be revealed. The main ingredient in Play-Doh is wheat flour (not mentioned on the label), to which your child might be allergic. Kilns should have negative pressure systems or be isolated in small rooms.
- Make sure teachers have training in the hazards of arts-and-crafts materials and use safe substitutes.
- Discourage school projects that include painting children's faces. "Nontoxic" art materials may contain heavy metals and other substances that are not FDA-approved for the skin.
- Finger painting should be used only as a safety lesson. Provide the children with vinyl gloves and instruct them in how not to get paint on their hands. Art students could use this lesson as well!

- Melting of crayons or wax is hazardous and can emit toxic fumes. Asthmatic children will suffer from anything burning as well as from all dusty procedures.
- Windows should be opened and schoolrooms aired every day. Art and science rooms should have local exhaust systems to remove highly toxic substances like formaldehyde.
- Let teachers and school administrators know that what's best for your asthmatic child is better for all the children as well as for school personnel.

Children's Asthma on the Rise

"I'm really concerned about toxins in the schools," says one midwestern school health supervisor. "I don't believe that most of the asthma I see comes from the school environment and air here is considered pretty clean. But I do notice that so many more products are perfumed and scented. I haven't been able to connect them to the kid's asthma but I've seen so much more asthma being noted on health cards. So I have to wonder because practically everything we pick up has a perfume in it.

"I've been doing this job for twenty-five years and as recently as 1988 there were only about thirty-five to forty kids with asthma in all five of my districts and now I've got almost one hundred."

THE PROBLEM OFFICE

Because "tight-building syndrome" has become a household word, many more office workers recognize that this environment can be a problem. But what to do about a large building with windows that don't open, and a ventilation system that circulates the same air from floor to floor, is not so easily solved.

Asthma in the Office

As many as one in five cases of asthma are work-related, and chemicals or biological work exposures may be the culprits. Substances that people work with or are exposed to at work can trigger an attack or worsen a preexisting condition. Triggers are everywhere. Offices and schools, says the Labor Coalition's Occupational Safety and Health Project, like other workplaces, may harbor the conditions for causing or worsening cases of asthma.[10]

Let's take a look at some common problems with "tight" office buildings, outgassing furniture, and other office equipment, and see what can be done.

IDENTIFYING PROBLEM AREAS

Water Damage

Some of the most common environmental problems in office buildings are due to water-damaged walls, floors, and ceiling tiles says Jay Danilczyk, President of Green Circle Solutions, Incorporated, indoor air-quality consultants who inspect and make recommendations for problem areas in commercial and residential buildings in and around New York City. "When water damage is not addressed immediately, it can harbor the growth of bacterial elements. In the majority of inspections we have performed, biological factors play a part. A number of common indoor bacteria and molds are seen, such as different species of aspergillus, penicillium, cladosporium, and gram negative bacteria."[11]

These problems often can be found in buildings with a history of water damage, from a fire sprinkler becoming activated, water from floods, plumbing leakage, or other water sources. Biological contaminants can result in allergies, asthma, and other health effects. "Contracting a building-related illness through bio-aerosol exposure can be devastating," says Jay Danilczyk. "The primary routes of exposure are inhalation, ingestion, or absorption through the skin. Each person reacts differently to different environmental exposures, but with each successive exposure the health effects become more severe. Over time permanent illness can develop."

Air Vents

Mold spores and bacteria can travel through ductwork. Most buildings don't maintain and service heating, venting, and air-conditioning systems (HVAC) ductwork as thoroughly as they address their other building areas. "If it's out of sight," says Danilczyk, "it tends to be out of mind. Ducts may be insulated with fiberglass, which becomes a breeding ground for contamination. And a biological problem in the machine room of an office space or a building can result in exposure in any office space served. Bio-aerosols can travel through the air duct system, and from floor to floor, depending on the system and design. When the mold spores settle they look for an opportunity to grow again. And that can result in the spread of biological problems."

According to one air handling system consultant for commercial buildings, "more molds are found in ducts that are used for both heating and cooling. You may be shocked if you look behind the return air grilles in the HVAC system of your home or office. Rather than being trapped by the filters in your unit, many of those airborne particles get trapped in the heating and cooling coils. Add a little moisture from condensation, murky drain pans, humidifiers, etc. and you now have the makings of a mold and bacteria farm in the ductwork, for future distribution to your breathing zone!" Fiberglass-lined ductwork found in most commercial buildings has even more problems, as it is porous and supports mold growth. Deteriorating fiberglass particles may be blown into the air.[12]

Researchers at Georgia State University collected and grew fungus samples from problem buildings in the Southeast. They found that volatile organic compounds (VOCs) that were emitted by the cultured fungi "were identical to those originating from solvent-based building materials and cleaning supplies." They recommend avoiding fiberglass lining and replacing cheap disposable air conditioning filters with more expensive efficient filters.[13]

Outgassing

If you have a newer, "tight" building that was constructed with less air leakage for energy-efficiency reasons in the 1970s, a time when there was also increased use of chemicals in building materials, you may be more likely to have a chemical outgassing problem or a ventilation efficiency problem. Newer offices constructed without adequate ventilation can have chemical contaminants build up to a point where they are noticeable, and adverse health effects may follow. But both old and new buildings could have biological or chemical and ventilation problems.

Three years before she developed her first symptoms of asthma, Roberta was an accountant working in a modern office building. "Then they redecorated our floor. They brought in brand-new carpeting and eventually my brain started to go. I stopped being able to add four plus four with a calculator; I would go to work and make horrendous mistakes and not understand why. I thought it was psychological—that I just didn't like the job. It was a tight building—the windows didn't open. And three years later I got Epstein-Barr. Then all the other problems and finally asthma."

Furniture and Carpets

Green Circle Solutions finds that biological contaminants are more common than outgassing furniture and carpet situations. However, many workers have problems from newer synthetic carpets, carpet backing, glues used for installation, and chemical stainproofing treatments. Older carpets may harbor molds and dust mites. Respiratory problems and other sensitivities can develop from exposure to cleaning fluids and perfumed rug shampoos.

Office partitions and ceiling tiles can offgas volatile organic chemicals (VOCs). Formaldehyde is often a component of building materials as well as of office furniture, partitions, and particleboard. A chronic exposure can sensitize people to any number of products containing formaldehyde, making life difficult.

OTHER TROUBLE SPOTS IN THE OFFICE

Ceiling tiles may have biological contamination such as molds and chemicals absorbed from pesticides and outgassing carpets, cabinets, and paneling.

Carbonless typewriter ribbons give off petroleum fumes.

Carbonless carbon paper should be eliminated or stored and used in well-ventilated areas; exposure to and contact with carbonless copy paper has been shown to result in upper respiratory congestion and upper airway obstruction.[14]

Photocopy machines emit ozone, hydrocarbons, and a host of other chemicals, both from the toner powder and the outgassing of plastics and plastic construction materials and electrical components. Copiers should be exhausted outside, be well maintained, and be in well-ventilated areas.

Laser printers emit hydrocarbons, respirable particulates, and ozone.

Computers' ozone, offgassing VOCs, and electromagnetic fields cause problems.

Office products such as felt-tip markers, inks and stamp pads, correction fluid, rubber cement, and spray adhesives and other aerosols can contribute significantly to the total pollutant load in office pollution. No one with asthma should be in an area where aerosols are being used. All of these materials should be stored in metal cabinets.

Fluorescent lights lack some wavelengths of light, causing headache and fatigue.

Coworkers' personal products, especially aftershave and perfume, can cause problems. Cigarette smoke in the air or on the clothes and in the hair of still-smoking coworkers is also a hazard.

Michael McCann, a health and safety consultant, says that in classic occupational asthma a person might be exposed to a sensitizing agent for a period of weeks or years before developing asthma symptoms. "Once sensitization occurs, exposure to even trace amounts can result in an asthmatic attack, usually within minutes of exposure. The susceptibility to asthma attacks can persist for years and even decades."[15]

WHAT THE OFFICE WORKER CAN DO

- Obtain as much information as possible about sick buildings.
- Keep an asthma diary:

If you have never had asthma but have started wheezing at work, if your asthma is returning, or if you notice a steady worsening of asthma symptoms at work, it is important to begin keeping a daily written record of what you are feeling. Document the symptoms every day as clearly as possible. If you can, note how and where you spend the most time as well as any unusual exposures. Try to learn what triggers your problem, and seek medical advice. If your family doctor is puzzled, an occupational health clinic is a good place to start. Early identification of sensitivity can be critical in preventing a chronic asthma condition or a serious asthmatic attack.

- Learn to be an Asthma Sleuth.

Here are a few sample questions for your diary. Remember that each workplace is unique.

Are you reacting to a material you are working with?
Do you spend a lot of time at the copy machine? How long? How do you
    feel during and after?
Is there a new laser printer or other new electronics in the office?
Are there windows that open? Are they ever opened?
Does the air seem particularly stuffy?
Are there new carpets or furniture in your department?
Is renovation going on in your area or in any part of the building?
Has anything been recently painted on your floor or on any other floor?
Are pesticides ever used?
Are you bothered by janitorial products?

- Document the incidents: Health symptoms? Frequency?

A certain time of day? That is an important factor.

- Find out how many coworkers experience unusual symptoms. They may experience "flulike symptoms," headaches, thirst, dizziness, disorientation, rashes, or eye irritation while you find wheezing and throat tightness increasing.

- The EPA has indoor air quality information as well as questionnaires. Obtain EPA forms that can be distributed throughout the office to additionally document that the situation is real.

- If there are well-documented complaints, a professional consultant should be called in to perform an inspection.

- You will have a better chance of being heard by management if you document carefully fellow workers' health problems.

- If your complaints are not being heard or you feel you cannot speak up, call the National Institute of Occupational Safety and Health (NIOSH) (800) 356-4674 or your local Occupational Safety and Health Administration (OSHA) office; experts there may be able to come and make a diagnosis of the building.

- Source problems and air contaminants should not be taken lightly, as there is the potential for long-term illness. Asbestos and lead-based paint fall into the category of indoor air quality.

- See a doctor—you must seek medical assistance in order for the indoor air quality to be considered a problem by management and the courts.

OUTSIDE SOURCES

You may have an outside source for an indoor air quality problem. A neighboring office activity can bring contaminants through your fresh air supply. If they are painting the fifth floor in your building and you are on the sixteenth floor, you may still be exposed to the fumes through your ventilation system if air is recirculated.

"It's common to find when construction is going on in one area of a building, another floor even ten floors above tends to have problems," says Green Circle. "We've also addressed problems where second-floor tenants have trouble with ground-floor storefronts, restaurants, or cafés, due to cooking odors or cigarette smoke infiltration."

Outdoor sources of indoor air problems include loading docks, trucks, cars, buses, and industrial activities. If these activities exist near your building, the fresh air intake location needs to be addressed.

People with asthma or allergies go into these buildings and get much sicker but they don't feel that they can quit their jobs. "Often," says consultant Michael McCann, "the only solution to asthma caused by a specific sensitizer is complete removal from exposure, involving a change of career."[16] If it is absolutely not economically feasible to change jobs or careers, you will want to redouble your efforts to work with fellow employees and management to make your workplace healthier.

SIMPLE THINGS TO DO

- Open a window if you have a window to open.
- Take breaks away from office equipment and cigarette smoke.
- Get outside if possible during the day.
- Replace fluorescent light with Vita-Light, which contains a range of light waves more like natural light.
- An air cleaner with a HEPA filter in your office will help with some pollution problems.

WHAT MANAGEMENT CAN DO

- The amount of fresh air entering the workplace should at least meet the standards of the American Society of Heating, Refrigeration, and Air-Conditioning Engineers (ASHRAE), to help dilute any indoor air contaminants.
- Reduce use of carpeting and particleboard office furnishings.
- Eliminate pesticide use by adopting Integrated Pest Management practices.
- Use less-toxic or nontoxic cleaning products.
- Reduce pollutants drawn into the air from outside the building or during renovation work.

Source Control

The best recommendation for any indoor air quality problem is eliminating the source. It doesn't work to build over the affected area. Water-damaged building materials have to be replaced. Encapsulation isn't recommended for biological contaminants such as molds because they will continue to grow.

Businesses should avoid purchasing products that have the potential to offgas. Material Safety Data Sheets (MSDS) should be obtained from the product manufacturer. The MSDS should identify the health hazards such as respiratory problems associated with chemicals used in manufacturing processes. Manufacturers are required to make the MSDS available. Formaldehyde-laden furniture and even carpets can be coated with a sealer (see Resources), although results may be problematical.

Properly maintain building ventilation systems.

One NIOSH study found photocopiers significantly correlated with symptoms such as mucous membrane irritation, flulike respiratory symptoms, headache, and fatigue.[17] Spaces that are used for copy machines or small presses should be designed specifically to exhaust fumes to the outside. Gases could be exhausted locally through the ductwork return register, which would be separate from the system itself.

In copy rooms the ventilation system should be well balanced with the proper cubic feet per minute, a fresh air supply, and adequate dilution. It should be distributed to all areas of the room, especially if there are no working windows and the ventilation system is not operating properly.

Kerry had a long battle with yeasts and molds. Her exposures worsened in her current job and she feels they may have caused her asthma. Her illness also coincided with the arrival of a color laser printer in the office. "I'm in advertising and I work with markers and with spray mount. At the time I started to get sick, I was using huge amounts of this spray adhesive in an aerosol can. I had so many chemical exposures that for a long time I had trouble concentrating long enough to read a newspaper article.

"If I use spray mount today I wear a mask and we have a booth that has a fan that sucks the spray glue under, plus a huge industrial air purifier. When I got sick, we were renovating and I demanded it.

"As much as possible I use watercolor markers instead of smelly design colors. I have a fan on my desk that blows the odor away. Every once in a while I will get up and take a walk. But this is a building in which you can't open the windows and air circulation is horrible. The vents may be full of molds. The air must circulate from all the other floors because there are days when I will get an allergic reaction and I'll have no idea why."

GET SMART ABOUT ART

Consider the fact that half of all Americans, many of them retirees, use artist and hobby materials, and one may have another clue as to the proliferation of cases of asthma in recent years.

Visual artists, craftspeople, photographers, and sculptors may use extremely toxic materials, often without any concern for the consequences. In fact, those who use toxic materials to make beautiful objects are often extremely defensive about their right to endanger themselves and others around them. "We're artists; this is what we do" is a statement I've heard more than once. This attitude may have been nurtured in school, especially art school, where students are made to feel special and privileged to have been "given" these abilities. In art school, career management is a vastly more popular subject than the consequences of exposure to artist materials.

Children, as we just saw, are often inadvertently exposed at school. And retired people pursuing their hobbies may not understand that innocent-looking materials can cause big health problems. For those with asthma this is more acutely felt. Here we deal with problem solving for these occupational hazards.

Arts and Crafts Materials — Use with Care

Monona Rossol, in *The Artist's Complete Health and Safety Guide,* writes about a time when she taught in a university chemistry department and decided to enter the graduate art program. Going back and forth between the schools she discovered that the same acids and chemicals were used in both places. While the chemists protected themselves with goggles, gloves, and fume hoods, she noticed that the artists used these chemicals "lovingly and intimately." They felt that any comment as to the health effects of the materials interfered with their creativity. "Unfortunately," she writes, "illness and death also interfere with creativity."[18] If you are one of the many who use artist's materials you need to become interested in information that will help you to protect your health. Pretend that you work in a chemistry lab— because you do!

OIL PAINT

Oil paints are traditionally made with pigments mulled into oils such as linseed oil. However, some well-known brands may contain other additives such as emulsifiers, antioxidants, small amounts of solvents, and foam retardants. Poppy seed oil and linseed oil in paints can also cause allergic reactions.

PIGMENTS

The beautiful array of color pigments available to us today would make an Old Master envious. But some of these colors contain heavy metals which can be absorbed through breaks in the skin or ingested if you eat or smoke while you paint. Benzadine pigments and dyes can be absorbed through the skin. There is also a danger of inhalation by artists who scrape or sand the paint as they work, or those who use pastels, heat processes, or spray paint, or do airbrushing. There are many impurities in paints, such as dioxins and PCBs, which can be absorbed through the skin.

Artist's paints are exempt from consumer paint lead laws, and lead is still found in such pigments as chrome yellow, chrome green, and some permanent whites. Naples yellow contains lead antimony. Cadmium, chromium, cobalt, and manganese are found in many colors. Vermilion contains mercury, veridian contains chromium. Rossol (whose book contains a complete list) suggests only buying from reputable companies who list the color index name and number on the label or on fact sheets.[19] Ask your art supply store for charts and information.

Nan, a painter, keeps her studio's air cleaner on all the time, even when she isn't there. "I've changed everything. I noticed that strong odors are irritants, so I leave nothing out in the open overnight—no rags, brushes, or turpenoid. For a couple of years I didn't work at all. I became very fussy out of necessity.

"My studio floor is made of terrazzo stone sealed with fifteen coats of environmental sealer. Any used furniture is also sealed. I buy metal or old formica which is completely outgassed. I bought an aluminum easel. When pollen season starts, the air conditioner is on as well as the air cleaner. I wash the filters once a week. I keep everything behind closed metal doors. At the end of the day I empty the garbage. Now that I have less of a total body load I don't have so much stress in mold season. Now I don't need drugs because I control my environment."

The major problem with oil paint is in thinning and cleaning up with solvents. Turpentine is a hazard and can cause asthmatics to have allergic reactions. Some find their airways closing when they use solvents. In these cases, refined cold-pressed linseed oil can be used as a medium. All solvents are respiratory irritants to varying degrees.

The safest way to paint is with just the paint itself. Protect your hands. Paints and solvents are sensitizers and can cause allergic reactions to the skin. Brushes can be put in mineral oil and washed later with soap and water.

If you must use a solvent, odorless paint thinner is the safest although it is still a petroleum distillate. Although solvents are dangerous for everyone, people with asthma may have an acute reaction. Solvents with "low odor" do not have the natural health warning signals associated with strong odors, so caution should be used. Some artists with asthma who react to terpenes may tolerate Natural Citrus Thinner, which contains d-limonene and other unknown ingredients. This is more toxic than terpentine and if used, should be used judiciously. One solvent product lists only limonene as an ingredient but it actually contains 8 percent turpentine. So if you are allergic to terpenes, that is not a good solution. Any ingredient that makes up less than 10 percent of a product doesn't have to be listed on the label.

Rossol points out that allergies can develop to anything used regularly and that *all* solvents are toxic to some degree although you may not feel the effects at low concentrations. However, they can damage the skin, eyes, liver, and kidneys, and depress the central nervous system as well as damaging your respiratory system. This damage may happen slowly over a long period of time.

If you must use a solvent request the Material Safety Data Sheet (MSDS) from the company or supplier of your product. It will list the chemical ingredients and the Threshold Limit Value (TLV), which will give a general indication of the toxicity. TLVs are allowable concentrations for exposure over an eight-hour day. A low TLV, 100 ppm or below, is highly toxic. Higher numbers show less toxicity, so that a number above 500 ppm is considered only slightly toxic. Look for a TLV of 300.

"Just Acrylics"

Water-based materials are, in general, safer than those employing solvents. For this reason many artists have switched to acrylic paint. Although there is little odor, most acrylic paints contain additives which give off ammonia and formaldehyde. As the paint dries, these are released into the air and can cause respiratory problems and allergy. Because formaldehyde is a known carcinogen, some ventilation is a must.

"To control my asthma and still do my work I made many changes in my studio and in my life," says Barbara, a sculptor. "I vacuum and damp mop regularly. When I do anything with a lot of dusts, such as sanding and grinding, I first lay down wet newspaper. I wear a dust mask for sweeping or simple dusts and a double respirator for everything else. I leave my dusty shoes and clothes in the studio so I don't track dust into the rest of the house.

"I don't work with solvents anymore. I hire people to do any spray-painting or plastering away from the house. I work in clay and have the work cast in bronze. I now work with oil-based clay instead of water-based because there is less dust and molds. I also do a lot of ink drawings for sculpture. The drawings are scanned by a computer and cut out of metal with a laser. I wear a mask and paint them with a water-based enamel. Someone else sprays the primer. I do any grinding in the garage.

"I take every precaution. My studio is not cluttered like my old studio. Everything is put away behind closed doors. And I mop regularly. I think it's difficult for artists to deal with keeping everything safe and clean. But I've totally changed my life and my family's life."

WELDING

Ozone, which Rossol calls "your original free radical," is present in electric arc welding and in the welding of aluminum and stainless steel. Nitrogen dioxide, an irritant that penetrates deeply into the lungs and slowly attacks the tissues, is developed in both electric arc and torch welding. According to the American Lung Association, "welding fumes rarely if ever contain just one contaminant."[20] And if cigarette smoke is also present, all of these diverse chemicals attack different parts of the respiratory system at the same time. "Toxic chemicals may result from the metal being welded, the coating on the metal, the contents of the rod including the fluxes, the products of incomplete combustion, or ozone and nitrogen dioxide."[21] Gases and metals may also be involved. Metal fumes and the acids and salts used in other processes involved in sculpting metal have also been implicated as lung irritants and as causing asthma.

Photography

The developers for black-and-white photography are mostly alkaline. "But the biggest problem with them," says Monona Rossol, "is that they need preservatives that are sulfites. As soon as you put them in water the sulfite starts offgassing sulfur dioxide. People who say they are allergic to sulfites are really allergic to sulfur dioxide, which is what it becomes. I've never seen color or black-and-white photography that does not have a sulfite in the process somewhere. Sometimes there are solvents in the color chemicals as well; that's why they can be more toxic. The manufacturers are working to make them safer. The color-developing chemical molecules are really complex chemicals. They've never really been studied for chronic hazards. We don't know how they break down or what they become in the body.

"Asthma and dermatitis are common problems for photographers. You can explain the asthma on the basis of the sulfur dioxide alone. But add to that acetic acid, which is in the fixers to neutralize the alkaline and stop the reaction.

"The paper used for photographs also gives out sulfur dioxide and acetic acid gasses for quite a while. After a week or so, when it is completely dry, nothing more is going to come off of them. Some people appear to be sensitive to the paper itself."

Dusty Procedures

- Never use any material in powdered form.
- Buy paint and clay ready made and don't grind your own pigments.
- Clay or Play-Doh should be used on a washable surface.
- Dried clay on newspaper creates clay dust when the newspaper is rolled up to be discarded.
- Many low-fire clays and slip-casting clays contain talc, which is contaminated with asbestos.
- Wet clay should be used and an exhaust fan and toxic dust respirator should be employed.
- Avoid sprinkling gold and silver dust into glue.
- If you must use pastels, a dust mask should be worn and disposed of at the end of the day. Check with your doctor about using a mask.
- Work areas including the floor should be damp mopped at the end of each work session.

Ventilation

- Make sure there is an open window and an exhaust fan. Exhaust stale air out of the work space while fresh air is brought in from another source.
- If there is only one window, fresh air can be brought in to dilute the noxious air and the whole thing exhausted out.
- A portable air cleaner with an HEPA filter and several pounds of charcoal may help keep the air free of vapors.
- In winter if you are shut up in a studio with art, hobby, or photography equipment, without benefit of an open window, a heat exchanger should be considered. It will remove some of the stale air and bring in fresh filtered air with very little heat loss. You will still need to ventilate at the end of the day.

Gloves

- Don't get paint or solvents on your hands.
- Stop work and wash hands regularly or wear rubber gloves. If you have a problem with the rubber or latex, buy white cotton gloves at the pharmacy and wear them as a liner.
- Many pigments used in art materials contain hazardous materials such as cadmium, lead, and arsenic. Skin contact can cause dermititis and paint may be absorbed through cuts and abrasions.

Woodworking

In working with wood the same dust rules apply.
- Masks and damp mopping are a must.
- Dust collectors should be used for woodworking machines.
- Be aware that certain kinds of wood and preservatives in the wood can cause allergic and even toxic reactions. Plywood and particleboard in particular contain formaldehyde and can outgas for years. Constant inhalation of sawdust-sensitizing wood such as African mahogany, mansonia, rosewood, cocobolo, and satinwood can cause major respiratory problems and allergy. Beech, teak, and especially Western red cedar are known to cause severe asthma.[22]

Spraying

Don't use an airbrush, spray paint, fixative, or anything in a spray can if you or anyone in the house has asthma. Many of these materials are quite toxic and the smaller the mist the more chance there is of inhaling it into your lungs. If you must spray your drawings, cover your mouth and nose and do it out-of-doors. Don't bring the drawings inside until they are completely dry.

Audrey's problems with asthma began when she worked with formal-dehyde-preserved fetuses while studying embryology. Later she got a job developing photographs. "I was using black-and-white chemicals with no ventilation in the darkroom, so there was sulfur dioxide in large amounts. Once I became allergic to sulfur dioxide, I would get asthma anytime there was a severe temperature change or bad air quality.

"Then I developed problems with ceramic materials and again when I worked as a potter. As soon as I changed my lifestyle I became healthy as a horse. I'm not a potter anymore. And I don't do all the other things I used to do such as repairing furniture. I can get away with doing one thing, but if I went back to exposing myself to wood dust or ceramic materials or paint strippers I would get into trouble.

"Today if there is an inversion I may feel uncomfortable but I won't get asthma because nothing else is adding to my load. I may hear a little rawl, but it won't progress because there are no other allergens in my life. I can handle it."

ENJOY YOUR WORK/MAINTAIN YOUR HEALTH

- Be careful about paints, clays, glazes, and markers labeled nontoxic. Many materials for children and hobbyists contain ingredients extremely irritating to the lungs. If you can smell it, don't use it. Rubber cement contains hexene and should not be used.
- Some poster paints have small amounts of preservatives such as formal-dehyde or phenol which can prove irritating.
- Heating wax can create fumes that are respiratory irritants.
- Fumes from kilns should be properly exhausted.
- Use tiny amounts of the least toxic solvents or none at all.
- Keep liquids, shellacs, varnishes, and finishes in tightly closed jars when not in use.
- Jars, bottles, and tubes can be wrapped in silver foil to prevent outgas-sing or contents can be poured into large mason jars with sealed lids.

- Don't leave brushes sitting in solvents. Let them sit in baby oil. Wipe off and wash them immediately after work.
- Don't have skin contact with pigments or solvents.
- Don't smoke or eat while painting.
- Avoid dusty procedures.
- Wear a disposable dust mask if your doctor agrees and you can get one that fits. The model with straps top and bottom is the best. For solvents and chemicals consult 3M for the correct mask and consult your doctor about wearing it.
- Store supplies in metal cabinets.
- Don't sleep or eat where you work.
- Use an exhaust fan but have another window open. Bring in fresh air and ventilate thoroughly at the end of the day.
- Dispose of all cans, bottles, and tubes no longer in use as hazardous waste.

"INNOCENT UNTIL PROVEN GUILTY"

In 1988 the Labeling of Hazardous Art Materials Act was passed. This law made it illegal to sell any art material in the United States whose label does not (1) reference a chronic hazard labeling standard, ASTM D-4236, and (2) list any hazard warnings required by this standard. According to Monona Rossol of Arts, Crafts and Theater Safety, no art materials without this label would ever be used in a school. And only products whose labels are in conformance with ASTM D-4236 and which have *no warnings at all* should be used in grade six and under.

But don't consider this label a guarantee of safety. Many chemicals which have never been tested for cancer and other chronic hazards can be labeled "nontoxic" by default. In particular, most organic pigments and dyes used in art materials, even those closely related to known carcinogens, can be labeled "nontoxic." Rossol says that currently, "hundreds of art materials containing untested and potentially hazardous chemicals are considered innocent until proven guilty." So we must use precautions with all art materials.

A Plea for Caution

Schools, offices, homes, and studios have only recently been taken into account as workplaces with "occupational" hazards. Asthma warns us that changes have to be made. Now we have some tools with which to do this. Are we listening to the warning? Are we making those changes?

CHAPTER 12

TRAVEL WITH ASTHMA

THE HOW, WHEN, WHY, AND WHERE
OF GOING PLACES

My lust for travel began at the age of four at my mother's knee as she read me a magic book from the Sunday school library. I still remember that moment when I reached up and unerringly picked it off the shelf. An American boy goes to France on a big ship and meets a new little friend, Pierre, who shows him, and us, Paris. There were charming watercolor illustrations of the Eiffel Tower, of children sailing boats in the Luxembourg Gardens, of the Grand Guignol puppet show, and artists in berets at their easels in Montmartre. I couldn't yet read, but I loved the pictures and I knew this was for me.

After college I had the good fortune to live abroad for three years and got to see everything pictured in that book and more. Since then I have really been hooked. This is all by way of explaining why I travel so much now without knowing what I will run into regarding food, water, air pollution, and strange outgassing materials.

Planning Ahead

Many of us had rich and varied lives before our activities were curtailed by asthma. While the limitations can make it particularly difficult to travel, with proper planning and precautions, we should still be able to have a wonderful trip.

Sometimes just being in a new environment stimulates the immune response. When we travel we spend more time out-of-doors, get more daylight in our eyes, look at nature, walk and exercise, and devote ourselves to having a good time. And, of course, this works best if we pick a place with a comfortable temperature, great vistas, activities that are special to us, loving friends or relatives, or new friends with whom to enjoy our leisure. And it works best in an unpolluted destination, free from allergens. But before you start looking at travel guides there are several things to take into consideration.

1. Your Physical State

• Is your asthma well under control? When you travel, especially abroad, pollutants or allergens may surface in the most unexpected places. Trains, cars, buses, and planes are difficult at best, and it is worse being ill in a country where you don't speak the language. Make sure your asthma is under good control before you plan a trip.

• Are you in a weakened condition? If so, unless it's absolutely necessary, postpone your trip until you get stronger and can deal with the exigencies of travel.

• Are you just starting to recover? Consider staying home a little longer to consolidate your gains. If you are doing well where you are now, happily ensconced with your air cleaners in your controlled environment, you may want to wait awhile to change locale or travel to a foreign country.

Which leads to the next consideration:

2. The Physical Condition of the Place to Which You Are Traveling

• Is there ragweed? Ragweed season in the United States varies. If you are going to the East Coast and you have a ragweed allergy, avoid mid-August to late September or October, when ragweed can be a problem. In the Northeast and Central Plains, August through October is peak ragweed time. On the West Coast, seasons vary from June to October in the California lowlands to July through September in the extreme Pacific Northwest. Plan accordingly. The seashore and the mountains may actually be the best bets to be ragweed-free. More good news for ragweed sufferers: the San Francisco Bay area, Seattle, southern Idaho, Vancouver, and Alaska have no ragweed seasons.[1]

• Are there molds? Molds can be found anywhere there is dampness. So any indoor accommodation may be moldy. Seaside air is great for people with asthma, and walking the beach when the prevailing winds come off the ocean can't be beat. The downside is that houses and tourist accommodations are more likely to be moldy and mildewy. That goes for lakeside cabins also. So choose your accommodations carefully. Watch out for "mold showers" in the Midwest when winds blow in off the fields.

High up in the mountains may be the best mold-free place in the Americas.[2] But if you are allergic to grasses and trees and are going to the mountains or coast, check the allergy season.

• Are there pollens? On the East Coast, tree pollens cause problems from March to May, grass pollens from May to August. Other parts of the country vary a lot. Many years ago people went to Arizona to escape the grasses and pollens of other locales. Eventually they brought all the greenery they had enjoyed back home with them for newly planted lawns. Now Arizona is not the refuge it once was. The seashore and the desert are the best bets for the pollen-sensitive. If you can't avoid the pollens and grasses, avoid foods that cross-react with whatever is in season (see chapter 7). Wyoming has a short tree pollen season from the end of March to the end of April, and a short grass allergy season in June and July. Kingman, Arizona, wins the prize, with no grass or tree pollen season at all! Ragweed checks in from August to late October.[3]

A cruise to nowhere will keep you pollen-free, but find a place on deck where you are not downwind from either cigarette smoke or smokestack exhaust to enjoy breathing out at sea. Check out smoke-free cruises on a ship that hasn't been recently renovated. And ask for a cabin that hasn't just been painted.

Send for a pollen calender for planning ahead. (See Resources.)

All These Dos and Don'ts

All these lists of precautions are not made to discourage you. Since everyone's condition is different, the lists will give you ideas about what to look out for and what to adapt to your own situation. Being well informed gives you options and control. And it may make the difference between a discouraging travel experience and a wonderful trip.

Although most asthmatics are sensitive to ragweed, pollens, or molds, they may be the least of your traveling problems. As we have already seen, these common allergens aren't fun but are not a danger to the nonallergic population. Taking the following precautions, however, would be an improvement in anyone's travel plans.

Traveling by automobile can be stressful but in a car you may have the most control over your environment.

- What kind of car is best? A few manufacturers have models that have a "max air" feature on the air-conditioning system. This completely closes off all outside air so that no fumes can enter. Check for this feature before you rent a car. For air pollution, exhaust fumes, roadwork, and pollens you will want to recirculate indoor air.
- Car air conditioners often harbor mold. Have the air-conditioning unit cleaned once a year and change filters regularly. Run the air conditioner or the heater for a few minutes before you get into the car.
- For non-air-conditioned cars, cover air vents with an air-conditioning filter, which can be cut to size and taped in place.
- You can buy a portable air filter that plugs into your cigarette lighter.
- Make sure your car is serviced regularly and have the exhaust system checked for leaks. Check your radiator and make sure that the gas cap, radiator, and brake fluid cap are well sealed before you leave town.
- Damp clean and vacuum the inside of your car.
- If the seats are made of smelly vinyl, find seat covers, or cover with cotton toweling. T-shirts are cute for seat backs and often fit well.
- Let someone else pump the gas. Don't go along for the ride when your traveling companion or friend takes the car to fill the gas tank.

PRECAUTIONS FOR ALONG THE WAY

- Avoid major highways with a lot of traffic. Take side streets instead. (Good advice for walking also.)
- Make sure the air-circulation system is closed when stopping behind cars and trucks with smelly exhaust systems and at gas stations.
- Avoid thruways full of buses and trucks. Parkways are reserved for cars and there are usually a lot of trees to buffer fumes.
- Avoid service station bathrooms. The less time spent near the gas pumps the better. Utilize rest rooms at restaurants or diners.
- Watch out for roadside pesticide spraying. Keep your windows closed and your face covered!
- Try to avoid freshly tarred highways.

- When stopping for gas, try to avoid long lines and waits.
- Don't pump your own gas. Stay put and roll up the windows.
- Make sure that the tank is not completely filled and *never* let them top it off.

Mobile Homes and Trailers

Trailers and mobile homes are sometimes a problem. Many elderly people who retire to or vacation in mobile homes have suffered asthma and other symptoms from the buildup of toxic chemicals in this very small space. Look for a trailer made of safer materials with no particleboard cabinets or paneling. Ventilate thoroughly. Keep the windows open. An air conditioner, even with the air vent open, may not provide enough fresh air. See chapter 10 and adapt house hints.

Going by Train

Trains vary greatly from car to car. Sometimes there is a burning brake smell, molds, or unidentifiable odors. Be alert to anything that may bother you, and move to another car.

Buses

An air-conditioned bus can be great unless you are stuck next to someone with strong perfume or hairspray. Don't sit where windows are open to exhaust fumes. Try a scarf over your mouth and nose. Avoid non-air-conditioned buses.

Air Travel

The greatest boon to travel in recent years has been the gradual banning of cigarettes on planes and in waiting areas in airports. However, there are still unexpected surprises, such as that which my friend and I experienced when flight attendants on a no-smoking flight from Crete to Athens smoked in the galley directly across from our seats.

CABIN FEVER

Before the mid-eighties, airplanes were designed to recirculate 100 percent fresh air every three minutes. This system was controlled by the pilot, who could save fuel by cutting down on fresh air. However, a person with respiratory problems could request that the air-conditioning be fully operative throughout the flight. Those days are gone now. Newer models are built to circulate half fresh air and half recirculated air that is freshened only every seven minutes or longer. When there is less fresh air circulation, all passengers suffer from higher levels of carbon dioxide, the outgassing of materials used to construct cabins, pesticides, and cleaning agents.[4] The pilot, however, still has some control over air circulation, which is also influenced by the plane's speed.

FLYING RIGHT

Cigarette Smoke

- Many airlines such as USAir now have some smoke-free international flights. *Ask* because you may not be told. Hopefully by the time you read this all airlines will be smoke-free.
- If you book on a mixed smoking/nonsmoking flight, make sure you will have use of a rest room in the nonsmoking section. There is nothing worse than having to wait in the rear of the plane where the smokers are.
- When you reserve your seat, request the *center* of the nonsmoking section away from first class and the galley.
- Request that the air-conditioning be used at full capacity. If you are stuck on the runway with the ventilation turned off tell them you have asthma and politely request that the pilot open the air packs. If you start to feel clammy in flight that's a good sign that you should inquire about the air packs.
- It's always important to let a flight attendant know if you are having difficulty breathing, says Diana Fairechild, a flight attendant for over twenty years and author of *Jet Smart: Over 200 Tips for Beating Jet Lag*. In this invaluable book she suggests that if your breathing becomes shallow and labored, ask the flight attendant for oxygen. Use language such as "I feel like I'm having difficulty breathing. May I have some oxygen, please?"[5]

Dehydration

- Use an atomizer to hydrate your face.
- Spray a weak saline solution into each nostril. Then coat with non-petroleum jelly.

- Drink plenty of water. Request spring water and bring your own just in case.
- Don't drink alcohol (you don't anyway, right?), which will dehydrate you further.

Comfort

- Eat lightly.
- Wear loose clothing.
- Stroll the aisles.
- Massage your feet.
- Do yoga stretches in your seat. (You'll figure out a way.) The Taoist exercises can be done in the rest room—when there isn't a line, of course. Or do a few now and the rest later.

Fumes

- Cover your face at takeoff and landing. If you don't want to use a face mask, a folded cotton handkerchief or scarf will help.

Health Precautions

- Get permission well in advance of trip for use of oxygen and nebulizers. Some interfere with radio signals.
- Call ahead to find out if your flight will be sprayed with pesticides. Bring a letter from your doctor so that you will be able to disembark before the spraying. Asthma and pregnancy are exceptions that are usually responded to.
- Medication and vitamins should always be in your carry-on luggage. No exceptions!

The Hotel Room — Your Home Away from Home

Now that you have taken elaborate precautions to arrive at your destination fairly unscathed, you want to make sure that your accommodations don't do you in. The wrong room can ruin an otherwise pleasant stay. The worst scenario is a room in which the windows don't open and new carpet and furniture have been recently installed.

CHECKLIST: BEFORE YOU LEAVE HOME

_____ On reserving your room ask for a nonsmoking room, or better yet, one on a nonsmoking floor.

_____ Request a room with a window that opens, but not over the pool or parking lot.
_____ Inquire as to whether the hotel is now being renovated or has recently undergone renovations.
_____ Choose an older unrenovated room that hasn't recently been sprayed with pesticides.
_____ If you are sensitive to chemicals ask that no cleaning products be used on preparing the room for day of arrival. Request that the room be cleaned with water and baking soda, vinegar and water (for mirrors and glass), and chlorine-free cleanser.
_____ They can't comply? Take your business elsewhere.
_____ Call again the day before arrival to talk to the housekeeper so that your instructions will be remembered.

Food for Travel

- Rice cakes with nut or sesame seed butter (whatever you are not allergic to) pack pretty well in the flight bag or carry-on. Pack several in a small plastic bag for early mornings in airports or breakfast on the plane. Extras come in handy for later, when you don't know where you will be or what you will find in the way of food.
- Packages of almonds, organic raisins, and seeds are small, unbreakable, and easy to put into a pocket. They provide extra energy for the long haul. Choose items safe for you.
- An apple or two will hold up very well and may prove welcome for travel if your diet allows.
- Rice balls don't sound too exciting but they are a useful travel strategy I learned in macrobiotic cooking class. And they are amazingly satisfying when you land in a strange country, are stuck at the airport, and haven't yet adjusted to the native cuisine.

RICE BALL RECIPE

Cut a sheet of pretoasted nori into four pieces. With dampened hands, press your cooked brown rice into a small firm ball. With a finger, make a hole in the center and press a small piece of umeboshi plum inside. This is crucial for keeping the rice ball from spoiling. Seal the hole with rice. Cover carefully with the pieces of nori, making sure all the rice is completely covered and that the nori sticks. Your hands need to be kept damp for this procedure. You can also roll the balls in toasted sesame seeds, which I find incredibly delicious. For a trip to Spain I got up at five in the morning to make my rice balls and lived on them the first two days abroad!

- Spring water. Former flight attendant Diana Fairechild says to carry your own bottled water just in case and drink eight to sixteen ounces for every hour of flight time. Those trips to the rest room, she says, are good exercise and will help with dehydration.[6]
- Bring several small bottles of spring water for long trips so that you can dispose of them as you travel. Save one small empty, refill in your hotel room (not with tap water) for use during the day.
- Tea bags are easy. Bring Taheebo tea to counter yeasty bread if you have a yeast problem.
- Dried unsulfured fruit may work for you. Small, light cardboard shakers of dehydrated parsley and sea vegetable sprinkles can add to the nutritional content of restaurant food.

The Travel Kit

- Organize your vitamins for the whole trip. If it's a week or less, use a vitamin tray organizer from the health food store. There are large flat ones with a number of compartments. Put different vitamins for different meals in each compartment or use them to separate each kind. Remember to label them with penciled stickers on the side of each compartment.
- For long trips use plastic Baggies tied in three or four sections, one for each day of the trip. Put your dinner vitamins in the bottom, put on a twisty, then the lunch vitamins, put on a twisty, then the breakfast vitamins on top. Put a package in your pocket in the morning and you are ready for anything.
- Bring your own nonfragrant soap.
- Bring a charcoal-and-gauze mask for fumes at takeoffs and landings. A cotton scarf helps if you are mask-shy.
- Pack a small plastic bag with scent-free laundry soap and baking soda for a softener. In foreign lands you can use this for hotel laundry or the Laundromat, so the rest of the trip isn't ruined by perfumey-smelling clothes.
- Try a small plug-in pot to heat water or soup, or an electric coil made for that purpose. There's nothing more comforting than the ability to make your own cup of tea.
- Bring extra Ziploc bags and a small bottle of citrus-seed extract. In situations where you need to take more precautions with uncooked

foods, just fill the plastic bag with bottled water, squeeze in a few drops of citrus-seed extract, and soak your fruit or veggies. This will kill off parasites and other strange unwanted creatures. Wash it off carefully and still peel everything before eating.

- The citrus-seed extract can double as a yeast fighter. You can drink it by adding a couple of drops to a glass of water. *Never* use it undiluted (it tastes bad enough), and please check with your doctor first!
- Tabasco brand pepper sauce is reputed to kill certain bacteria on food, including *V. cholerae,* which is responsible for cholera, according to researchers on antimicrobial agents.[7] Other hot sauces, horseradish, and lemon were said to be less potent but also effective.

On Arrival

- If the room smells from mold or mildew or anything strange, ask to see another one. Even year-old carpets, furniture, and drapes can still be outgassing.
- Check the air conditioner filter for dust and mold. If it is simple to dismantle, you can wash out the filter yourself.
- Chlorine can be a problem, so make sure your room isn't near or above a pool or sauna whose chlorine fumes may waft down the corridor or up the stairs or in the window.
- Look for and remove deodorizers in closets and bathroom. Bring your own nonscented soap.
- A cotton pillowcase from home is always welcome. Some people bring their own cotton sheets if they are bothered by chlorine or scented laundry detergents. But don't let them end up in the hotel laundry!

BED-AND-BREAKFASTS AND APARTMENT HOTELS

Bed-and-breakfasts and apartment hotels may be the best bets for controlling your own travel environment. Call first to inquire about pets, air fresheners, or new construction. See if they will accommodate your request for no chlorine or fabric softener in the sheets, a nonallergenic room, etc. In B and B's you may be able to request a special breakfast; in apartment hotels you have your own kitchen.

THE MEDICINE KIT

I always wanted to go to Mexico but was worried about becoming ill. For my first trip I went to a small vegetarian spa where they grew their own vegetables and the water was purified.

Since then I have made several trips to Mexico although many of my "well" friends worry about parasites and such. Now before I take this kind of a trip I start preparing my gut several weeks before with acidophilus and garlic in the mornings and digestive enzymes after meals. (Check with your nutritionally oriented doctor and find the combination that is best for you.) Then I pack my "secret weapons" in the bag with the vitamins:

- **Curing Pills.** This is a Chinese formula which can help eliminate what herbalist Letha Hadady calls "travel critters." Not only are curing pills strengthening and balancing for digestion, they are also good for motion sickness, MSG reactions, jet lag, diarrhea, and other travel woes. The authors of *Between Heaven and Earth: A Guide to Chinese Medicine* recommend the use of these with each meal where water is questionable.[8] They come in vials, ten to a box, and are inexpensive. You take one vial with each meal.
- **Po Chai Pills** are good for diarrhea and help with stomach cramps, nausea, and similar travel woes.[9] There are those in my family who swear by Po Chai Pills. They come in bottles of one hundred tiny pills. Recommended are one to two bottles four times a day.
- **Intestinalis** is a combination of twenty-two herbs that offers protection against parasites. This is recommended by Ann Louise Gittleman, in *Natural Healing for Parasites.*[10]
- **Yin Chiao Pills.** Avoidance of colds is of utmost importance when traveling with asthma. I always take these along. Six tablets every three hours are recommended at the first sign of a cold.[11] They are only taken for the first couple of days. Be sure to get the green-and-white box that says "Yin Chiao Chieh Tu Pien." There are twelve bottles to a box.

  These Chinese tablets and pills are mild herbal formulas and can be chewed. Best taken thirty minutes before or after a meal with warm water.
- **Echinacea** liquid drops in a small bottle are good to have for the first sign of a cold. Take only for the duration.

All of the Chinese remedies can be purchased by mail. (See Resources.) The boxes are small and can be easily packed. When I'm abroad I put a tiny bottle of Curing Pills in my pocket on my way to dinner.

For those traveling in India, Letha Hadady suggests Maha Sudarshan Churna, a bitter powder with which you fill empty capsules to protect yourself from worms, parasites, and liver inflammation. However, if you contract amoebas, Hadady says they must be treated with antibiotics. She carries Dr. Christopher's PK Combination for travel in India and China; it contains herbs to help rid the body of worms and to attack amoebas. She also takes digestive enzymes with hydrochloric acid.[12]

Everyone may not be able to take these combinations of herbs because everyone's allergy problems are different. But they may be worth a try. Check with your practitioner and see if you can do a small trial at home first to make sure they agree with you.

EAT CAREFULLY

- Don't eat an airplane dinner if you are flying at night. Eat lightly and wait till your arrival to have a real meal.
- Don't overeat the first day of a trip, especially where the altitude is high.
- Always drink bottled water. Continue to drink a lot of water the first few days. Hotels often provide safe water which is drinkable. That is *not* water out of the tap.
- In countries where the water is questionable don't eat salads or unpeeled fruit. And don't eat *anything* sold by a vendor on the street.
- Don't eat dairy or creamy desserts. Eggs completely cooked are fine.
- Stay away from sugary desserts just like you would at home. They create phlegm and will interfere with digestion.
- Stay away from yeasty breads. Mexico has tortillas which are a wonderful alternative (even at home). Other countries have their own unyeasted breads. Try matzos and chapatis.

IN PURSUIT OF CLEAN AIR

For news about the weather or the exchange rate abroad we can consult our local newspaper, but there are few sources to consult for a pollution report. Exhaust fumes are a major source of pollution at home and abroad, but outside the United States a cheaper grade of petrol is used and emission control from cars, buses, and trucks is nonexistent. And smoking is even more widespread than in the United States. You may find bank tellers, museum guards, police, and hotel operators all smoking on duty. People also smoke in elevators and other enclosed spaces. In Spain everyone seems to smoke on the street, in coffee bars, and in restaurants. There is no such thing as a nonsmoking section in a restaurant.

The Magic Word

If you are using medication don't forget to bring along a brand-new inhaler and a prescription for any necessary medications from your doctor. Abroad know how to ask for your medication in the trade name of that country just in case. If you are not making yourself clear, put the box or canister on the counter, point to your chest, and say, "Asthma."

In fact "asthma" can sometimes be the magic word. On a trip to Paris I was going through the turnstile at the Louvre when a guard spotted my bottle of Evian water and pointed to the No Food or Drink Allowed sign written in English. "Asthma," I said, hand to my chest. "Pardon!" said the guard, extremely apologetic as he waved me through. "Asthma," I said in a very crowded restaurant when the party at the next table lit their cigarettes. The manager quickly and cheerfully moved our party to another table. "Asthma," I said on another occasion, when a woman eating nearby held her cigarette slightly behind her (as smokers do) so that the smoke went into my face instead of her own. "Oh pardon," said she, "excusez-moi!" and hurriedly put out her cigarette as she continued to apologize. A note: This probably won't work in the U.S.

City Strategies

You can avoid lodgings downtown in big cities and stay in a suburb or in the hills outside of town. Watch out for cities that are ringed by mountains, even those with mountains on three sides that look out to sea.

One traveler reported, "Arizona has this incredibly clear, bright atmosphere but when you drive into that bowl down where Phoenix is, much like Mexico City there's this awful haze and your eyes water, your chest tightens, and your throat gets dry." Here are some clues for better breathing in the big cities:

- Stay outside of town, preferably up high.
- Sightsee early in the morning when the air is still fresh and avoid sightseeing during rush hour.
- Take advantage of siesta hours to walk around town. Even if most everything is closed at that time it's a lot more peaceful. And you can strategize for when things open.
- Find air-conditioned restaurants in which to rest and watch your diet. Sugar and alcohol and foods to which you are allergic make everything worse.
- Examine maps and guidebooks carefully to make sure your hotel isn't

on a main shopping street or thoroughfare and is in the uphill part of town.

- Ask for a room off the street on a courtyard.
- Consult the telephone book for health food restaurants with smoke-free meals.

Hiking the Gorge

I had been to Greece once in the days when the skies were blue and clear, and I always longed to return. So when I read of a *downhill* eleven-mile hike in the Samaria Gorge ending on the Libyan Sea, I went for it. Not being a hiker, I practiced walking New York instead of riding the subway. Four months of Tai Chi class helped with balance. Far from exhaust fumes and man-made products down in the gorge, with the varying terrain of rock, trees, rushing water, and flowering bushes, it was extremely clean, clear, and invigorating. Although stones and rocks on the descent made going tough, the clean pure air and fresh water made up for it. Did I ever think I could walk that far? No I did not. But I had a feeling that walking the gorge would be different than trekking the trafficky streets of Manhattan and I was right!

Spas, Retreats, and Yoga Camps

There are a number of facilities designed for vacations that will implement good health. These camps, spas, and retreats have wonderful features such as fresh air, exercise, meditation, stress-free living, vegetarian food, and like-minded people bent on improving their health and well-being. Lots of interesting information is exchanged.

However, there can be problems for someone with asthma, even in the most idyllic of settings. Before you go, call ahead and get as much information as possible.

CHECKLIST

_____   Is it damp and mildewy?
_____   How cold does it get at night at that time of year?
_____   Are there new carpets, construction, or new furnishings?
_____   Is there a fireplace in the cabin?
_____   Do they build fires or incinerate garbage nearby?
_____   Is there a heavily chlorinated swimming pool?

_____ Is there a wood-fired sauna?
_____ Are there cats, molds, ragweed, or other allergens? Ask about your own worst triggers.
_____ What kind of food is available?
_____ Is access to the kitchen available at certain times? Can food needs be accommodated?
_____ Do they spray with pesticides?

The Conservative Side

Everyone's condition is different and everyone has a different attitude about traveling. So all these dos and don'ts are precautions on the most conservative side. One thirty-five-year-old woman with asthma took a trip around the world backpacking. "My greatest fear was that I would have an attack in some remote faraway place but it didn't happen. And I was very careful to avoid colds."

Fifty-five-year-old Annette, who has had asthma off and on since she was twenty, found that traveling, hiking, and climbing are "the best medicine" for her asthma. She always takes along her inhaler, which she doesn't like to use. "If I find that I don't have it with me I get in a panic. I may be in denial about my asthma but I like to feel that I can take care of myself." She has noticed that just being away from the stress of city life makes her feel much better.

But when Annette travels she is smart enough to pick places where the air is very pure. She has been to the Southwest and all over New Mexico. "It's dry and really good for people with asthma. I've been to all the pueblos and archaeological sites. Arches in Utah is beautiful but my favorite place is south of there, at Canyonlands, a large national park. It offers a lot of opportunities for people who like to climb. I went with a friend for three weeks, camped out, and every day explored a different direction. Hiking and climbing are great, not just for the heart, but for the lungs. When I came back I felt the benefit for six months. My lungs were perfectly clear and I felt a lot of energy. Living outside was wonderful for me." She also goes hiking, climbing, and rock scrambling on weekends at home.

"I'm planning a trip to Nevada in September. I can't say I'm asthma-free but I haven't had an attack in ten years. My advice to people is go where you want to go and do what makes you happy."

I hope this travel section has provided inspiration. Just remember that not everyone is ready or able to go around the world or climb a mountain. You and your doctor are the best judge of what you can and can't do. But it may be better to visit a new and interesting environment than to stay home and mope, particularly if you go where the air is cleaner.

Travel for an asthmatic can be difficult. You have to love it to the point where you can put up with whatever may come along. But as one traveler remarked, one of the pleasures is simply to be in a place where breathing is easier. If you love it, then do it, don't let the asthma stop you. But you really have to love it because there is no *must go* here.

If you have started a new regimen as outlined in the rest of the book, you now have important tools for getting strong, taking care of yourself, and going places. So:

- Choose your destination wisely and plan carefully.
- Leave time to make trains, planes, and buses without last-minute rushing and stress.
- Travel light or use baggage on wheels so you don't have to carry heavy suitcases.
- Be prudent about food.
- Camping outside and/or spending a lot of the time out-of-doors is a good way to avoid stressful hotel rooms.
- Schedule rest times into your travel plans.

The practical advice contained in this chapter is not designed to make you crazily cautious but to give you tools with which to control the situation so that you can relax and enjoy yourself. The pleasure of being in a new place can create a great state of mind which will affect your health for the better.

Be prudent . . . spread your wings . . . have a wonderful time. And don't forget to send me a postcard!

CHAPTER 13

THE ESSENCE

A DAY IN THE LIFE

W e are still "asthmatics" in the sense that our airways may continue to be capable of responding to "triggers." But now that we know how to pay attention to every aspect of our lives, we should no longer have to suffer asthma "attacks." And if for unforeseen reasons we do have an attack, we now have tools for dealing with it successfully.

As we noted in Chapter 1, the Chinese say, "A long journey begins with the first step." The question is, Will we take that step? Remember, this is your life. How do you want to live it? How do you see yourself this time next year? How will you get there?

In the Present, Paying Attention

The master of self-defense teaches that if you're in the present, paying attention, and have skills with which to respond, then a threat doesn't immediately cause panic. It's a sign to stay awake and respond. But if one is faced with a threat and is *not* in the present, taken by surprise, and has no skills with which to respond—the response is fear. And fear can immobilize you and make it more difficult to respond appropriately.

Being awake, paying attention, and developing skills is what we are aiming for. Paying attention and addressing what needs attention is different than being ready to fight with a constant automatic flight-or-fight response.

So let's create a plan for a future in which asthma can't exist. This includes a qualified practitioner who addresses your total health. However, going from doctor to doctor looking for a "cure" isn't the answer either. Our participation in this process is crucial: proper rest, proper breathing, proper exercise, proper nourishment, and a proper toxin-free environment. And remembering to exhale completely!

Here is a plan for incorporating what we have learned in this book into our day. You already have an innate awareness of which of these to choose to make the most significant difference.

- *Getting enough sleep* and rising at a regular time.
- *Stretching in the morning,* leaving time when you awake.
- *Breathing* into the abdomen.
- *Meditating,* even for a few minutes, to have strength and peace for the rest of the day.
- *Eating breakfast*—whole grains, oatmeal, soup with vegetables, a steamed green, a boiled egg, something that "sticks to the ribs."
- *Taking vitamins and/or herbs* or comparable nutrients.
- *Wearing natural fabrics.* Choosing personal products with care. Nothing that makes you feel suddenly tired, itchy, wheezy.
- *Bringing your lunch and snacks to work.* Avoiding allergens. Every bite bringing nourishment and balance. Being as good to yourself as you are to your car.
- *Keeping a food/symptom diary.* Reviewing it from time to time.
- *Being aware. Becoming an asthma sleuth*—chemical-free at home and at work. Being an advocate for better ventilation and clean air.
- *Getting outside during the day* for a change of air, and light in the eyes. The shade will do. Getting some sun for vitamin D. Protect eyes from glare.
- *Exercising* during the day.
  Park several blocks from where you are going. Get off the bus or subway a stop or two early, and walk the rest of the way.
  Use the stairs instead of the elevator for a few floors.
  Close the office door or use the rest room to do the Taoist exercises.
  Join a yoga or Tai Chi class.
  Swim.
  Dance. Any kind, anytime, anywhere.

- *Feeling chest tightness?*
  Use your pressure points.
  Stretch and lift the rib cage.
  Sip spring water, room temperature, regularly.
  Watch what you eat—no sugar, white flour, caffeine.
  Try a medicinal tea.
  Put eucalyptus drops (essential oils) in a pot with purified water and inhale the steam. (Don't get too close.) Heat water with ginger or eucalyptus, soak and wring out a washcloth, and use as a compress on your chest.
  Do the sun salutations. Do your three-part breathing. Become expert at these before you have an emergency.
  Take up a wind instrument.
- *Feeling panic?*
  Do your hara or belly breathing.
  Take your B vitamins, especially pantothine.
  Get someone to massage your feet or work on the pressure points on your back.
  Work with your nutritional doctor on cutting back medication.
- *Buying organic food.*
- *Eating a nourishing dinner* based on whole grains, legumes, and vegetables.
  If you are not a strict vegetarian include fish or organic meat or chicken occasionally.
  Develop a "special relationship" to ground-growing vegetables.
  Plan your menus ahead of time. As you feel better you will have more enthusiasm for this.
- *Taking some time for quiet enjoyment.*
  Talk to a friend.
  Read a book for pleasure.
  Listen to music.
  Cultivate friends and activities that make you smile and laugh.
- *Cultivating love in your life.* It can be for a friend, relative, or child.
- *Developing a spiritual life.* Seek the company of like-minded friends. Pray, chant, sing God's praises.
- *Develop gratefulness.* Contemplate what you have to be thankful for. Do a kindness for someone worse off.
- *Before retiring:*
  Skin brushing—with a natural brush for lymphatic system.
  Soak feet in hot water and baking soda.

Massage feet before bedtime.
- *Retiring in a dark room.*
Long, deep breathing and meditation.
White light meditation.
Get a good night's sleep.

Become an Advocate for Clean Air

It's been about ten years since my terrible asthma years began, and in that time a car "emissions" law was passed in New York making the air noticeably cleaner. There is no smoking now in most restaurants, schools, and public spaces. Health food stores have proliferated. There is a heightened awareness about toxins where I work and live. Has it been easy? No. But you've got to develop awareness for your own sake and for others who may not get interested until they become ill themselves. Once you clean up your own work and living spaces you can do your bit to make sure that strong environmental laws are passed and enforced.

A wise person once said, "A mountain is an obstacle but it's also a challenge."

Preserving the Essence

We have seen how the Essence that we receive from food and air combines with our Original Essence to give us reserve energy. In *The Stress of Life* Hans Selye writes that all of the stressors, from emotions to viruses to chemicals, cause the adrenals to release adrenaline. When this happens constantly we exhaust our reserves. We may be able to get by from day to day, but we have nothing extra for a stress emergency. We are living beyond our means.

If we live beyond our physical means, according to Chinese medicine, not getting enough Essence from our food and the air that we breathe, we have to dip into our Original Essence. And if we spend that, we exhaust our reserves, and our lives end before they have to. We must only spend what we make.

"Maladaptation"

"In Chinese medicine, health is the ability of an organism to respond appropriately to a wide variety of challenges in a way that insures maintaining equilibrium and integrity," write the authors of *Between Heaven and Earth; A Guide to Chinese Medicine.*[1] Throughout history we have been called on to adapt and respond to every new stress, but we finally seem to have become "maladaptive." There is simply too much to adapt to. No other generation has had the challenge of having to adapt to the thousands of new chemicals that are produced every year. When I ask doctors why the rise in asthma, the consensus is that chemicals and misuse of antibiotics are the major stressors overcoming our ability to adapt.

Chemical exposure is on the rise, in the food, air, and water. In a recent incident in a poor inner-city neighborhood, in a school near a toxic sludge dump, half of the children had asthma attacks and nosebleeds. Are inhalers going to fix this condition? Are more asthma drugs really helping us to adapt? Allergist Doris Rapp, M.D., writes, "The impact of the global total disregard for our environment affects us all. The problem of world wide chemical pollution can no longer be ignored by the public, physicians, educators or legislators."[2]

What Is Puzzling?

- Heavy metal toxicity depresses the immune response.
- More products than ever outgas chemical vapors.
- The symptoms of asthma are treated with more chemicals.
- Food no longer supplies us with needed nutrients. Pesticide-laden food, fast food, and junk food further injure immunity.
- Antibiotics, overused, cause destruction of friendly flora and lead to candida and parasites. Inappropriate antibiotic use also causes infectious diseases such as antibiotic-resistant malaria, cholera, and tuberculosis to make comebacks.[3]

If we further pollute the planet, aren't we using up the Prenatal Essence of the universe? If we don't start conserving what we have, will the planet have any resources on which to draw? We are running out of essence and running out of time.

The worldwide galloping rise of asthma may be the symptom, the wake-up call that says "Pay attention, now!" and change what you can.

"LIFE IS LIVING THROUGH ME"

Sometimes people complain about how much there is to do to get well. That one would feel "paranoid" living like this all the time. But many of us feel that making changes is a small price to pay for health and normalcy. Personally, I am grateful to my asthma for showing me a healthier way to live. As I become stronger and vigilance isn't as necessary, I understand that maintaining good habits for life is the long-term goal. I am thrilled that I now have tools with which to work on every aspect of my health. Rather than having "too much to do," I feel empowered knowing this asthma will not creep up on me again at some later date. And by making me change my life, asthma may have saved me from other, more serious illness.

I recently had an interesting discussion about vigilance and "having too much to do" with acupuncturist, teacher, and author Dianne Connelly.

"I don't think we are trained in this culture to say that this may have something to do with life as it is living through me," said Dianne. "The Chinese would say that this notion that we are living life is too small. It's more like life is living us. This is how life lives, it lives through us. Life is not a finished happening; like Walt Whitman said, we get to contribute a verse."

I shared with her my experiences with people who resist the idea of making changes, even small changes that could affect their lives for the better.

"That notion that we get to contribute something to this dance," Dianne replied, "is, for some people in this culture, a brand-new idea. An idea that we get to personally offer to the rest of us. The Chinese say that life is living each of us for the sake of all the rest of us. You can then say that, if I have asthma, it's not my asthma. It's that call from life that says 'Pay attention here to *that we breathe*,' and then become the teacher and the offering for all the rest of us not to take it for granted."

"Asthma Is My Friend"

Dianne has a patient who says, "Asthma is my friend." He had struggled with his breathing for a number of years, and had been taking cortisone and other steroids. In the course of treatment, he began to observe his asthma in a new way. Whenever he would get asthma, he would stop and say, "Hold on, here's my teacher. What am I meant to be learning or paying attention to here?" He never thought asthma would be a friend. He was too busy fighting to get rid of it rather than seeing what it was saying—what meaning he could make of it. Now he lives with ease and peacefulness and when he has breathing problems, he becomes an inquirer. "What's happening here? This is my friend, my teacher."

"The Chinese associate the lungs with the element of precious metals," explains Dianne. "It's the element that deals with the great jewels of life and remembering that life is a jewel, that it is multifaceted. The breath of life is really a call to the great jewel that we are, the great value and worth of each of us. Attention must be paid; the bow to the value, worth, and wonder of life. In the presence of a gorgeous jewel, we are *breath-taking.* That moment of awe is very much associated with the lungs.

"There's a Chinese saying: 'My barn having burned to the ground, I can now see the moon.' If a person is suffering from asthma, they can look to the other side and say, 'Here's the suffering, what's the gift? What must I bear and what can I let go of that I don't have to bear?'

"Breath is crucial to every being. That there are more instances of asthma now may be a giant wake-up call for the culture. Asthma may be a reminder that we need to breathe together."

In my suffering I found the gift. By writing this book I've attempted to take the worst years of my life and turn them into a positive offering for the rest of us. I hope we can all find meaning in our illness, use asthma as a friend and teacher, and find the strength and ability to listen. This is the wake-up call for the breath of life itself.

APPENDICES

CAT-WASHING INSTRUCTIONS

(From the Division of Allergy and Clinical Immunology, Department of Medicine, Washington University School of Medicine. Courtesy of Dr. James Wedner)

B oth kittens and adult cats can be bathed. It is easier to introduce bathing to a kitten because adult cats do not like to be wet. But they can be introduced to bathing if it's gentle.

Trial cats were bathed in distilled water from the supermarket, which was effective. Tap water or soapy water was not used but might also work.

The water should be warm but not too hot. It is easier to introduce the cat to bathing if the water is nice and warm.

Cats are washed from ten to fifteen minutes, rubbing the entire cat, including a gentle wash of the face.

When finished, get as much water out as possible, then towel dry with soft cloth. You can then blow-dry the fur using a low setting—not too hot. Don't touch the wet cat with the dryer.

If bathing is too difficult (trial cats were bathed under "light anesthesia") or you are too sensitive to do this yourself, a pet groomer could do it for you.

Understand that cat washing is not a substitute for medical care for your cat allergies. A visit to an allergist is recommended to determine whether you are actually allergic to cats.

GUIDELINES FOR DENTAL CARE

INFORMATION FOR HYPERSENSITIVE PATIENTS

(Dr. Alfred V. Zamm's guidelines for dental care for hypersensitive people, including those with asthma.)

I. *Hypersensitive patients do not tolerate certain organic molecules commonly found in dental offices*

    A. Local anesthetic

       1. If a local anesthetic is required, 3% carbocaine without epinephrine in a single-dose disposable "carpule" with no preservative should be used.

       2. Epinephrine: Epinephrine comes with a bisulfate preservative, which is often very disruptive to hypersensitive patients. In addition, the epinephrine itself is often degraded more slowly by an inefficient cytochrome p-450 system (detoxification enzyme system); hence, small doses give large effects to these patients.

    B. Other organic molecules

       1. Avoid eugenol or substances containing eugenol. Even in small quantities, eugenol can be devastating to many patients.

       2. Avoid the use of "varnish" to coat the inside of the tooth prior to treatment.

       3. Avoid protective plastic tooth coatings, as they are often not tolerated.

       4. Plastic tooth-filling materials should be chosen carefully (See sections III and IV).

5. Root Canals: Root canal "caulking" paste is often not tolerated by chemically sensitive patients. This paste contains cytotoxic substances such as eugenol and halogenated hydrocarbons such as chlorothymol and iodothymol, as well as resins. These substances frequently produce insidious chronic reactions.

II. *Substances which have almost always been well tolerated*

    A. "ZOP" (zinc oxyphosphoric acid) cement (be careful not to have ZOE inadvertently substituted, as ZOE contains eugenol).

    B. Gold (high gold alloy such as Sterngold brand, Bio-C, and Bio-H). These gold alloys do not contain palladium.

    C. Gold foil for small fillings.

III. *Some choices for replacement of mercury-containing amalgam dental fillings*

    A. A modality which utilizes an inorganic cement: Gold (use ZOP cement without eugenol). Flecks brand (Mizzy Co.) is recommended. The "snow white" (no color added) ZOP should be used.

    B. A modality which utilizes an organic (plastic) material is "composite resin." However, organic compounds are not tolerable for some patients. They must use inorganic compounds. Some individuals are intolerant to the plastic. To find out if you are intolerant to fillings containing plastic, replace one small filling and wait two weeks. Watch for any reactions over this two-week period. If you have not had any adverse reactions during this two-week period, replace a second small filling and wait another two weeks and watch for any possible reactions. This is done as a check to make absolutely sure that you can tolerate the plastic.

IV. *Toxic reactions to mercury versus allergic reactions to plastic*

It is common to have a toxic reaction to mercury vapors resulting from the removal of the mercury-containing fillings. This toxic reaction takes place during the first week, and over the second week it gradually lessens. Do not confuse this with an allergic reaction to the plastic, which starts during the first few days and will not lessen, but will worsen over the next one to two weeks. If you determine that you are reacting to the plastic, have the dentist remove this test plastic filling immediately. In this case, do not proceed to the second trial. Your only choice will be gold and ZOP cement without eugenol.

V. *Care of the xenobiotically sensitive patient before and after the removal of dental mercury*

    A. Vitamin C is somewhat protective against foreign (xenobiotic) molecules.

1. Don't take vitamin C between the time you awaken in the morning and your dental appointment, as it will lessen the effect of anesthesia.
2. Do take vitamin C right after the dental work, while you are in the dental office (don't forget to bring it with you). It will help you deal with the xenobiotic substances that are unavoidably encountered during a dental visit, even though no dental work may have been done. Every dental office is unavoidably polluted.

B. Take chemically pure liquid selenium solution as previously prescribed; however, take it in a double dose (if tolerated) with food. This is to be done three days before and three days after each dental visit. The selenium will help protect you against unavoidable exposure to mercury during the removal process. Selenium will also help protect you against the unavoidable exposure to xenobiotic substances in the dental office.

To find a mercury-free dentist, write to this foundation and ask for the names of mercury-free dentists in your area:

The Foundation for Toxic-Free Dentistry
P.O. Box 60810
Orlando, FL 32860-8010
Include a self-addressed stamped envelope

ABOUT THE DRUGS

The mainstay of asthma "management" programs in orthodox medicine is the use of pharmaceuticals. If you are being treated by an orthodox physician, your asthma is undoubtedly being treated with one or more of these drugs. Hopefully, while using this book, you and your doctor were able to reduce your dependence on medication. Still, it is important to know some facts about the pharmaceuticals you may still use.

The Asthma Paraphernalia

THE METERED-DOSE INHALER (MDI)

Your doctor probably prescribed a bronchodilator, an anti-inflammatory, or an anticholinergic drug, all of which are inhaled into the lungs by means of a metered-dose inhaler (MDI). The most common form of drug therapy for asthma is the bronchodilating inhaler.

You may be interested to know that the idea for the metered-dose inhaler was conceived by an eight-year-old girl who, tired of struggling with her bulky hand bulb contraption, asked her father, who worked for a lab, to "put it in a spray thing like mom has for her hair."[1]

How to Use Your Metered-Dose Inhaler

The inhaler should not touch your lips. Despite the illustration that comes with your medication, it is better not to put the inhaler directly into your mouth. If you are holding your inhaler between your lips to puff you are probably getting a lot of medication at the back of your mouth and throat and not enough into your lungs. This may be irritating to the throat. Holding the mouthpiece a few inches from your mouth enables a fine spray to get where it's supposed to go, deep into the airways.

Shake the inhaler. If you do not shake your inhaler well, you may be inhaling more propellant than medication. Or you may reach a point at which you run out of medication before you run out of propellant.[2]

You may have seen instructions for floating your inhaler in a container of water. The theory is that if it sinks it's full; if it floats, it's empty; and if it tilts on an angle, there is still medication left. However, what is left in the half-full inhaler could be mostly propellant. To avoid that possibility:

1. Remove the cap from the inhaler. Supporting the inhaler with your thumb underneath and second and third fingers on top of the canister, shake the inhaler vigorously ten or twelve times to thoroughly mix the medication with the propellant.

2. Tilt your head back slightly and, holding the tube about two inches *away* from your mouth, exhale, then take a deep inhalation as you squeeze the canister.

3. Hold your breath for ten seconds, then let it out slowly through pursed lips as you relax.

4. Sit down and relax! Don't use your inhaler on the run.

5. If your doctor has prescribed two puffs, wait at least one minute (five may even be better) and then repeat the process.

6. If you are using a bronchodilator, the first puff opens the large passageways (the bronchial tubes) and the second puff opens the small airways (the bronchioles).

7. If you are using a bronchodilator plus a second inhalant (steroid, cromolyn sodium, or cholinergic drugs) use the bronchodilator first, wait one to three minutes, and then use the second inhaler.

8. Remember to *vigorously* shake the canister first. Make sure you always have one brand-new inhaler on hand in case the one you are using becomes ineffective.

9. Rinse your inhaler every day and wash it in warm, soapy water often. Use a toothpick to keep the small hole in the inhaler open and free of inhalant debris.

SPACERS

A spacer puts the proper distance between you and the inhalant. It allows the medication to be held in a chamber for a few seconds until it's inhaled. It is easier to use than the canister alone because the timing of the inhalation doesn't have to be perfect. It prevents the large particles of the inhalant from hitting the back of the throat and reduces bad taste and irritants. It can double the delivery of the drug to the lungs compared to the amount delivered by the metered dose inhaler.[3] It helps you get the most from the inhalation. When using a spacer allow only one puff to enter at a time. Inhale before two seconds have elapsed and hold the breath for ten seconds for the full effect.

Spacers available at the pharmacy are:

Aerochamber. A long tube into which fits the entire metered dose inhaler.

Inspirease. A collapsible canister which allows you to see more clearly how you are doing.

Inhalaid. May be the most effective. Both Inspirease and Inhalaid provide feedback to the user via a flow-sensor device that tells when you are inhaling too fast. The spacer allows more medication to be delivered to the alveoli.

NEBULIZERS

A nebulizer is a machine that draws liquid up through a tube by air compression, breaks liquid medication into droplets, and delivers it over a longer period of time, usually about ten to fifteen minutes. The ultrasonic version breaks up the droplets into tiny particles, which can be inhaled more deeply. You may get a better effect from your medication using an ultrasonic nebulizer, but be sure to check the dosage on the package with the one that is in your metered-dose inhaler. The nebulizer version may produce effects of shorter duration.

Pharmaceuticals

BRONCHODILATORS

Bronchodilating inhalers are the most commonly used pharmaceutical for people with asthma. Bronchodilators open the airways when they begin to close. They are great as rescue remedies but should not be overused.

1. ADRENERGIC AGENTS, called beta-agonists, or beta$_2$- agonists bronchodilators.

Beta$_2$- agonists open the airways when they begin to close by relaxing the smooth muscle. They work fast and last from four to six hours. This action may break the descent toward an asthma attack and lessen the severity of an attack. It has no effect on inflammation in the airway. It can also mask underlying symptoms of inflammation, creating false confidence. Because relief is usually immediate it gives the illusion that everything is well. However, if the bronchodilator opens the airways and you are still exposed to allergens or environmental irritants that can be inhaled, the open airways may promote the deeper inhalation of even more irritants. This could lead to the "late response"—a new and more serious attack several hours later. The ability to open the airways with bronchodilators can provide a rescue remedy, but will do nothing for the mucus plugs and inflammation—other symptoms that must be addressed so that the condition doesn't continue to worsen. When you use a bronchodilator regularly, you are applying emergency therapy over a long period of time.

Malcolm Sears, M.D., is a New Zealand doctor who has been a leader in researching drawbacks of beta-agonist therapy. He was one of the researchers involved in the much publicized study of the B-agonist fenoterol in which it was unexpectedly found that regular use of inhaled fenoterol had deleterious effects on asthma. This, researchers found, held true even when subjects also used inhaled corticosteroids.[4] In a symposium devoted to investigating this problem at the Royal Society of Medicine in London, in February of 1992, Dr. Sears said that his study showed that mild and moderate asthma may become more severe through the use of regular short-acting B-agonist therapy.

Subsequently the Executive Committee of the American Academy of Allergy and Immunology issued a position statement recommending that patients withdraw nonessential doses slowly "until the patient ideally is only using the medication as needed before exercise or for 'breakthrough' acute asthma symptoms."[5]

ALBUTEROL is the most common bronchodilating drug used in this country. You probably know it as Proventil or Ventolin. TERBUTALINE is sold as Brethaire and METAPROTERENOL is sold as Alupent. These drugs stimulate $beta_2$-receptors, which help relax the airway muscles. These beta-agonists act fast and imitate the action of adrenaline. SALMETEROL, sold as Serevant, is slow-acting but longer lasting. Problems arise when patients misunderstand or are not informed as to correct use.

Side Effects of Beta-agonists
    increased or irregular heart rate
    restlessness and nervousness

panic attacks or anxiety
headache
muscle tremor
difficulty in urination
dry mouth

There is some evidence that terbutaline can cause loss of magnesium, which can increase muscle spasms.[6]

If you overuse the bronchodilator you might experience breathlessness and assume that you need to use your inhaler again. This breathlessness may be from overmedication. As one emergency-room nurse put it, the bronchodilator can "create need."

EPINEPHRINE or adrenaline is also a bronchodilator, but it causes even more negative reactions, making it an unreliable drug for asthmatics.[7] Epinephrine is powerful and works fast, but its effects are short-lived. Epinephrine is marketed over the counter, but self-treating with over-the-counter drugs can be dangerous.

COMBINATION DRUGS

EPHEDRINE mixed with THEOPHYLLINE and HYDROXYZINE, a tranquilizer, is marketed under the name Marax.

EPHEDRINE mixed with THEOPHYLLINE and a sedative, PHENO-BARBITAL, becomes Tedral.

Add GUAIFENESIN, an expectorant, to this mix, and you get Bronkotabs.

Side Effects of Epinephrine

Disturbance of heart's normal rhythm
Increased blood pressure
Urine retention
Headaches and overstimulation of the brain.

In Europe epinephrine and isoproternol are rarely used because they are associated with a very high incidence of cardiac side effects.[8]

Is Your Inhaler Upside Down?

Dr. D. W. Cockcroft writes in the *Annals of Allergy* that in his experience coordinating the activator with the inhaler is often a problem. One patient inhaled through the nose while activating the inhaler in the mouth; another held the inhaler upside down or sideways (like a harmonica). One patient

used the beta-agonist inhaler four times a day without ever activating it.[9]
Dr. Ambrose A. Chiang in a letter to the *New England Journal of Medicine*
writes that one forty-three-year-old didn't get better or worse although she
had increased her beta-agonist dose to forty puffs a day. When she was asked
to demonstrate, "she fired the aerosol twice with the dust cap on, then
quickly removed the cap, placed the mouthpiece between her lips, and inhaled."[10] This is all very amusing unless you were one of those who couldn't
breathe and was never instructed in the correct use of the metered-dose
inhaler. Dr. Chiang says that studies show that respiratory therapists are
better than doctors and nurses at instructing patients in inhaler use.

2. METHYLXANTHINES, THEOPHYLLINE

For many years the mainstay of most asthma medication programs in the
United States was a theophylline product. Theophylline was found to be a
convenient means to stabilize hyperactive airways.[11] As a result of the NIH
1991 Guidelines for the Diagnosis and Management of Asthma theophylline
is no longer at the top of the list. Unfortunately, some doctors have not
caught up and are still prescribing this oral medication.

There is a lengthy list of theophylline products, some of the most common
being Slo-Bid, Theo-Dur, Elixophyllin, Constant-T, and Choledyl. The liquids may contain sugar. Check with your pharmacist as to correct usage.
They are not interchangeable.

Theophylline works by stimulating the heart and relaxing smooth muscles
around the airways. It may also help keep airways clear of mucus.

It is very important to know that this drug has a very narrow therapeutic
range—a very limited range between having enough medication in the
bloodstream to keep the airways open, and so much medication that dangerous side effects such as tremors and even convulsions develop.

In 1990 the Association of Trial Lawyers of America told the Food and
Drug Administration that it knew of twenty-six preventable theophylline-
related incidents of death or serious injury since 1975. The association
claimed that theophylline products can cause serious complications, including seizures and permanent brain damage, and should be banned for sale
without a prescription.[12] In January 1996, the FDA banned the sale of cough/
cold combinations containing theophylline.

Those using theophylline are advised to have a test to monitor the level
in the bloodstream. Age and weight are also taken into consideration for the
amount prescribed. When I was taking theophylline my blood level was only
monitored in the hospital emergency room. Has your doctor suggested monitoring yours?

Theophylline and Metabolism

The level of theophylline in the bloodstream depends on how the drug is being metabolized.

a. Children and the elderly metabolize medication quite differently than those in the prime of life, on whom these drugs are usually tested.

b. The way theophylline is metabolized will change daily depending on the amount of protein or carbohydrates being eaten or the effects of other medication or conditions. Low carbohydrate, high-protein foods decrease the body's ability to assimilate the drug.[13]

c. Cigarette smoking and enzyme-activating drugs like phenobarbital clear the body of theophylline faster, so that higher doses would be needed.[14]

d. During the course of viral infections theophylline remains in the body longer and can lead to toxicity.[15]

e. Erythromycin prolongs the life of theophylline, which makes for potential toxic interaction.[16]

Side Effects of Theophylline

If you use theophylline you may have experienced these side effects:

Nausea
Headache
Trembling
Diarrhea
Sleeplessness
Inability to concentrate
Spaciness
Restlessness

It can also cause cardiac arrhythmia and seizures.[17]

Theophylline depletes the body of vitamin B_6, which may already be deficient in asthmatics.[18] (See chapter 9.)

Back in 1989 Dr. Donald Aaronson, then president of the American College of Allergy and Immunology, said, "Theophylline's days as a first-line therapy are over."[19]

3. ANTICHOLINERGICS

According to the Guidelines for asthma, anticholinergic agents may be most effective in patients with chronic obstructive pulmonary disease and partially reversible airflow obstruction.[20] They block bronchoconstriction caused by some inhaled irritants. ATROPINE, an early anticholinergic drug (found in plants and used in traditional medicine), was popular in Europe until the 1800s when it stopped being used because of its many adverse effects. However, the development of IPRATROPIUM BROMIDE, whose side effects are said to be minimal, has renewed interest in this drug. Unlike atropine, it can dilate the bronchi without being absorbed into the other organs of the body. Ipratropium is marketed under the name of Atrovent.

I was surprised to read that anticholinergic drugs will not increase "hypoxemia," subnormal oxygen content in the arterial blood, as do adrenergic drugs.[21] Does this mean that regular use of fast-acting bronchodilating drugs might be worsening asthma and creating dependence by reducing the amount of oxygen in the bloodstream?

Anticholinergic agents can both prevent and reverse beta blocker-induced bronchospasm.[22] However, they are less effective against histamines, antigens, and exercise-induced asthma than adrenergic agents. Because they are slower acting, in severe asthma it is recommended that this drug be augmented by albuterol.

Side effects of ipratropium are said to be few—mostly coughing. However, the lack of published side effects might simply reflect the fact that the drug hasn't been as widely used as others with documented side effects.[23]

4. ANTI-INFLAMMATORY PREVENTIVE INHALANTS

In 1991, the treatment of asthma was turned upside down when the National Heart, Lung, and Blood Institute published new asthma guidelines advising first-line use of steroidal and nonsteroidal anti-inflammatory inhalants for controlling asthma.

INHALED STEROIDS

Inhaled corticosteroid therapy became popular in the early 1970's with the development of BECLOMETHASONE DIPROPIONATE.

Inhaled corticosteroids are the primary anti-inflammatory drugs for addressing asthma, but they *cannot* be used during an asthma attack. Rather, they are for regular use as a preventive measure. The steroids in this inhaler help relieve inflammation but may have to be used for two to four weeks before they begin to take effect. Inhaled steroids are usually begun when asthma is under good control.

If you are using a bronchodilator, this inhaler is used several minutes later, when the airways are dilated.

The steroids utilized via an inhaler are said not to get into the bloodstream and cause the side effects of steroids taken internally. They are considered a great advance in the management of asthma. Nevertheless, inhaled steroids are potent drugs. Low doses are said to be free from "important systemic effects."[24] Some of the most common names for inhaled steroids are Vanceril, Aerobid, Azmacort, and Beclovent.

The literature accompanying the Vanceril inhaler, a brand of beclomethasone dipropionate, states that the anti-inflammatory mechanism by which this steroid inhaler addresses inflammations is unknown, as is the drug's action in the lung. Also unknown are the possible long-term effects of the drug.

ORAL STEROIDS

You may be familiar with synthetic steroids manufactured as PREDNISONE, PREDNISOLONE, OR METHYLPREDNISONE. If you are taking steroids orally they are best administered in the morning or every other morning to coincide with the body's own production of steroids.[25] This gives the adrenals some recovery time before the next dose.

Side Effects

   Osteoporosis
   Weight gain
   Hypertension
   Diabetes
   Myopathy
   Psychiatric disturbance
   Skin fragility
   Cataracts
   Ulcers

A 1982 study entitled "Corticosteroids: Many of Their Side Effects Are Really Their Actions" by Kenneth L. Becker, M.D., of George Washington University, reports that this list of side effects of corticosteroids should surprise no one, as they are "just part and parcel of the action of these drugs." His list includes Cushingoid features, susceptibility to infection, and hypothalamic-pituitary-adrenal dysfunction.[26]

A new steroid drug, Deflazacort, in use in Italy, Spain, and Portugal, supposedly has less systemic side effects.[27]

CROMOLYN SODIUM (INTAL)

SODIUM CROMOGLYCATE is a bioflavonoid-like substance derived from an herb used for centuries in Egyptian medicine. It was discovered from investigations of an antispasmodtic agent, *khellin*, which was derived from the Mediterranean plant *Ammi visnaga*. Sodium cromoglycate is one of the three major drugs which were then synthesized from the active ingredient, khellin.[28] Sodium cromoglycate is one of the asthma drugs with the fewest side effects.

It used to be believed that sodium cromoglycate (Intal) and nedocromil sodium (Tilade) work by preventing mast cells from releasing histamines when they come in contact with an allergen. However it is now thought that they are effective because they inhibit eosinophils and lessen airway inflammation. They also reduce bronchial constriction in both early- and late-phase reactions.[29]

Now that Intal is available in inhaler form, doctors claim to know of almost no negative side effects. However, some mild common side effects include irritation of the throat, hoarseness, dry mouth, coughing, chest tightness, and bronchospasm.

Cromolyn sodium can be used before exposure to an allergen such as pets, pollens, or molds, or to a sensitizer such as cold air.

Intal is now also used for its anti-inflammatory effect in the treatment of asthma. According to a Boston study, "Emergency visits for epinephrine and other therapy for an acute asthmatic attack were reduced 96% after cromolyn sodium was introduced into the treatment regimen."[30]

Tilade works along a different pathway than Intal. In 127 clinical trials Tilade was found to have the optimal effect with patients with moderate asthma who were also using inhaled or oral bronchodilators. A trial with Tilade in Europe found it to be more effective than cromolyn sodium (Intal) in treating moderately severe asthma.[31] Patients treated with nedocromil sodium were able to significantly reduce their day- and nighttime use of beta-agonist inhalers as compared with either the placebo or cromolyn groups.

An Italian study found that nedocromil sodium (Tilade) is not effective in adults when given after an asthma attack has started. It should only be used as a long-term preventive treatment.[32]

Drugs Can Cause or Worsen Asthma

When visiting the doctor, dentist, or pharmacist, be sure to tell them you have asthma. Many drugs worsen asthma and some actually cause asthma.

DRUGS AND THE ELDERLY

Many drugs are unsuited for elderly people, and millions of older Americans are hospitalized or die each year because of prescription drugs.[33] The prevalence of late-onset asthma, worsening of symptoms, and death from asthma are also on the rise among people over fifty-five years of age.[34]

Some of the drugs implicated in worsening asthma include:

Beta-blockers such as TIMOPTIC for glaucoma. The insert says loud and clear not to use if you have asthma. Nevertheless, it is sometimes prescribed by disbelieving practitioners.

TIMOPTIC for glaucoma can cause very severe bronchoconstriction and acute asthma attacks.[35] In several patients even a few drops in the eye have been responsible for worsening asthma attacks.[36] Timolol maleate (timoptic) is also marketed as Blocadren, which has been associated with pneumonia and bronchitis as well as with bronchospasm.

Beta-blockers for hypertension, high blood pressure, irregular heart rate, and glaucoma. PROPRANOLOL, marketed as Inderal, is best known. It is used to treat hypertension, angina, cardiac arrhythmias, and migraine. Inderal can cause wheezing, shortness of breath, and bronchospasm.

BETA-BLOCKERS, THEOPHYLLINE and EPINEPHRINE are three of the drugs which may account for increased asthma-related deaths among people over fifty-five.[37]

THEOPHYLLINE and EPINEPHRINE may exacerbate existing heart conditions. Toxic concentrations are reported to cause increased rate of respiration and cardiorespiratory arrest.[38]

HEPARIN, an anticoagulant used for conditions such as cerebral thrombosis and pulmonary embolism, has also been associated with shortness of breath, wheezing, and asthma.[39]

ASPIRIN: Five to 20 percent of asthmatic adults experience severe or fatal reactions from aspirin. People with aspirin-sensitive asthma are advised to use Tylenol (acetaminophen). However, recent studies show that many asthma sufferers also react to acetaminophen. Check with a doctor about the best alternative for you.[40]

OVER-THE-COUNTER PREPARATIONS. Aspirin is the most common cause of drug-induced asthma.[41] Aspirin is an ingredient in hundreds of over-the-counter preparations. Common ones include Bufferin, Alka-Seltzer, Anacin, Pepto-Bismol, Coricidin, Excedrin, and Empirin with Codeine.

OTHER COMMON NONSTEROIDAL ANTI-INFLAMMATORY DRUGS (NSAID) that should be avoided include Motrin, Advil, Nuprin (ibuprofen), Naprosyn, and Indocin. Percodan will have the same effect. Do not let your doctor or dentist give you this drug if you know you are allergic to aspirin.

OTHER DRUGS to avoid include antibiotics such as penicillins and tetracycline; beta-blockers, both systemic and topical; antihypertensives; and ophthalmic cholinergic agonists such as methacholine and ophthalmic cabachol.

TAMOXIFEN: Doctors in Great Britain reported on a fifty-three-year-old woman with asthma taking tamoxifen for breast cancer. Within an hour after taking the drug her forced expiratory volume fell by nearly 70 percent.[42]

The Essential Guide to Prescription Drugs, by James W. Long and James J. Rybacki, contains a complete list of drugs that may cause lung dysfunction or damage. This HarperCollins publication is revised and updated every year. If you are taking drugs for asthma and/or another condition this book should be consulted.

NIH NURSES HEALTH STUDY

In spite of all the new research and guidelines for more effective use of medication, the National Institutes of Health Nurses Health Study revealed some surprising statistics. During 1994–95, 63 percent of study subjects reported using beta-agonists, 56 percent used theophylline, 52 percent used inhaled steroids. Thirty percent had used oral or intravenous steroids. Only 19 percent reported using cromolyn sodium,[43] the safest of all of these medications.

NOTES

CHAPTER 1

1. M. Kaliner and R. Lemanske, "Rhinitis and Asthma," *Journal of the American Medical Association* 268: 2807–29 (1992).
2. Kenneth M. Moser, "Multiple Contexts," in *Bronchial Asthma: Mechanisms and Therapeutics,* ed. Earle B. Weiss and Myron Stein, 3d ed. (Boston: Little, Brown, 1993), 11.
3. "Asthma Toll Is Up Sharply, U.S. Reports," *New York Times,* 3 May 1996.
4. *Guidelines for the Diagnosis and Management of Asthma* (Bethesda, Md.: National Heart, Lung, and Blood Institute; National Institutes of Health, August 1991), 35.
5. Robert Lin, personal communication, 1995.
6. Lawrence K. Altman, "Rise in Asthma Deaths Is Tied to Ignorance of Many Physicians," *New York Times,* 4 May 1993.
7. Donald Drake and Marian Uhlman, *Making Medicine, Making Money* (Kansas City, Mo.: Andrews and McMeel, 1993), 86.
8. Edward N. Teall, ed., *New Concise Webster's Dictionary* (New York: Modern Promotions, 1980), 336.
9. Gerald Epstein, personal communication, 1995.
10. Robert Atkins, *Dr. Atkins' Health Revolution: How Complementary Medicine Can Extend Your Life* (Boston: Houghton Mifflin, 1988), 7.

CHAPTER 2

1. Leon Hammer, *Dragon Rises, Red Bird Flies: Psychology and Chinese Medicine* (Barrytown, N.Y.: Station Hill Press, 1990), 37.
2. N. B. Pride, "Physiology: Changes in Pulmonary Function in Asthma," in *Asthma,* 3rd ed., ed. T. J. H. Clark, S. Godfrey, and T. H. Lee (New York: Chapman & Hall Medical, 1992), 52–53.
3. Michael Winn, personal communication, 1996.

4. Drew Di Vittorio, personal communication, 1994.

5. Deborah Valentine Smith, personal communication, 1995.

6. Dianne Connelly, personal communication, 1996.

7. Iona Marsaa Teeguarden, *Acupressure Way of Health: Jin Shin Do* ® (Tokyo and New York: Japan Publications, 1978), 9.

8. Iona Marsaa Teeguarden, *Student Handbook #3 for Jin Shin Do* ®. For further information contact Jin Shin Do Foundation for Bodymind Acupressure, P.O. Box 1097, Felton, CA 95018.

CHAPTER 3

1. "The American Asthma Report 11," *Air Currents* 4 (1993). A national survey conducted by Glaxo/Allen & Hansburys.

2. N. Hogshead, "Exercise-Induced Asthma and the Athlete," *American Journal of Asthma and Allergy for Pediatricians* 5 (4): 221–22 (1992).

3. Reed Moscowitz, personal communication, 1995.

4. Irvin Caplin, *The Allergic Asthmatic* (Springfield, Ill.: Thomas, 1968), 81, 83–84.

5. P. G. J. Burney, L. A. Laitinen, S. Perdrizet, et al., "Validity and Repeatability of the IUATLD (1984) Bronchial Symptoms Questionnaire: An International Comparison," *European Respiratory Journal* (2): 940–45 (1989).

6. P. M. Yellowlees and R. E. Ruffin, "Psychological Defenses and Coping Styles in Patients Following a Life-Threatening Attack of Asthma," *Chest* 95 (6): 1298–1303 (1989).

7. Robert Lin, personal communication, 1995.

8. M. Haida, K. Ito, S. Makino, and T. Miyamoto, "Psychological Profiles of Patients with Bronchial Asthma," *Arerugi Japanese Journal of Allergology* 44 (1): 16–25 (1995).

9. Iona Marsaa Teeguarden, *The Joy of Feeling: Bodymind Acupressure, Jin Shin Do* ® (New York and Tokyo: Japan Publications, 1987), 231.

10. Ibid.

11. Ibid., 59.

12. Ibid., 232.

13. Gerald Epstein, personal communication, 1995.

14. Teeguarden, 233.

15. Andrew Weil, *Health and Healing* (Boston: Houghton Mifflin, 1985), 236.

16. Mike Samuels and Nancy Samuels, *Seeing with the Mind's Eye: The History, Techniques, and Uses of Visualization* (New York and La Jolla, Calif.: Random House, The Bookworks, 1993), 66.

17. Carol E. McMahon, "The Role of Imagination in the Disease Process: Pre-Cartesian History," *Journal of Psychological Medicine* 6 (2): 179–84 (1976).

18. Gerald Epstein, personal communication, 1995.

19. William Fezler, *Creative Imagery: How to Visualize in All Five Senses* (New York: Simon & Schuster, Fireside, 1989), 37.

20. Gerald Epstein, *Healing Visualizations: Creating Health through Imagery* (New York: Bantam Books, 1989), 66.

21. Serafina Corsello, personal communication, 1996.

CHAPTER 4

1. George W. Bray, "The Hypochlorhydria of Asthma in Childhood," *Quarterly Journal of Medicine* (1931): (24) 182–87. Refers to H. Donnally, who in 1929 showed that foreign proteins can be eliminated in breast milk.

2. Dr. Michael Weitzman quoted in Jane E. Brody, "Allergies in Infants Are Linked to Mothers' Diets," *New York Times,* 30 August 1990, B14.

3. Sandra Blakeslee, "Research on Birth Defects Shifts to Flaws in Sperm," *New York Times,* 1 January 1991, 1, 36.

4. Ted Kaptchuk, *The Web That Has No Weaver* (New York: Congdon & Weed, 1983), 36.

5. F. Haas and S. S. Haas, *The Essential Asthma Book: A Manual for Asthmatics of All Ages* (New York: Ivy Books, 1987), 61.

6. Martin Feldman, personal communication, 1995.

7. Martin Feldman, introduction to *No More Allergies,* by Gary Null (New York: Villard Books, 1992), xi.

8. Martin Feldman, all quotes from personal communication, 1995.

9. Steven Schechter, *Fighting Radiation and Chemical Pollutants with Foods, Herbs, and Vitamins* (Encinitas, Calif.: Vitality, Ink, 1990), 42.

10. W. R. Beisel, R. Edelman, K. Nauss, and R. M. Suskind, "Single Nutrient Effects on Immunologic Functions," *Journal of the American Medical Association* 245 (1): 53–58 (1981).

11. Gary Null, *The Complete Guide to Health and Nutrition* (New York: Delacorte Press, 1984), 281.

12. R. F. Cathcart III, "Vitamin C: The Nontoxic, Nonrate-Limited, Antioxidant Free Radical Scavenger," *Medical Hypotheses* 18: 61–77 (1985).

13. Robert Atkins, *Dr. Atkins' Health Revolution: How Complementary Medicine Can Extend Your Life* (Boston: Houghton Mifflin, 1988), 342.

14. Sheldon Saul Hendler, *The Doctor's Vitamin and Mineral Encyclopedia* (New York: Simon & Schuster, 1990), 102–3.

15. Michael Murray and Joseph Pizzorno, *Encyclopedia of Natural Medicine* (Rockland, Calif.: Prima Publishing, 1991), 161.

16. D. F. Horrobin, "Gamma-Linolenic Acid in Medicine," in *1984–85 Yearbook of Nutritional Medicine,* ed. J. Bland (New Canaan, Conn.: Keats Publishing, 1985), 31.

17. Schechter, 122–23.
18. Null, 477.
19. Martin Feldman, personal communication, 1996. Citation from P. J. Babidge and W. J. Babidge, "Determination of Methylmalonic Acid by High-Performance Liquid Chromatography" in *Analytical Biochemistry* 216 (2): 424–26 (1994).
20. Murray and Pizzorno, 54.
21. Schecter, 122.
22. Murray and Pizzorno, 59.
23. Beisel et al., 53–58.
24. Louise Tenney, *Health Handbook* (Provo, Utah: Woodland Books, 1987), 198.
25. Michael K. Farrell, "Gastroesophageal Reflux and Esophageal Dysfunction," in *Bronchial Asthma: Mechanisms and Therapeutics,* 3d ed., ed. E. B. Weiss and M. Stein (Boston: Little, Brown, 1993), 1023–29.
26. Kaptchuk, 57.
27. John Floyer, *A Treatise of the Asthma* (London, 1698), quoted in George W. Bray, "The Hypochlorhydria of Asthma in Childhood," *Quarterly Journal of Medicine* (January 1931): 181–96.
28. Leo Galland, personal communication, 1995.
29. Leo Galland, "Leaky Gut Syndrome: Breaking the Vicious Cycle," *Townsend Letter for Doctors and Patients* (August-September 1995): 62–68.
30. Ibid.
31. Christopher Hobbs, *Foundations of Health: The Liver and Digestive Herbal* (Capitola, Calif.: Botanica Press, 1992), 117–18.
32. William G. Crook, *The Yeast Connection and the Woman* (Jackson, Tenn.: Professional Books, 1995), 25.
33. Murray and Pizzorno, 185.
34. Gary Null, *Healing Your Body Naturally: Alternative Treatments to Illness* (New York: Four Walls Eight Windows, 1992), 217.
35. Warren Levin, personal communication, 1994.
36. Crook, 47–49.
37. E. B. Collins and P. Hardt, "Inhibition of Candida albicans by Lactobacillus acidophilus," *Journal of Dairy Science* 63 (5): 830–32 (1980).
38. Serafina Corsello, personal communication, 1995.
39. David C. Jamison, ed., "Air Pollution and Asthma: Questions and Answers," *Asthma Update* (summer 1990).
40. Kurt W. Donsbach, *Oxygen, Hydrogen Peroxide, Magnesium Peroxide, Chlorine Peroxide* (Rosarito Beach, Baja Calif., Mexico: Wholistic Publications, 1991), 26.
41. William J. Rea, "The Effect of the Environment on the Individual" (talk given at the Foundation for the Advancement of Innovative Medicine [FAIM] New York City, 10 May 1994).

42. N. Zamel, N. A. Molfino, S. C. Wright, et al., "Effect of Low Concentrations of Ozone on Inhaled Allergen Responses in Asthmatic Subjects," *Lancet* 338: 199–203 (1991).

43. Samuel H. Watson and Charles S. Kibler, "Drinking Water as a Cause of Asthma," *Journal of Allergy* 5 (1): 197 (1934).

44. Alfred V. Zamm with Robert Gannon, *Why Your House May Endanger Your Health* (New York: Touchstone Simon & Schuster, 1982), 129.

45. Alfred V. Zamm, personal communication, 1995.

46. Alfred V. Zamm, "Candida albicans Therapy, Is There Ever an End to It? Dental Mercury Removal: An Effective Adjunct," *Journal of Orthomolecular Medicine* 1 (4): 261–62 (1986).

47. Alfred V. Zamm, *Mercury and Dentistry Newsletter Quarterly* 1 (1): 2 (1986).

48. Gerald E. Poesnecker, *Chronic Fatigue Unmasked: What You and Your Doctor Should Know About the Adrenal Syndrome, Today's Most Misunderstood, Mistreated, and Ignored Health Problem,* 2d ed. (Richlandtown, Pa.: Humanitarian Publishing, 1993), 162–63.

49. William J. Rea, *Chemical Sensitivity,* vol. 1 (Boca Raton: Lewis Publishers, 1993), 321.

50. Fred Soyka, *The Ion Effect* (New York: Bantam Books, 1991), 21.

51. C. J. Kensler and S. P. Batrista, "Chemical and Physical Factors Affecting Mammalian Trachea," *American Review of Respiratory Disease* 93: 93–102 (1966), and A. P. Krueger and R. F. Smith, "The Effects of Air Ions on the Living Mammalian Trachea," *Journal of General Physiology* 42: 69–82 (1958).

52. Jeffrey S. Bland, "Food and Nutrient Effects on Detoxification," *Townsend Letter for Doctors and Patients* 149: 40–44 (1995).

53. D. V. Godin and S. A. Wohaieb, "Nutritional Deficiency, Starvation, and Tissue Antioxidant Status," *Free Radical Biology and Medicine* 5: 165–66 (1988).

54. L. J. Smith, J. Anderson, M. Shamsuddin, and W. Hsueh, "Effect of Fasting on Hyperoxic Lung Oxgen in Mice," *American Review of Respiratory Disease* 141: 141–49 (1990).

55. F. Batmanghelidj, *Your Body's Many Cries for Water: You Are Not Sick, You Are Thirsty* (Falls Church, Va: Global Health Solutions, 1995), 116.

56. Ibid., 119.

57. Jerry Hogan, ed., "Ways to Feel Better: A Talk by Carolyne Cesari," *The Healer* (fall 1994), 8.

58. Schechter, 42.

59. Ibid., 49–50.

60. Ibid., 47.

61. Ibid., 49.

62. Eric R. Braverman and Carl C. Pfeiffer, *The Healing Nutrients Within: Facts, Findings, and New Research on Amino Acids* (New Canaan, Conn.: Keats Publishing, 1987), 13.

63. Ibid., 90.

64. Andrew Chevallier, *Natural Taste Herbal Teas: A Guide for Home Use* (Surry, England: Amberwood Publishing, 1994), 17.

65. Michael T. Murray, *The Healing Power of Herbs: The Enlightened Person's Guide to the Wonders of Medicinal Plants* (Rocklin, Calif.: Prima Publishing, 1995), 332.

66. Hobbs, 123.

CHAPTER 5

1. Gretchen Finney, "Medical Theories of Vocal Exercise and Health," *Bulletin of the History of Medicine* 50 (5): 395–406 (1966).

2. Ravi Singh, personal communication, 1996.

3. L. Hoffman-Goetz, R. Keir, R. Thorne, et al., "Chronic Exercise Stress in Mice Depresses Splenic T Lymphocyte Mitogenesis in Vitro," *Clinical and Experimental Immunology* 66 (3): 551–57 (1986).

4. J. P. Finnerty, et al., "Role of Leukotrienes in Exercise-Induced Asthma. Inhibitory Effect of ICI 204219, a Potent Leukotriene D4 Receptor Antagonist," *American Review of Respiratory Disease* 145 (4, part 1): 746–69 (1992).

5. Iona Marsaa Teeguarden, *The Joy of Feeling: Bodymind Acupressure, Jin Shin Do®* (Tokyo and New York: Japan Publications, Inc., 1987), 338.

6. For further description of Pal Dan Gum see *The Joy of Feeling,* 337–48. Audiotapes and videotapes of the Pal Dan Gum exercises are available from the Jin Shin Do Foundation for Bodymind Acupressure, P.O. Box 1097, Felton, CA 90518.

7. *Kundalini Yoga/Sadhana Guidelines: Exercise and Meditation Manual* (Pomona, Calif.: Kundalini Research Institute, 1978), 36.

CHAPTER 6

1. R. T. Frank, "The Hormonal Causes of Premenstrual Tension," *Archives of Neurology and Psychiatry* 26: 1053 (1931).

2. Jon R. Luoma, "New Effect of Pollutants: Hormone Mayhem," *New York Times,* 24 March 1992.

3. Serafina Corsello, all quotes from personal communication, 1995.

4. D. Lieberman, G. Kobernik, et al., "Subclinical Worsening of Bronchial Asthma during Estrogen Replacement Therapy in Asthmatic Post-menopausal Women," *Maturitas* 21 (2): 153–57 (1995).

5. Rebecca J. Troisi, Frank E. Speizer, Walter C. Willett, et al., "Menopause, Postmenopausal Estrogen Preparations, and the Risk of Adult-Onset Asthma," *American Journal of Respiratory and Critical Care Medicine* 152 (4, part 1): 1183–88 (1995).

6. D. W. Morrish, B. J. Sproule, T. H. Aaron, D. Outhet, and P. M. Crockford,

"Hypothalamic-Pituitary-Adrenal Function in Extrinsic Asthma," *Chest* 75: 2 (1979).

7. R. G. Townley, I. L. Trapani, and A. Szentivanyi, "Sensitization to Anaphylaxis and to Some of Its Pharmacological Mediators by Blockade of the Beta-adrenergic Receptors," *Journal of Allergy* 39 (3): 177–97 (1967).

8. Peter Barnes, "Neural Mechanisms in Asthma," in *Asthma,* 3d ed., ed. T. J. Clark, S. Godfrey, and T. H. Lee (London: Chapman & Hall Medical, 1992), 143.

9. Henry Gray, *Gray's Anatomy,* eds. T. Pickering Pick and Robert Howden (New York: Gramercy Books, 1977), 985.

10. John W. Tintera, "What You Should Know About Your Glands and Allergies," *Women's Day* (February 1959): quoted in G. E. Poesnecker, *Chronic Fatigue Unmasked: What You and Your Doctor Should Know About the Adrenal Syndrome, Today's Most Misunderstood, Mistreated, and Ignored Health Problem,* 2d ed. (Richlandtown, Pa.: Humanitarian Publishing, 1993), 16–18.

11. Hans Selye, *The Stress of Life* (New York: McGraw-Hill, 1956, rev. ed. 1976), 395. Selye writes that all data from stressor effects of various occupations are in *Stress in Health and Disease Reading* (Boston: Butterworths, 1976).

12. Leon Hammer, *Dragon Rises, Red Bird Flies: Psychology and Chinese Medicine* (Barrytown, N.Y.: Station Hill Press, 1990), 13.

13. Warren Levin, personal communication, 1996.

14. Paavo Airola, *Hypoglycemia: A Better Approach* (Sherwood, Ore.: Health Plus, 1977), 119.

15. Ron Teeguarden, *Chinese Tonic Herbs* (New York: Japan Publications, 1994), 105.

16. Susun S. Weed, *Wise Woman Herbal: Healing Wise* (Woodstock, N.Y.: Ash Tree Publishing, 1989), 173.

17. Michael T. Murray, *The Healing Power of Herbs: The Enlightened Person's Guide to the Wonders of Medicinal Plants* (Rocklin, Calif.: Prima Publishing, 1995), 270.

18. Ibid.

19. N. R. Farnsworth et al., "Siberian Ginseng (Eleuthercoccus senticosus): Current Status As an Adaptogen," *Economic and Medical Plant Reseach* 1, 156–215 (1985).

20. Gerald E. Poesnecker, *Chronic Fatigue Unmasked: What You and Your Doctor Should Know About the Adrenal Syndrome, Today's Most Misunderstood, Mistreated, and Ignored Health Problem,* 2d ed. (Richlandtown, Pa.: Humanitarian Publishing, 1993), 110.

21. Richard J. Wurtman, "Effects of Light on the Human Body," *Scientific American* 233: 68–77 (1975).

22. See John N. Ott, *Light, Radiation, and You* (Greenwich, Conn.: Devin-Adair Publishers, 1985).

23. "The Plowboy Interview—John Ott: The 'Light' Side of Health," *Mother Earth News* (January-February 1986): 17–22.

CHAPTER 7

1. Ralph Bookman, quoted in *Rodale's Allergy Relief Newsletter* 3 (7) (1988).
2. Patrick Young, *Asthma and Allergies: An Optimistic Future* (Washington D.C.: U.S. Department of Health and Human Services, National Institutes of Health, March 1980) publication no. 80–388, xi.
3. Alfred V. Zamm with Robert Gannon, *Why Your House May Endanger Your Health* (New York: Touchstone Simon & Schuster, 1982) 40–41.
4. M. P. Carroll, C. Gratziou, and S. T. Holgate, "Inflammation and Inflammatory Mediators in Asthma," in *Asthma*, 3d ed., ed. T. J. H. Clark, S. Godfrey, and T. H. Lee (New York: Chapman & Hall Medical, 1992), 189.
5. N. Zamel, N. A. Molfino, S. C. Wright, et al., "Effect of Low Concentrations of Ozone on Inhaled Allergen Responses in Asthmatic Subjects," *Lancet* 338: 199–203 (1991).
6. Zamm and Gannon, 98.
7. Doris Brunza, "Tea Tree Oil," *Heal* newsletter, ed. Joy Rothenberg, New York City, April 1994.
8. G. L. Sussman, S. Tarlo, and J. Dolovich, "The Spectrum of IgE-Mediated Responses to Latex," *Journal of the American Medical Association* 265 (21): 2844–47 (1991).
9. G. L. Sussman and D. H. Beezhold, "Allergy to Latex Rubber," *Annals of Internal Medicine* 122 (1): 43–46 (1995).
10. G. Brugnami, A. Marabini, A. Siracusa, and G. Abbritti, "Work-Related Late Asthmatic Response Induced by Latex Allergy," *Journal of Allergy and Clinical Immunology* 96: 457–64 (October 1995).
11. Elizabeth C. Barton, "Latex Allergy: Recognition and Management of a Modern Problem," *Nurse Practitioner* 18 (11): 54–58 (1993).
12. Brugnami et al., 457–64.
13. Sussman and Beezhold, 43–46.
14. Y. Tan and C. Collins-Williams, "Aspirin-Induced Asthma in Children," *Annals of Allergy* 48 (1): 1–5 (1982).
15. Andrew Szczeklik and Krzysztof Sladek, "Aspirin, Related Non-steroidal Anti-inflammatory Agents, Sulfites, and Other Food Additives as Precipitating Factors in Asthma," in *Bronchial Asthma: Principles of Diagnosis and Treatment*, 3d ed., ed. M. E. Gershwin and G. M. Halpern (Totowa, N.J.: Humana Press, 1994), 563.
16. Jane E. Brody, "Food Allergy Called Unseen Asthma Villain," *New York Times*, 21 February 1996.
17. K. A. Ogle and J. D. Bullock, "Children with Allergic Rhinitis and/or Bronchial Asthma Treated with Elimination Diet: A Five-Year Follow-up," *Annals of Allergy* 44: 273–78 (1980).
18. Jacqueline A. Krohn, "Adverse Food Reactions Part I: IgE Food Allergy and Non-IgE Mediated Food Intolerance," *The Human Ecologist* 65: 1–6 (1995).

19. "Instant Action Is the Answer When Foods May Be Fatal," *Rodale's Allergy Relief Newsletter* 3 (10) (1988) 2.
20. Michio Kushi, *Allergies*, ed. M. Mead and J. D. Mann (Tokyo and New York: Japan Publications, 1985), 62–63.
21. Paul Pitchford, *Healing with Whole Foods: Oriental Traditions and Modern Nutrition* (Berkeley, Calif.: North Atlantic Books, 1993), 225–26.
22. "Hideous or Harmless, MSG: It's Hard to Avoid," *Rodale's Allergy Relief Newsletter* 3 (9) (1988) 3.
23. R. Garrison and E. Somer, "Vitamin Research: Selected Topics," chapter 5 in *The Nutrition Desk Reference* (New Canaan, Conn.: Keats Publications, 1985), 93–94.
24. "Itchy Mouth? Fresh Fruit May Be the Cause," *Rodale's Allergy Relief Newsletter* 3 (2) (1988) 1, 7.
25. J. L. Cousergue, "L'Allergie aux Produits Terpéniques chez les Asthmatiques," *Revue Francaise de Allergologie* 5 (3): 160–68 (1965).
26. "Don't Put Too Much Stock in Food Families," *Rodale's Allergy Relief* 3 (2) (1988) 7.
27. John H. Boyles Jr., "The Validity of Using the Cytotoxic Food Test in Clinical Allergy," *Ear, Nose, and Throat Journal* 56 (4): 168–173 (1977). Also: Robert C. Atkins, *Dr. Atkins's Health Revolution: How Complementary Medicine Can Extend Your Life* (Boston: Houghton Mifflin, 1988), 114.
28. Paavo Airola, *Hypoglycemia: A Better Approach* (Sherwood, Ore.: Health Plus, 1977), 24.
29. Ibid., 75.
30. Ibid., 76.

CHAPTER 8

1. M. P. A. Cosman, "Feast for Aesculapius," *Annual Review of Nutrition* 3 (1): 1–33 (1983).
2. Steven R. Schechter, *Fighting Radiation and Chemical Pollutants with Foods, Herbs, and Vitamins* (Encinitas, Calif.: Vitality, Ink, 1990), 74.
3. Paul Pitchford, *Healing with Whole Foods: Oriental Traditions and Modern Nutrition* (Berkeley, Calif.: North Atlantic Books, 1993), 549.
4. Aveline Kushi, *Aveline Kushi's Complete Guide to Macrobiotic Cooking for Health, Harmony, and Peace.* (New York: Warner Books, 1985), 289.
5. Pitchford, 547.
6. Henry C. Lu, *The Chinese System of Food Cures: Prevention and Remedies* (New York: Sterling Publishing, 1986), 14.
7. Mike Samuels and Nancy Samuels, *Seeing with the Mind's Eye: The History, Techniques, and Uses of Visualization* (New York and La Jolla, Calif.: Random House, Bookworks, 1993), 93.

CHAPTER 9

1. Warren Levin, personal communication, 1994.
2. Robert C. Atkins, *Dr. Atkins' Health Revolution: How Complementary Medicine Can Extend Your Life* (Boston: Houghton Mifflin, 1988), 6, 35.
3. William R. Beisel, Robert Edelman, Kathleen Nauss, and Robert Suskind, "Single-Nutrient Effects on Immunologic Functions. Report of a Workshop Sponsored by the Department of Food and Nutrition and Its Nutrition Advisory Group of the American Medical Association," *Journal of the American Medical Association* 245 (1): 53–58 (1981).
4. Jean H. Humphrey and Keith P. West Jr., "Vitamin A Deficiency: Role in Childhood Infection and Mortality," in *Micronutrients in Health and in Disease Prevention* ed. Adrianne Bendich and C. E. Butterworth Jr. (New York: Marcel Dekker, 1991), 312–13.
5. "The Effect of Vitamin E and Beta Carotene on the Incidence of Lung Cancer and Other Cancers in Male Smokers," *New England Journal of Medicine* 330 (15): 1029–35 (1994).
6. G. S. Omenn, G. Goodman, M. Thornquist, et al., "The B-carotene and Retinol Efficacy Trial (CARET) for Chemoprevention of Lung Cancer in High Risk Populations: Smokers and Asbestos-Exposed Workers," *Cancer Research* (Suppl.) 54: 2038s–43s (1994).
7. Jeffrey Bland, "The Beta-Carotene Controversy in Perspective" (editorial), *Townsend Letter for Doctors and Patients* 154: 100–102 (May 1996). He cites H. Sies, W. Stahl, and A. R. Suncquist, "Antioxidant Functions of Vitamins: Vitamins E and C, Beta-carotene, and Other Carotenoids," *Annals of the New York Academy of Science* 669: 7–20 (1992).
8. Ibid.
9. Beisel et al., 53–58.
10. Ibid.
11. P. J. Collipp, S. Goldzier III, N. Weiss, et al., "Pyrodoxine Treatment of Childhood Bronchial Asthma," *Annals of Allergy* 35: 93–97 (1975).
12. R. Delport, J. B. Ubbink, W. J. Serfontein, P. J. Becker, and L. Walters, "Vitamin B_6 Nutritional Status in Asthma: The Effect of Theophylline Therapy on Plasma Pyridoxal-5'-Phosphate and Pyridoxal Levels," *International Journal for Vitamin and Nutrition Research* 58 (1): 67–72 (1988).
13. R. D. Reynolds and C. L. Natta, "Depressed Plasma Pyridoxal Phosphate Concentrations in Adult Asthmatics," *American Journal of Clinical Nutrition* 41 (4): 684–88 (1985).
14. Gary Null, *The Complete Guide to Health and Nutrition* (New York: Delacorte Press, 1984), 282.
15. R. Garrison and E. Somer, "Vitamin Research: Selected Topics," in *The Nutrition Desk Reference* (New Canaan, Conn.: Keats Publications, 1985), 93–94.

16. Ronald Hoffman in *New Life* (March-April 1991).

17. R. F. Cathcart III, "Vitamin C: The Nontoxic, Nonrate-limited, Antioxidant," *Medical Hypotheses* 18 (1): 61–77 (1985).

18. W. I. Aderele, S. I. Ette, O. Oduwole, and S. J. Ikpeme, "Plasma Vitamin C (Ascorbic Acid) Levels in Asthmatic Children," *African Journal of Medicine* 14: 115–20 (1985).

19. C. C. Anah, L. N. Jarike, and H. A. Baig, "High Dose Ascorbic Acid in Nigerian Asthmatics," *Tropical and Geographical Medicine* 32: 132–37 (1980).

20. C. J. Doelman and A. Bast, "Oxygen Radicals in Lung Pathology," *Free Radical Biology and Medicine* 9 (5): 381–400 (1990). See also J. E. Heffner and J. E. Repine, "Pulmonary Strategies of Antioxidant Defense: State of the Art," *American Review of Respiratory Disease* 140: 531–54 (1989).

21. S. N. Meydani and J. B. Blumberg. "Vitamin E and Immunity in the Aged," in *Micronutrients in Health and in Disease Prevention* (New York: Marcel Dekker, 1991), 295.

22. R. J. Troisi, W. C. Willett, S. T. Weiss, et al., "A Prospective Study of Diet and Adult-Onset Asthma," *American Journal of Respiratory and Critical Care Medicine* 151 (5): 1401–8 (1995).

23. J. N. Roehm, J. G. Hadley, D. B. Menzel, "The Influence of Vitamin E on the Lung Fatty Acids," *Archives of Environmental Health* 24 (4): 237–42 (1972).

24. M. McCarty, "Can Dietary Selenium Reduce Leukotriene Production?" *Medical Hypotheses* 13 (1): 45–50 (1984).

25. Ibid.

26. L. Hasselmark, R. Malmgren, O. Zetterman, and G. Unge, "Selenium Supplementation in Intrinsic Asthma," *Allergy* 48: 30–36 (1993).

27. J. Stone, L. J. Hinks, R. Beasley, S. T. Holgate, and B. E. Clayton, "Selenium Status of Patients with Asthma," *Clinical Science* 77: 495–500 (1989).

28. Doelman and Bast, 381–400.

29. Sheldon Saul Hendler, *The Doctors' Vitamin and Mineral Encyclopedia* (New York: Simon & Schuster, Fireside, 1991), 192.

30. Sherry A. Rogers, *Tired or Toxic* (Syracuse, N.Y.: Prestige Publishing, 1990), 159.

31. Editors of *Prevention* magazine, *Complete Book of Vitamins and Minerals for Health* (Emmaus, Pennsylvania: Rodale Press, 1988), 197.

32. V. G. Haury, "Blood serum," *Journal of Laboratory and Clinical Medicine* 26: 340–44 (1940).

33. E. H. Brunner et al., "Effect of Parenteral Magnesium on Pulmonary Function, Plasma cAMP, and Histamine in Bronchial Asthma," *Journal of Asthma* 22 (1): 3–11 (1985).

34. E. M. Skobeloff, W. H. Spivey, R. M. McNamara, and L. Greenspon, "Intravenous Magnesium Sulfate for the Treatment of Acute Asthma in the Emergency Department," *Journal of the American Medical Association* 262 (9): 1210–13 (1989).

35. G. Marone et al., "Physiological Concentrations of Zinc Inhibit the Release of

Histamine from Human Basophils and Lung Mast Cells," *Agents Actions* 18: 103–6 (1986).

36. Michael Murray and Joseph Pizzorno, *Encyclopedia of Natural Medicine* (Rocklin, Calif.: Prima Publishing, 1991), 131.

37. Eric R. Braverman and Carl C. Pfeiffer, *The Healing Nutrients Within* (New Canaan, Conn.: Keats, 1987), 337.

38. C. Picado, J. A. Castillo, N. Schinca, et al., "Effects of a Fish Oil Enriched Diet on Aspirin Intolerant Asthmatic Patients: A Pilot Study," *Thorax* 43 (2): 93–97 (1988).

39. J. P. Arm and T. H. Lee, "The Use of Fish Oil in Bronchial Asthma," *Allergy Proceedings* 10 (3): 185–87 (1989).

40. Braverman and Pfeiffer, 92–93.

41. G. Boman, U. Backer, U. S. Larsson, B. Melander, and L. Wahlander, "Oral Acetylcysteine Reduced Exacerbation Rate in Chronic Bronchitis: Report on a Trial Organized by the Swedish Society for Pulmonary Diseases," *European Journal of Respiratory Diseases* 64: 405 (1983), cited by I. Ziment in "Acetylcysteine: A Drug with an Interesting Past and a Fascinating Future," *Respiration* 50, suppl. 1: 26–30 (1986).

42. I. Ziment, "Acetylcysteine: A Drug That Is Much More Than a Mucokinetic," *Biomedicine and Pharmacotherapy* 42 (8): 513–19 (1988).

43. Patricia Hopkinson, Diane Miske, Jerry Parsons, Holly Shimizu, *Herb Gardening* (New York: Pantheon Books, 1994), 72.

44. Stephan T. Chang, *The Great Tao* (San Francisco, Calif.: Tao Publishing, 1985), 169.

45. Sue Minter, *The Herb and Medicinal Gardens at the Chelsea Physic Garden* (n.p.: Trustees of the Chelsea Physic Garden Company, 1993).

46. William K. Stevens, "Shamans and Scientists Seek Cures in Plants," *New York Times,* 28 January 1992.

47. Hendler, 294.

48. Andrew Weil, *Health and Healing* (Boston: Houghton Mifflin, 1985), 101–2.

49. *Chinese Herbal Medicine: Materia Medica,* rev. ed., comp. and trans. Dan Bensky and Andrew Gamble with Ted Kaptchuk (Seattle, Wash: Eastland Press, 1993), 29.

50. Ibid.

51. Ron Teeguarden, *Chinese Tonic Herbs* (New York and Tokyo: Japan Publications, 1994) 136–37.

52. Hendler, 294.

53. Teeguarden, 98–99.

54. Bensky and Gamble, 319.

55. Murray, 145.

56. A. G. Palma-Carlos, "Basic Aspects of Therapy in Intrinsic Asthma," *Agents Actions* 28: 263–77 (1989).

57. J. Kleijnen and P. Knipschild, "Ginkgo Biloba," *Lancet* 340: 1136–39 (1992).
58. Bensky and Gamble, 76.
59. Murray and Pizzorno, 500.
60. M. Kubo, Y. Kimura, and T. Odani, "Studies on Scutellariae Radix Part II: The Antibacterial Substance," *Planta Medica* 43 (2): 194–201 (1981).
61. C. P. Sung, A. P. Baker, et al., "Effects of Angelica Polymorpha on Reaginic Antibody Production," *Journal of Natural Products* 45: 793 (1982).
62. Teeguarden, 91.
63. Murray and Pizzorno, 154.
64. M. Homma, K. Oka, et al., "Impact of Free Magnolol Excretions in Asthmatic Patients Who Responded Well to Saiboku-To, a Chinese Herbal Medicine," *Journal of Pharmacy and Pharmacology*. 45: 844–46 (1993).
65. M. Homma, K. Oka, et al., "A Novel 11B-Hydroxysteroid Dehydrogenase Inhibitor Contained in Saiboku-To, a Herbal Remedy for Steroid-Dependent Bronchial Asthma," *Journal of Pharmacy and Pharmacology* 46: 305–9 (1994)
66. Chang, 168.
67. D. G. Massey, Y. K. Chien, and G. Fournier-Massey, "Mamane: Scientific Therapy for Asthma?" *Hawaii Medical Journal* 53 (12): 350–51, 363 (1994).
68. Michael T. Murray, *The Healing Power of Herbs: The Enlightened Person's Guide to the Wonders of Medicinal Plants* (Rocklin, Calif.: Prima Publishing, 1995), 101–2.
69. Letha Hadady, personal communication, 1996.
70. Murray and Pizzorno, 217–18.
71. C. Gopalakrishnan, et al., "Effect of Tylophorine, a Major Alkaloid of Tylophora Indica, on Immunopathological and Inflammatory Reactions," *Indian Journal of Medical Research* 71, 940–48.
72. W. Farrar, "Tcuitalal: A Glimpse of Aztec Food Technology," *Nature* 211: 341–42 (1966).
73. J. C. Dillon, A. P. Phuc, and J. P. Dubacq, "Nutritional Value of the Alga Spirulina," *World Review of Nutrition and Dietetics* 77: 32–46 (1995). Originally published in A. P. Simopoulos, ed., *Plants in Human Nutrition* (Basel: Karger, 1995).
74. O. Hayashi, T. Katoh, and Y. Okuwaki, "Enhancement of Antibody Production in Mice by Dietary *spirulina platensis*," *Journal of Nutritional Science and Vitaminology* 40 (5): 431–41 (1994).

CHAPTER 10

1. William J. Rea, "Indoor Air Pollution," *Human Ecologist* (Summer 1990): 16.
2. Mike Thomas, *Indoor Air Review* (April 1993).

CHAPTER 11

1. Ellen Swallow Richards quoted by Katherine Keenan in *Healthy Home and Workplace* newsletter, ed. Mimi Weisbord, 2 (3) (1992).
2. Irene Wilkenfeld. Unless otherwise noted, all quotes are from personal communication, February 1996.
3. "Asthma and Our Schools," *FYI: A Health and Safety Newsletter for School Employees* Ithaca, N.Y.: The Labor Coalition, October 1995.
4. R. E. Binder, C. A. Mitchell, H. R. Hosein, and A. Bouhuys, "Importance of the Indoor Environment in Air Pollution Exposure," *Archives of Environmental Health* 31 (6): 277–79 (1976).
5. Ibid.
6. "Contaminated Classrooms," *Public Citizen's Report,* 1988.
7. Theron G. Randolph and Ralph W. Moss, *An Alternative Approach to Allergies,* rev. ed. (New York: Harper & Row, 1989), 110–11.
8. Angela Babin, Perri Peltz, and Monona Rossol, *Children's Art Supplies Can Be Toxic,* 1984, 1988, 1989. Published by the Center for Safety in the Arts.
9. *Occupational Health and Safety,* January 1996, 13–14.
10. "Asthma and Office Work," *FYI: A Health and Safety Newsletter for Office Workers* Ithaca, N.Y.: The Labor Coalition, September 1995.
11. Jay Danilczyk, personal communication, 1995.
12. Cited in *Healthy Home and Workplace* 2 (2) (1992).
13. *Occupational Health and Safety,* January 1996, 13–14.
14. M. S. Morgan and J. E. Camp, "Upper Respiratory Irritation from Controlled Exposure to Vapor from Carbonless Copy Forms," *Journal of Occupational Medicine* 28: 415–19 (1986), cited in *EPA Research and Development Manual — Office Equipment: Design, Indoor Air Emissions, and Pollution Prevention Opportunities,* EPA-600/R-95-045, March 1995. Prepared for Office of Radiation and Indoor Air by Air and Energy Engineering Research Laboratory, Research Triangle Park, NC 27711.
15. Michael McCann, "Occupational Asthma," *FYI,* NY Foundation for the Arts 7 (2) 1991.
16. Ibid.
17. National Institute of Occupational Safety and Health, *Indoor Air Quality and Work Environment Study,* HETA 88-364-2104, 1991. Library of Congress, Madison Building, Health Hazard Evaluation Report, Washington, D.C. Cited in the *EPA Research and Developmental Manual — Office Equipment: Design, Indoor Air Emissions, and Pollution Prevention Opportunities.*
18. Monona Rossol, *The Artist's Complete Health and Safety Guide* (New York: Allworth Press, 1990), 9.
19. Monona Rossol. Unless otherwise noted, all quotes are from personal communication, 1995.
20. "Lung Hazards on the Job, Welding," *The American Lung Association,* 1984.

21. Ibid.
22. Michael McCann, "Occupational Asthma."

CHAPTER 12

1. *The United States Pollen Calendar,* American Academy of Allergy and Immunology Allergen Network, 1993.
2. "25 Breathe-Easy Tips from America's Top Allergists," *Prevention,* August 1989.
3. *The United States Pollen Calendar.*
4. *New York Times,* June 1993, cited in *Healthy Home and Workplace* 3 (3) (1993).
5. Diana Fairechild, *Jet Smart: Over 200 Tips for Beating Jet Lag* (Berkeley, Calif.: Celestial Arts Publishing, 1992), 75.
6. Ibid. 62–63.
7. David Williams, "A Spicy Solution to a Slippery Problem," *Alternatives,* January 1994, 53.
8. Harriet Beinfield and Efrem Korngold, *Between Heaven and Earth: A Guide to Chinese Medicine* (New York: Ballantine Books, 1992), 317.
9. Jake Fratkin, *Chinese Herbal Patent Formulas: A Practical Guide* (Santa Fe, N.M.: Shya Publications, 1986), 155.
10. Ann Louise Gittleman, *Natural Healing for Parasites* (New York: Healing Wisdom Publications, 1995), 11.
11. Beinfield and Korngold, 316.
12. Letha Hadady, "Travel Critters," *Free Spirit,* June, 1990, 59–61.

CHAPTER 13

1. Harriet Beinfield and Efrem Korngold, *Between Heaven and Earth: A Guide to Chinese Medicine* (New York: Ballantine Books, 1992), 36.
2. Doris Rapp, in *Is This Your Child?* quoted in William G. Crook, *The Yeast Connection and the Woman* (Jackson, Tenn.: Professional Books, Inc., 1995), 390.
3. "Infectious Diseases Resistant, Study Finds," *New York Times,* 20 May 1996.

APPENDIX III

1. Thomas L. Petty, *Second Wind Newsletter,* September 1992.
2. "Death Rates in Asthmatic Patients (letter)," *Medical Journal of Australia* 147 (9): 469 (1987).
3. S. P. Newman et al., "Effect of Inspirease on the Deposition of Metered Aerosols in the Human Respiratory Tract," *Chest* 89: 55 (1986). J. H. Toogood et al.,

"Use of Spacers to Facilitate Inhaled Corticosteroid Treatment of Asthma," *American Review of Respiratory Disease* 129: 723–9 (1984).

4. M. R. Sears, "Should We Be Using B-agonists for Treatment of Chronic Asthma?" *Beta Agonists in the Treatment of Asthma: The Proceedings of a Symposium Held at the Royal Society of Medicine, London, February 1992,* ed. J. F. Costello and R. D. Mann (Pearl River, N.Y.: Parthenon Publishing Group, 1992), 79–87.

5. "Executive Committee of the American Academy of Allergy and Immunology Position Statement," *Journal of Allergy and Clinical Immunology* 91: 1234–37 (1993).

6. L. A. Cannon, D. E. Heiselman, J. M. Dougherty, and J. Jones, "Magnesium Levels in Cardiac Arrest Victims: Relationship between Magnesium Levels and Successful Resuscitation," *Annals of Emergency Medicine* 16: 11, 1195–99 (1987).

7. F. Haas and S. S. Haas, *The Essential Asthma Book: A Manual for Asthmatics of All Ages* (New York: Ivy Books, 1987), 108.

8. A. G. Palma-Carlos and A. L. Jordao, "Aspects of 'International' Asthma," in *Bronchial Asthma,* 3d ed., ed. M. E. Gershwin and G. M. Halpern (Totowa, N.J.: Humana Press, 1994), 458–59.

9. D. W. Cockcroft, "Practical Issues in Asthma Management: Correct Use of Inhalation Device" (editorial), *Annals of Allergy* 71 (2): 83–84 (1993).

10. A. A. Chiang, "Misunderstandings about Inhalers (letter)," *New England Journal of Medicine* 330 (23): 1690–91 (1994).

11. M. M. Weinberger, "Methylxanthines," in *Bronchial Asthma: Mechanisma and Therapeutics,* 3d ed., ed. E. B. Weiss and M. Stein (Boston: Little, Brown, 1993), 764.

12. "Popular Asthma Drug Dangerous, Lawyers Say," *Miami Herald,* 31 October 1990, 5B.

13. A. Kappas, et al., "Influence of Dietary Protein and Carbohydrate on Antipyrine and Theophylline Metabolism in Man," *Clinical Pharmacology and Therapeutics* 20: 634 (1976).

14. Palma-Carlos and Jordao, 463.

15. G. Koren and M. Greenwald, "Decreased Theophylline Clearance Causing Toxicity in Children During Viral Epidemics," *Journal of Asthma* 22 (2): 75–79 (1985).

16. Palma-Carlos and Jordao, 463.

17. Ibid.

18. P. G. J. Burney, "Epidemiology," in *Asthma,* 3d ed., ed. T. J. H. Clark, S. Godfrey, and T. H. Lee (London: Chapman & Hall, 1992), 279.

19. M. L. Zoler, "Doctors Still Buck Asthma Advice," *Medical World News,* 25 September 1989, 12.

20. *Guidelines for the Diagnosis and Management of Asthma* (Bethesda, Md.: National Heart, Lung, and Blood Institute; National Institutes of Health, 1991), 41.

21. N. J. Gross, "Anticholinergic Agents," in *Bronchial Asthma: Mechanisms and Ther-*

apeutics, 3d ed., ed. E. B. Weiss and M. Stein (Boston: Little, Brown, 1993), 882.

22. P. W. Ind, "Anticholinergic Blockade of Beta-Blocker Induced Bronchoconstriction," *American Review of Respiratory Disease* 139: 1390 (1989).

23. Gross, 876–79.

24. R. M. Brodgen et al., "Beclomethasone Dipropionate: A Reappraisal of Its Pharmacodynamic Properties and Therapeudic Efficacy After a Decade of Use in Asthma and Rhinitis," *Drugs* 28: 99 (1984).

25. H. Herxheimer, *A Guide to Bronchial Asthma* (London: Academic Press, 1975), 84.

26. K. L. Becker, "Corticosteroids: Many of Their Side Effects Are Really Their Actions," *Drug Therapy* January 1982, 131–33, 137, 139.

27. R. Gray, C. Harrington, L. Coulton, J. Calloway, M. de Broe, and J. Kanis, "Long-Term Treatment of Chronic Inflammatory Disorders with Deflazacort," Journal of Orthopedic Rheumatology 3: 15–27 (1990).

28. S. Minter, *Plants in Medicine* (London: Chelsea Physic Garden, 1991).

29. Palma-Carlos and Jordao, 467.

30. R. N. Ross, M. Morris, S. R. Sakowitz, and B. A. Berman, "Cost-effectiveness of Including Cromolyn Sodium in the Treatment Program for Asthma: A Retrospective, Record-Based Study," *Clinical Therapeutics* 10 (2): 188–203 (1988).

31. S. Lal, P. D. Dorow, K. K. Venho, and S. S. Chatterjee, "Nedocromil Sodium Is More Effective Than Cromolyn Sodium for the Treatment of Chronic Reversible Obstructive Airway Disease," *Chest* 104 (2): 438–47 (1993).

32. E. Crimi, B. Violante, R. Pellegrino, and V. Brusasco, "Clinical Aspects of Allergic Disease: Effect of Multiple Doses of Nedocromil Sodium Given After Allergen Inhalation in Asthma," *Journal of Allergy and Clinical Immunology* 92 (6): 777–83 (1993).

33. "Prescriptions Often Harmful to the Elderly, GAO Warns," General Accounting Office Study, *Syracuse Post Standard,* 9 August 1995, c-10.

34. *Executive Summary: Guidelines for the Diagnosis and Management of Asthma* (Bethesda, Md.: National Asthma Education Program; Office of Prevention, Education, and Control; National Heart, Lung, and Blood Institute; National Institutes of Health, July 1994) publication no. 94–3042A, 43.

35. S. D. Lockey, "Bronchospasm Precipitated by Ophthalmic Instillations of Timolol," *Annals of Allergy* 46: 267 (1981).

36. R. B. Schoene, T. R. Martin, N. B. Charan, et al., "Timolol Induced Bronchospasm in Asthmatic Bronchitis," *Journal of the American Medical Association* 245: 1460–61 (1981).

37. *Guidelines for the Diagnosis and Management of Asthma,* 129.

38. S. J. Matthews, F. Schneiweiss, and R. J. Cersosimo, *A Clinical Manual of Adverse Drug Reactions* (Norwalk, Conn.: Appleton-Century-Crofts, 1986), 589.

39. Ibid., 315.

40. R. A. Settipane, P. J. Schrank, R. A. Simon, et al., "Prevalence of Cross-

Sensitivity with Acetaminophen in Aspirin-Sensitive Asthmatic Subjects," *Journal of Allergy and Clinical Immunology* 96: 480–85 (1995).

41. I. B. Iamandescu, "NSAIDs-Induced Asthma: Peculiarities Related to Background and Association With Other Drug or Non-Drug Etiological Agents," *Allergologia et Immunopathologia* 17 (6): 285 (1989).

42. R. B. Smith, J. A. Dewar, and J. H. Winter, "Tamoxifen-Induced Asthma (letter)," *Lancet* 341 (8847): 772 (1993).

43. R. J. Troisi, W. C. Willett, S. T. Weiss, "A Prospective Study of Diet and Adult-Onset Asthma," *American Journal of Respiratory and Critical Care Medicine* 151 (5): 1401–8 (1995).

BIBLIOGRAPHY

ALLERGIES

Crook, W. G., *Detecting Your Hidden Allergies*. Jackson, Tenn.: Professional Books, 1988.

Faelten, Sharon. *The Allergy Self-Help Book*. Emmaus, Pa.: Rodale Press, 1983.

Golos, Natalie, and Frances Golos Golbitz. *Coping with Your Allergies*. New York: Simon & Schuster, 1986.

Krohn, Jacqueline. *The Whole Way to Allergy Relief and Prevention: A Doctor's Complete Guide to Treatment and Self-Care*. Point Roberts, Wash.: Hartley & Marks, 1991.

Kushi, Michio. *A Natural Approach: Allergies*. New York: Japan Publications, 1985.

Null, Gary. *No More Allergies: Identifying and Eliminating Allergies and Sensitivity Reactions to Everything in Your Environment*. New York: Villard Books, 1992.

Null, Gary, with Martin Feldman. *Good Food, Good Mood: Treating Your Hidden Allergies*. New York: St. Martin's Press, 1988.

Randolph, Theron G., and Ralph W. Moss. *An Alternative Approach to Allergies*. New York: Harper & Row, 1989.

Swartz, Harry. *The New Allergy Guide Book: A Practical Program of Prevention and Control*. 3d ed. New York: Continuum Publishing, 1987.

CANDIDA AND PARASITES

Chaitow, Leon. *Candida Albicans: Could Yeast Be Your Problem?* Rochester, Vt.: Healing Arts Press, 1987.

Crook, W. G. *The Yeast Connection and the Woman*. Jackson, Tenn.: Professional Books, 1995.

Gittleman, Ann Louise. *Natural Healing for Parasites*. New York: Healing Wisdom Publications, 1995.

Truss, C. Orian. *The Missing Diagnosis*. 1986. (Available from The Missing Diagnosis, P.O. Box 26508, Birmingham, AL 35226)

ASTHMA AND ALLOPATHIC MEDICINE

Caplin, Irvin. *The Allergic Asthmatic*. Springfield, Ill.: Thomas, 1968.
Clark, T. J. H., S. Godfrey, and T. H. Lee, eds. *Asthma*. 3d ed. New York: Chapman & Hall Medical, 1992.
Gershwin, M. Eric, and Georges M. Halpern. *Bronchial Asthma: Principles of Diagnosis and Treatment*. 3d ed., Totowa, N.J.: Humana Press, 1994.
Haas, F., and S. S. Haas, *The Essential Asthma Book: A Manual for Asthmatics of All Ages*. New York: Ivy Books, 1987.
Hannaway, Paul J. *The Asthma Self-Help Book*. Rocklin, Calif.: Prima Publishing, 1992.
Herxheimer, Herbert. *A Guide to Bronchial Asthma*. New York: Academic Press, 1975.
National Heart, Lung, and Blood Institute of the National Institutes of Health, *Guidelines for the Diagnosis and Management of Asthma*. Bethesda, Md.: National Institutes of Health, 1991. Publication no. 91–3042.
Weiss, Earle B., and Myron Stein, eds. *Bronchial Asthma: Mechanisms and Therapeutics*. 3d ed. Boston: Little, Brown, 1993.

MIND-BODY, MEDITATION, AND VISUALIZATION

Epstein, Gerald. *Healing Visualizations: Creating Health through Imagery*. New York: Bantam Books, 1989.
———. *Healing into Immortality*. New York: Bantam Books, 1994.
Fezler, William. *Creative Imagery: How to Visualize in All Five Senses*. New York: Fireside, 1989.
Muktananda, Swami. *Meditate*. South Fallsburg, N.Y.: SYDA Foundation, 1979.
———. *Mystery of the Mind*. South Fallsburg, NY: SYDA Foundation, 1981.
Rossi, Ernest Lawrence. *The Psychobiology of Mind-Body Healing: New Concepts of Therapeutic Hypnosis*. New York: W. W. Norton & Company, 1993.
Samuels, Mike, and Nancy Samuels. *Seeing with the Mind's Eye: The History, Techniques, and Uses of Visualization*. New York and La Jolla, Calif.: Random House, Bookworks, 1993.

ORIENTAL HEALING

Beinfield, Harriet, and Efrem Korngold. *Between Heaven and Earth: A Guide to Chinese Medicine*. New York: Ballantine Books, 1991.
Chang, Stephen T. *The Great Tao*. San Francisco, Calif.: Tao Publishing, 1985.
Chia, Mantak. *Transform Stress into Vitality*. Huntington, N.Y.: Healing Tao Books, 1985.

298

Connelly, Dianne M. *All Sickness Is Home Sickness.* 2d ed. Columbia, Md.: Traditional Acupuncture Institute, 1993.

————, *Traditional Acupuncture: The Law of the Five Elements.* 2d ed. Columbia, Md.: Traditional Acupuncture Institute, 1994.

Gach, Michael Reed. *Acupressure's Potent Points: A Guide to Self-Care for Common Ailments.* New York: Bantam, 1990.

Hammer, Leon. *Dragon Rises, Red Bird Flies: Psychology and Chinese Medicine.* Barrytown, N.Y.: Station Hill Press, 1990. (psychology and acupuncture)

Kaptchuk, Ted. *The Web That Has No Weaver.* New York: Congdon and Weed, 1983. (Chinese medicine clearly explained)

Kushi, Michio. *A Natural Approach: Allergies.* New York: Japan Publications, 1985.

Maciocia, Giovanni. *Foundations of Chinese Medicine.* New York: Churchill Livingston, 1989.

McNamara, Sheila. *Traditional Chinese Medicine.* New York: Basic Books, 1996.

Teeguarden, Iona Marsaa. *Acupressure Way of Health: Jin Shin Do®.* Tokyo and New York: Japan Publications, 1978.

————. *The Joy of Feeling: Bodymind Acupressure, Jin Shin Do.* Tokyo and New York: Japan Publications, 1987.

————, ed. *Complete Guide to Acupressure.* Tokyo and New York: Japan Publications, 1996.

CHINESE HERBS AND PATENT MEDICINES

Bensky, Dan, and Andrew Gamble, with Ted Kaptchuk. *Chinese Herbal Medicine: Materia Medica.* Seattle, Wash.: Eastland Press, 1986.

Fratkin, Jake. *Chinese Herbal Patent Formulas: A Practical Guide.* Portland, Oreg.: Institute for Traditional Medicine, 1986.

Hadady, Letha. *Asian Health Secrets.* New York: Crown, 1996.

Naeser, Margaret A. *Outline Guide to Chinese Herbal Patent Medicines in Pill Form—An Introduction to Chinese Herbal Medicines.* 2d ed. Boston, Mass.: Boston Chinese Medicine, 1996.

Teeguarden, Ron. *Chinese Tonic Herbs.* New York: Japan Publications, 1984.

CHINESE FOOD ENERGETICS

Flaws, Bob, and Honara Wolfe. *Prince Wen Hui's Cook: Chinese Dietary Therapy.* Brookline, Mass.: Paradigm Publishing, 1985.

Jilin, Liu, and Gordon Peck, eds. *Chinese Dietary Therapy.* New York: Churchill Livingston, 1995.

Leggett, Daverick. *Helping Ourselves: A Guide to Traditional Chinese Food Energetics.* Devon, England: Meridian Press, 1994.

Lu, Henry C. *The Chinese System of Food Cures: Prevention and Remedies*. New York: Sterling Publishing, 1986.

————. *Chinese Foods for Longevity: The Art of Long Life*. New York: Sterling Publishing, 1990.

Pitchford, Paul. *Healing with Whole Foods: Oriental Traditions and Modern Nutrition*. Rev. ed. Berkeley, Calif.: North Atlantic Books, 1996.

MACROBIOTICS

Gallinger, Shirley, and Sherry A. Rogers. *Macro Mellow, Recipes for Macrobiotic Cooking*. Syracuse, N.Y.: Prestige Publishing, 1992.

Kushi, Aveline. *Aveline Kushi's Complete Guide to Macrobiotic Cooking for Health, Harmony and Peace*. New York: Warner Books, 1985.

Kushi, Michio. *The Macrobiotic Way: The Complete Macrobiotic Diet and Exercise Book*. Wayne, N.J.: Avery Publishing Group, 1985.

Rogers, Sherry A. *You Are What You Ate: A Macrobiotic Way*. Syracuse, N.Y.: Prestige Publishing, 1988.

————. *The Cure Is in the Kitchen: A Guide to Healthy Eating*. Syracuse, N.Y.: Prestige Publishing, 1990.

Turner, Kristina. *The Self-Healing Cookbook: Macrobiotic Primer for Healing Body, Mind, and Moods with Whole, Natural Foods*. Grass Valley, Calif.: Earthtones Press, 1987.

VEGETARIAN COOKING

Brown, Edward Este, and Deborah Madison. *The Greens Cookbook: Extraordinary Vegetarian Cuisine from the Celebrated Restaurant*. New York: Bantam, 1987.

Colbin, Annemarie. *Food and Healing*. New York: Ballantine Books, 1986.

VITAMINS AND HERBS

Atkins, R. C. *Dr. Atkins' Health Revolution: How Complementary Medicine Can Extend Your Life*. Boston: Houghton Mifflin, 1988.

Braverman, Eric R., and Carl C. Pfeiffer. *The Healing Nutrients Within*. New Canaan, Conn.: Keats, 1987.

Hendler, Sheldon Saul. *The Doctor's Vitamin and Mineral Encyclopedia*. New York: Simon & Schuster, 1990.

Hobbs, Christopher. *Foundations of Health: The Liver and Digestive Herbal*. Capitola, Calif.: Botanica Press, 1992.

Hoffman, David. *The Elements of Herbalism*. Dorset, England: Element Books, 1990.

Hopkinson, Patricia, Diane Miske, Jerry Parsons, and Holly Shimizu. *Herb Gardening*. New York: Pantheon Books, 1994.

Lad, Vasant, and David Frawley. *The Yoga of Herbs*. Santa Fe, N.M.: Lotus Press, 1986. (Ayurvedic approach)

Murray, Michael, and Joseph Pizzorno. *Encyclopedia of Natural Medicine*. Rocklin, Calif.: Prima Publishing, 1991.

Murray, Michael T. *The Healing Power of Herbs: The Enlightened Person's Guide to the Wonders of Medicinal Plants*. Rocklin, Calif.: Prima Publishing, 1995.

Null, Gary. *The Complete Guide to Health and Nutrition*. New York: Delacorte Press, 1984.

Schechter, Steven R. *Fighting Radiation with Foods, Herbs, and Vitamins*. Brookline, Mass.: East-West Health Books, 1988.

Tierra, Michael. *Planetary Herbology*. Santa Fe, N.M.: Lotus Press, 1988. (Eastern and Western traditions)

Weed, Susun S. *The Wise Woman Herbal: Healing Wise*. Woodstock, N.Y.: Ash Tree Publishing, 1989.

YOGA AND BREATHING

Devananda, Swami Vishnu. *The Complete Illustrated Book of Yoga*. New York: Crown Publishing, Julian Press, 1988.

Loehr, James E., and Jeffrey A. Migdow. *Take a Deep Breath*. New York: Villard Books, 1986.

Singh, Ravi. *Kundalini Yoga for Strength, Success, and Spirit*. New York: White Lion Press, 1991.

Sorvino, Paul. *How to Become a Former Asthmatic*. New York: New American Library, 1985.

OTHER HEALTH BOOKS OF INTEREST

Airola, Paavo. *Hypoglycemia: A Better Approach*. Sherwood, Oreg.: Health Plus Publishers, 1977.

Batmanghelidj, F. *Your Body's Many Cries for Water: You Are Not Sick, You Are Thirsty*. Falls Church, Va.: Global Health Solutions, 1995.

Campbell, A. H., ed. *Natural Health Handbook*. Secaucus, N.J.: Chartwell Books, 1984.

Davis, Albert Roy, and Walter C. Rawls Jr. *The Magnetic Effect*. Kansas City, Mo.: Acres U.S.A., 1990.

Haas, Elson M. *Staying Healthy with the Seasons*. Berkeley, Calif.: Celestial Arts, 1981.

Illich, Ivan. *Medical Nemesis: The Expropriation of Health*. New York: Pantheon Books, 1976.

Ott, John N. *Light, Radiation, and You*. Greenwich, Conn.: Devin-Adair, 1985.

Poesnecker, Gerald E. *Chronic Fatigue Unmasked: What You and Your Doctor Should Know About the Adrenal Syndrome, Today's Most Misunderstood, Mistreated, and Ignored Health Problem*. 2d ed. Richland, Pa.: Humanitarian Publishing, 1993.

Rogers, Sherry A. *The E.I. Syndrome: An Rx for Environmental Illness. Are You Allergic to the 21st Century?* Syracuse, N.Y.: Prestige Publishing, 1986.

Selye, Hans. *The Stress of Life*. Rev. ed. New York: McGraw-Hill, 1976.

Soyka, Fred, with Alan Edmonds. *The Ion Effect: How Air Electricity Rules Your Life*. New York: Bantam, 1991.

Weil, Andrew. *Health and Healing*. Rev. ed. Boston: Houghton Mifflin, 1995.

———. *Natural Health, Natural Medicine*. Rev. ed. Boston: Houghton Mifflin, 1995.

HEALTHY HOMES

Becker, Robert O. *Cross Currents: The Perils of Electropollution, the Promise of Electromedicine*. Los Angeles: Jeremy P. Tarcher, 1990.

Berthold-Bond, Annie. *Clean and Green: The Complete Guide to Nontoxic and Environmentally Safe Housekeeping*. Woodstock, N.Y.: Ceres Press, 1990.

Dadd, Debra Lynn. *The Non-Toxic Home: Protecting Yourself and Your Family from Everyday Toxics and Health Hazards*. Los Angeles: Jeremy P. Tarcher, 1986.

———. *The Nontoxic Home and Office*. Los Angeles: Jeremy P. Tarcher, 1992.

Hunter, Linda Mason. *The Healthy Home: An Attic to Basement Guide to Toxin-Free Living*. Emmaus, Pa.: Rodale Press, 1989.

Lawson, Lynn. *Staying Well in a Toxic World*. Chicago: Noble Press, 1993.

Rousseau, David, with W. J. Rea and Jean Enwright. *Your Home, Your Health and Well-Being: What You Can Do to Design or Renovate Your House or Apartment to Be Free of Outdoor and Indoor Pollution*. Vancouver, B.C.: Hartley & Marks, 1987.

Schoemaker, Joyce M., and Charity Y. Vitale. *Healthy Homes, Healthy Kids*. Washington, D.C. and Covelo, Calif.: Island Press, 1991.

Waldbott, George L. *Health Effects of Environmental Pollutants*. Saint Louis: C. V. Mosby, 1973.

Winter, Ruth. *A Consumer's Dictionary of Cosmetic Ingredients*. New York: Crown, 1989.

———. *A Consumer's Dictionary of Household, Yard, and Office Chemicals*. New York: Crown, 1992.

Zamm, Alfred V., with Robert Gannon. *Why Your House May Endanger Your Health*. New York: Touchstone, 1980.

HEALTHY SCHOOLS

Jacobson, Lauren. *Children's Art Hazards*. Booklet available for $2 from the Natural Resources Defense Council Inc., 40 West Twentieth Street, New York, N.Y. 10011, Attention: Publications.

Miller, Norma L., ed. *The Healthy School Handbook*. Washington, D.C.: National Education Association, 1995. It includes nearly two dozen chapters on topics including pesticides, cleaning products, floor covering, ventilation, EMFs, and more. Available free on loan, or buy it for $20 from NCEHS, 1100 Rural Ave., Voorhees, NJ 08043.

Rapp, Doris. *Is This Your Child?* New York: William Morrow, 1991.

ARTS AND CRAFTS

McCann, Michael. *Health Hazards Manual for Artists*. N.Y.: Nick Lyons, 1985.

Rossol, Monona. *The Artist's Complete Health and Safety Guide*. N.Y.: Allworth Press, 1990.

———. *Stage Fright: Health and Safety in the Theater*. N.Y.: Allworth Press, 1991.

———. *Keeping Claywork Safe and Legal*. 2d ed. Brandon, Oreg.: National Council on Education in the Ceramic Arts, 1996. Call 800-99-NCECA to purchase.

Rossol, Monona, and Susan D. Shaw. *Overexposure: Health Hazards in Photography*. N.Y.: Allworth Press, 1990.

TRAVEL

Fairechild, Diana. *Jet Smart: 200 Ways to Beat Jet Lag*. Berkeley, Calif.: Celestial Arts Publishing, 1992. Call 1-800-841-2665 to purchase.

RESOURCES

To Find Qualified Physicians and Health Care Providers:

American Academy of Environmental Medicine
4510 W. 89th Street
Prairie Village, KS 66207

American Holistic Medical Association
4101 Lake Boone Trail, Suite 201
Raleigh, NC 27607
Fax (919) 787-4916

Pan American Allergy Society
P.O. Box 947
Fredricksburg, TX 78624
Fax (210) 997-8625

Foundation for the Advancement of Innovative Medicine (FAIM)
2 Executive Boulevard, Suite 404
Suffern, NY 10901

American Association of Naturopathic Physicians
2366 Eastlake Avenue E, Suite 322
Seattle, WA 98102

To Find a Homeopath:

National Center for Homeopathy
810 N. Fairfax #306
Alexandria, VA 22314

Homeopathic Educational Services
2124 Kittredge Street
Berkeley, CA 94704
(510) 649-0294

To Find an Acupuncturist:

To find a graduate practitioner in your area:
The Traditional Acupuncture Institute
American City Building
10227 Wincopin Circle, Suite 100
Columbia, MD 21044-3422

For a list of member practitioners:
American Association of Acupuncture and Oriental Medicine
4101 Lake Bone Trail #201
Raleigh, NC 27607-6518
(919) 787-5181

Information about Jin Shin Do

The Jin Shin Do Foundation is an international network of authorized teachers and registered acupressurists founded by Iona Marsaa Teeguarden. To find a practitioner in your area or for information about studying Jin Shin Do contact:
Jin Shin Do® Foundation for Bodymind Acupressure™
P.O. Box 1097
Felton, CA 95018

Information about Kundalini Yoga

3HO Foundation
International Headquarters
1620 Preuss Road
Los Angeles, CA 90035

To Order Books on Eastern and Western Natural Healing:

Redwing Book Company
44 Linden Street
Brookline, MA 02146
(800) 873-3946
Ask for complete catalog.

ACTS FACTS (Arts, Crafts and Theatre Safety)
181 Thompson Street, #23
New York, NY 10012

Ten issues per year
Editor: Monona Rossol

Asthma Update
123 Monticello Avenue
Annapolis, MD 21401

Quarterly—latest drug and other information
Editors: Helen and David Jameson

Delicate Balance
National Center for Environmental Health Strategies
1100 Rural Avenue
Voorhees, NJ 08043

News and information on legislation
Editor: Mary Lamielle

Health Facts
Center for Medical Consumers
237 Thompson Street
New York, NY 10012

Monthly up-to-date health information
Editor: Maryann Napoli

ALTERNATIVES for the Health Conscious Individual
Mountain Home Publishing
P.O. Box 829
Ingram, TX 78025

Editor: Dr. David Williams

TOWNSEND LETTER for Doctors & Patients
Townsend Letter Group
911 Tyler Street
Port Townsend, WA 98369
(360) 385-6021
Fax (360) 385-0699

Magazine—ten issues per year, alternative medical information

Health and Environmental Organizations

Human Ecology Action League (HEAL)
P.O. Box 29629
Atlanta, GA 30359
(404) 248-1898

Membership includes quarterly publication and list of meetings in your area with talks by progressive doctors.

Bio Integral Resource Center
P.O. Box 7414
Berkeley, CA 94707
(510) 524-2567

Information about Integrated Pest Management (IPM)

The National Center for
Environmental Health Strategies
1100 Rural Avenue
Voorhees, NJ 08043

The Delicate Balance environmental newsletter includes information about occupational illness.

Northwest Coalition for
Alternatives to Pesticides (NCAP)
P.O. Box 1393
Eugene, OR 97440
(503) 344-5044

NY Coalition for Alternatives
to Pesticides (NYCAP)
33 Central Ave.
Albany, NY 12210
(518) 426-8246

Membership includes informative newsletter.

Mail-Order Cooking Supplies
Chinese Cooking Herbs and Patent Herbal Medicines

Lin's Sisters Associates Corp.
4 Bowery
New York, NY 10002
(800) 228-3822 ask for Susan
(212) 962-5417

Large and small orders

Yeung Cheng Co.
154 Mott Street
New York, NY 10013
(212) 925-8098 ask for Lisa

Large and small orders

Mayway Trading Co.
622 Broadway
San Francisco, CA 94133
(415) 788-3646

Large orders only

Health care providers can order Medicine Works Herbal Formulas from:
K'an Herb Co.
(800) 543-5233

308

Ryan Drum
Wildcrafted Medicinal Herbs
Waldron Island, WA 98297

Eleanor and John Lewallen (Sea Vegetable Gourmet Cookbook)
P.O. Box 372
Navarro, CA 95463

Macrobiotic Supplies

Mountain Ark Traders
120 SE Avenue
Fayetteville, AR 72701
(800) 643-8909

Organic Food

Walnut Acres
Walnut Acres Road
Penns Creek, PA 17862
(717) 837-0601

Nutritional Supplements (write for catalogs)

Freeda Pharmaceuticals
36 E. 41st Street
New York, NY 10017
(212) 685-4980

For more than fifty years have manufactured own vitamins, which are free of most allergens.

Klaire Laboratories, Inc.
P.O. Box 618
Carlsbad, CA 92008
(714) 438-1083

N.E.E.D.S.
527 Charles Avenue, 12-A
Syracuse, NY 13209
(800) 634-1380

Large selection of vitamins, homeopathic, and herbal products

The Vitamin Shop
(800) 223-1216

N.E.E.D.S.
527 Charles Avenue, 12-A
Syracuse, NY 13209
(800) 634-1380 (for free catalog)

National Ecological and Environmental Delivery System—books, air cleaners, water filters, and quality environmental products

Befit Enterprises Ltd.
P.O. Box 5034
Southampton, NY 11969

EMF protection, light and magnet therapies, and other health products

Healthy Hardware
P.O. Box 3217
Prescott, AZ 86303
(520) 445-8225

Electromagnetic field shielding and videotape that tells how to reduce high EMF

Nontoxic Environments, Inc.
P.O. Box 384
Newmarket, NH 03857
(800) 789-4348

Building and household products for sensitive people

Well Being Ranch
P.O. Box 435
Harper, TX 78631

High-grade tea tree oil and other products

Mail-Order for Allergy Products

Allergy/Asthma Technology Ltd.
Bio-Tech Systems
P.O. Box 25380
Chicago, IL 60625
(800) 621-5545

Acarosan Dust Mite Remover
peak-flow meters

Allergy Control Products
96 Danbury Road
Ridgefield, CT 06877
(800) 422-DUST

Allergy Control Solution, which inactivate mites and cat dander
peak-flow meters

N.E.E.D.S.
527 Charles Avenue, 12-A
Syracuse, NY 13209
(800) 634-1380

Austin and Enviracaire Air Cleaners

The Practical Allergy Research Foundation
P.O. Box 60
Buffalo, NY 14223-0060
(800) 787-8780
(716) 875-5578

NEO-Life Cleaning Products

NEO-Life Green—contains kelp, can be used as soap, shaving cream, shampoo, laundry soap, and stain remover. Use as a washable glove for protecting hands.

NEO-Life Rugged Red—for heavy-duty use, contains added detergents. General cleaner for office, home, linoleum, screens, glass, etc.

To order, call (716) 875-0378.

Mail-Order Cotton write for free catalogs

The Cotton Place
P.O. Box 59721
Dallas, TX 75229
(800) 451-8866

Naturalguard Barrier Cloth, cotton bedding, clothing, fabrics, yarn, and more

Janice Corp.
198 Route 46
Budd Lake, NJ 07828
(800) JANICES

Made-to-order cotton mattresses, bedding, and padding

Pure Podunk
RR1 Box 69
Thetford Center, VT 05075
(802) 333-4505

Organic cotton, linens, and bedding

Mother Hart's
3300 S. Congress Ave.
Unit 21
Boynton Beach, FL 33424
(407) 738-5866

Untreated bath towels and sheets

Terra Verde Trading Company
77 Spring Street
New York, NY 10012
(212) 925-4533

Untreated bedding, books, and more

Seventh Generation   Cottons, laundry supplies, and more
49 Hercules Drive
Colchester, VT 05446
(800) 444-7336

Mail-Order Air Cleaners

Austin Air Cleaner   HEPA filter plus twenty pounds of zeo-
701 Seneca Street   lite or activated charcoal
Buffalo, NY 14210
(716) 856-3704

E. L. Foust Company, Inc.   All stainless steel—contains HEPA filter
P.O. Box 105   and added charcoal
Elmhurst, IL 60126
(800) 225-9549

Bio-Tech Systems   Portable air cleaners with HEPA filter
P.O. Box 25380
Chicago, IL 60625
(800) 621-5545

Mail-Order Heat Exchangers

Air X Change   Air-to-air heat exchangers
401 V.F.W. Drive
Rockland, MA 02370
(617) 871-4816

Therma-Stor Products   Inexpensive plastic duct to out-of-doors
P.O. Box 8050
Madison, WI 53708
(800) 533-7533

The U.S. Pollen Calendar

This month-by-month guide points out peak pollen periods for fourteen common
weeds, trees, and grasses around the country. To order, call the American Academy
of Allergy and Immunology at (800) 822-2762.

American Environmental Health Foundation, Inc.
8345 Walnut Hill Lane, Suite 205
Dallas, TX 75231
(214) 361-9515
    Call or write for a catalog. They sell a Pollutant Detection Kit for home testing. Their deluxe kit includes tests for formaldehyde, carbon monoxide, and radon, and an organic water test that tests for sixteen items.

The Safer Home Test Kit allows you to test for carbon monoxide, radon gas, lead poisoning, microwave oven radiation, and ultraviolet radiation. Available from N.E.E.D.S. (800) 634-1380.

Hazardous Substances Resource Guide

This publication explains the risks associated with twelve hundred chemicals. It is available from:
Gale Research Inc.
P.O. Box 33477
Detroit, MI 48232-5477
(800) 877-GALE

Lead Testing

University of North Carolina Environmental Studies Program
29½ Page Avenue
Asheville, NC 28801
(704) 251-0518

Lead dust kits and lead analysis for paint chips, water, soil, and ceramics. Takes three weeks.

Pace Environs
81 Finchdene Square
Scarborough, Ontario
Canada M1X 1B4
(800) 359-9000

Frandon Lead Alert Kit tests ceramics and china

Mercury Testing

ChemCheck
P.O. Box 1210
Framingham, MA 01701
(800) 262-5323

Northeast Center for Environmental Health P.O. Box 2716 Syracuse, NY 13220	Spot tests for furniture and fabrics
AFM Enterprises 11 40 Stacy Court Riverside, CA 92507 (714) 781-6860	AFM Water Seal for sealing formaldehyde vapors
Mortell Co. Department HC 550 N. Hobble Avenue Kankakee, IL 60901	Hyde-Chek Formaldehyde Vapor Sealer

Mold Plates

Northeast Center for Environmental Health Box 2716 Syracuse, NY 13220	Find out what kind of molds and where they are.

Laboratory Testing

ELISA/ACT immunology test:
Serammune Physicians Lab
1890 Preston White Drive, Suite 201
Reston, VA 22091
(800) 533-5472

Comprehensive digestive stool analysis:
Great Smokies Diagnostic Laboratory
18A Regent Park Boulevard
Asheville, NC 28806
(800) 522-4762

Hair analysis:
TEI Trace Elements
P.O. Box 514
Addison, TX 75001-0514

For the two-hour workshop *How Environmentally Safe Are Our Schools?* by environmental medical writer Irene Wilkenfeld, write to Safe Schools, 205 Paddington Drive, Lafayette, LA 70508.

FYI: A Health and Safety Newsletter for School Employees
Labor Coalition
109 West State Street
Ithaca, NY 14850
(800) 804-8252
(607) 277-5670

For answers to questions about chemicals and arts, crafts, and photography materials, call (212) 777-0062, E-mail to 75054.2542a compuserve.com, or write:
Monona Rossol
Arts, Crafts and Theater Safety
181 Thompson Street, #23
New York, NY 10012

Problem Office Information

The Labor Coalition
109 West State Street
Ithaca, NY 14850
(607) 277-5670

Chemical Injury Information Network
P.O. Box 301
White Sulphur Springs, MT 59645
(406) 547-2255

Building Air Quality, S/N 055-000-00390, Government Printing Office, 1991. A 229-page loose-leaf book with recommended procedures for developing an "indoor air quality profile" and blank forms to be used for establishing an indoor air quality program and compiling information on pollution sources. Write for information:
New Orders
Superintendent of Documents
Box 371-954
Pittsburgh, PA 15250-7954

EPA Research and Development Manual—*Office Equipment: Design, Indoor Air Emissions, and Pollution Prevention Opportunities*, EPA-600/R-95-045, March 1995. Prepared

for Office of Radiation and Indoor Air by Air and Energy Engineering Research Laboratory, Research Triangle Park, NC 27711.
Write to:
National Technical Information Service
Springfield, VA 22161
(703) 487-4650
Fax: (703) 321-8547

For more information about a specific product or chemical call the Hazardous Material Information Hotline at (800) 334-2467.

Safe Arts and Crafts Resources

The Palette with Lid provides an airtight storage box for your acrylic or oil paints. The Sta-Wet Palette will keep all paint odor inside the box. Comes with disposable palette sheets for each kind of paint. Refills are available.
Masterson Art Products
P.O. Box 10775
Glendale, AZ 85318

Photosuds is a nonalkaline hand cleaner for photographers. It has a slightly acid pH and is free of oils that can spoil negatives. The acid quality helps restore the skin's pH balance and counteract the effects of strongly alkaline photochemicals. To order in the United States, call (716) 382-3256. To order in Canada:
Envision Compliance, Ltd.
150 Clark Boulevard, Unit 132
Bramalea, Ontario L6T 4Y8
(416) 453-2159

Sprint less-toxic photo chemicals are available through the mail from:
B & H Photo
119 W. 17th Street
New York, NY 10011
(212) 807-7474
or call Sprint (800) 356-5073

Nitro-Pro Gloves have an extra tough nitrile coating and jersey liner for use with solvents and other chemicals. Also available are Cotton Flock-lined Nitrile Gloves and SafeAir Badges to wear or hang to measure carbon monoxide, sulfur dioxide, ozone, or a host of other chemicals in your workplace. To order, call Lab Safety Supply (800) 356-0783, fax (800) 543-9910. Ask for their Personal and Industrial Safety Catalog. Technical help is available at (800) 356-2501.

316

Masks and respirators are available from H. G. Pasternack, who will suggest the correct 3M respirator for your job. To order, contact:

H. G. Pasternack, Inc.
OH & SP Division
New York, NY
10011
(800) 433-3330

Travel Information

Hospitality Plus is a travel guide for sensitive travelers published by the Human Ecology Action League (HEAL). It provides information about safe, smoke-free accommodations and facilities in the United States for people with asthma and other sensitivities. The guide also includes a reading list and tips for travelers.
Human Ecology Action League
P.O. Box 29629
Atlanta, GA 30359

International Association for Medical Assistance to Travelers
This volunteer group compiles an annual list of doctors in 125 countries who speak English, agree to take a specified fee, and meet the group's criteria. You also receive a chart of climate information and a world immunization chart. For a contribution of $25 they also send all twenty-four world climate charts.
417 Center Street
Lewiston, NY 14092
(716) 754-4883

Medic Alert
For an annual fee you receive a bracelet identifying any health problems, medications, and allergies, such as penicillin, plus a twenty-four hour emergency number that can be called collect from home or abroad to receive your vital medical facts, information about medications, etc.
2323 Colorado Avenue
Turlock, CA 95382
(800) 763-3428

Environmental Stress Index
Rates 204 cities in the United States for air and water quality, toxic releases, and more.
Zero Population Growth
1400 16th Street, N.W., Suite 320
Washington, DC 20036

(202) 332-2200

Information about Prevailing Winds
National Climatic Data Center
National Environmental Satellite
Data & Information Service
NOAA
151 Patton Avenue, Room 120
Asheville, NC 28801-5001

The Green Index
    This state-by-state guide to the nation's environmental health ranks the fifty states
for two hundred environmental health indicators, including air pollution, toxic waste,
and agricultural pollution.
Institute for Southern Studies
P.O. Box 531
Durham, NC 27702
(919) 419-8311
Fax (919) 419-8315

Topographical maps
U.S. Geological Survey Information Services
P.O. Box 25286
Denver Federal Center
Denver, CO 80225

Easy Trips
Green River canoeing in Utah and hiking in Arches
National Park are arranged by:
Women in the Wilderness
566 Ottawa Avenue
St. Paul, MN 66107
Phone and fax: (612) 227-2285

For information on Sivananda Yoga Camps in Quebec; Nassau, Bahamas; Kerala,
India; New York State, and California: contact Sivananda Ashram Yoga Camp Head-
quarters
Eighth Avenue
Val Morin, Quebec
Canada J0T 2R0
(819) 322-3226

INDEX

breathing exercises
  alternate nostril, 80–81
  and the lymphatic system, 52
  three-part yoga, 81–82
bronchodilator inhalers (Proventil), 10,
    116, 269–71
  adrenergic agents, 269–72
  anticholinergics, 273–74
  anti-inflammatory preventive inhalants,
    274–76
  methylxanthines, theophylline, 272–73
brown rice, 168–69
Bufferin, 277
burdock (herb), 161
  and the lymphatic system, 52
buses, traveling by, 242

caffeine
  and the adrenal function, 120
  on the plus side, 155–56
  why cut down, 155
Candida albicans, 58
  allergy to, 58–59
  case history, 144–46
  getting rid of, 60
  parasites and, 61
Caplin, Irvin, 32–33
Cathcart, Robert, 192–93
cat-washing instructions, 263
Cesari, Carolyne, 75
ch'c (chi). See Qi
chemical allergens, 146–50
  chemicals and asthma, 146–47
  cigarette smoke, 149, 225
  developing awareness, 149–50
  Multiple Chemical Sensitivity (MCS),
    147
  synthetic material offgassing, 149
  vapors, 147–49
chemicals and asthma, 146–47
Chi Kuan Yen Wan (Chinese patent
    herbal), 199
Chiang, Ambrose A., 272
Chinese herbal healing, 165, 180, 196–
    200
  angelica polymorpha, 198–99
  ashwagandha (Ayurvedic herb), 201

astragalus, 198
boswellin (Ayurvedic herb), 201
chi kuan yen wan, 199
Chinese herbs used in Japan, 199–200
Chinese licorice root, 199
Chinese patent herbals, 199
echinacea angustifolia (Native
    American herb), 200
ephedra (ma huang), 197–98
ginkgo biloba, 198
herbs from Hawaii, 200
magnolia officinalis, 200
Ping Chuan Wan (or Ping Chuan Pill),
    199
purpurea (Native American herb), 200
skullcap (or scutellaria), 198
spirulina (blue-green algae), 201
tylophora asthmatica (Ayurvedic herb),
    200
See also minerals; vitamins
Chinese licorice root, 199
Chinese medicinal cooking, 161–65
  bacteria, 164–65
  color, 163–64
  cooking pots, 164–64
  digestion, 165
  doctrine of signatures, 163
  five tastes or flavors, 162
  food energies, 162–63
  oils, 164
  unusual ingredients, 165
  yin and yang, 162
Chinese medicine
  acupuncture, 10, 16–19
  acupressure, 15, 16, 19–29
  asthma, 13–15
  eight pillars, 13
  harmonious balance and, 10
  a western experience with, 10–12, 18–
    19
  See also Jin Shin Do®
Chinese patent herbals, 199
Chinese System of Food Cures, The (Lu), 162
chiropractic
  and the lymphatic system, 52
chlorine, 67
cigarette smoke, 149, 225

I Ching
  as one of the eight pillars of Chinese
    medicine, 13
Ibiki-Ken (skin brushing method), 53
IgE (immunoglobin E) allergy antibody,
    124–25
immune nutrients, 51
  testing for, 52
immune systems, 47–57
  allergic component, 48–50
  balancing, 49
  breakdown, 50
  detoxification, 72–75
  digestion, 53–56
  heavy metals, 67–71
  lymphatic system, stimulating,
    52–53
  nutritional correction, 50–52
  other immune suppressors, 71–72
  rain barrel total load theory (Rea), 61–
    62
  rebalancing, 49–50
  restoring, 60–61
  thymus and lymph glands, enhancing,
    52
  yeast connection, 57–64
Inderal (propranolol), 277
Intal (cromolyn sodium), 84, 275–76
intestine. *See* large intestine
ions (positive)
  as immune suppressor, 71
  ion balance, 71–72
Irish moss, 160

Japan, Chinese herbs used in, 199–200
Jet Smart: Over 200 Tips for Beating Jet Lag,
    (Fairechild), 243
Jin Shin Do® (acupressure), 15, 19–29
  acu-points, 20–28
  stopping attacks before they start, 28
Journal of Orthomolecular Medicine, 68–69
Journal of Psychological Medicine, 39
Joy of Feeling, The (Teeguarden), 36–37
juice fasting, 73–74

kasha, 169
kelp, 160

kidney
  acu-point combination, 26
  connection to asthma, 15
Kidney Essence, 15, 122, 152
kidney meridian-related asthma, 15
Kidney Qi, 152
kidney-related problems
  what to eat and not eat, 184–85
kombu, 160
Krohn, Jacqueline, 136
kuzu, 161

Labeling of hazardous Art Materials Act,
    237
Lachman, Leigh J., 134–35
large intestine
  acu-point combination, 25
  yin and yang pairing, 13, 37
laughing, as exhalation practice, 78
laundry products, 207
latex allergies, 132–33
  if sensitive to, 133
lead, 70–71
  detoxifying with vitamins, 75
  in schools, 216
Lee, Carleton H., 143
legumes, and a macrobiotic diet, 159
Levin, Warren, 58, 61, 115, 117–19, 119–
    20, 120, 123, 126, 189
licorice (herb), and the lymphatic system, 52
Light, Radiation and You (Ott), 121
Lin, Robert Y., 6, 34, 132
Lippman, Morton, 66
liver
  acu-point combinations, 24–25
  and digestion, 56–57
liver meridian-related asthma, 15
Long, James W., 278
lotus root, 161
Lu, Henry, 162
lung-related problems
  what to eat and not eat, 184–85
lungs
  acu-point combinations, 21–23
  Chinese medicine's view of, 13–15
  contacting through Taoist visualization,
    44–45

morning exercises, 85–88
Moscowitz, Reed, 32, 35, 36
Moser, Dr. Kenneth, 5
Motrin, 277
moxa, 18
MSG, reaction to, 138
mucus, 54
dispersing, 185
mugwort (Artemesia vulgaris), 18
Multiple Chemical Sensitivity (MCS), 147
Murray, Michael, 120

National Heart Lung and Blood Institute, 6
National Institute of Occupational Safety and Health, 227
National Institutes of Health, 7
natural light
and the hormonal system, 121, 121–22
and the pituitary gland, 121
proper light, what to do for, 121–22
nebulizers, 269
New Zealand, asthma death rate in, 7
night sweats, what to eat and not eat, 183–84
nightshades, as an allergen, 157
nori (porphyra family), 160
Nurses' Health Study (NHS), 114, 278
nutrition
and the lymphatic system, 52
nutritional cooking. See medicinal cooking

Occupational Safety and Health Administration, 227
office (trigger free)
asthma in the office, 222–23
carbonless carbon paper, 225
carbonless typewriters, 225
ceiling tiles, 225
coworkers' personal products, 225
fluorescent lights, 225
furniture and carpets, 225
laser printers, 225
Material Safety Data Sheets (MSDS), 228–29
National Institute of Occupational Safety and Health, 227

occupational asthma, 203
Occupational Safety and Health Administration, 227
office products, 225
outgassing, 224
outside sources, 227
photocopy machines, 225
simple things to do, 228
water damage, 223
what management can do, 228
what the office worker can do, 226–27
See also arts and crafts; home; school; traveling
Office of Alternative Medicine (National Institutes of Health), 7
omega-3 fatty acids, 195
optimism, importance of, 45–46
Osler, Sir William, 30
Ott, John, 121, 121–22
outside influences (toxic substances), 65–72
air, 66
detoxification, 72–75
food, 65
heavy metals, 67–71
water, 67
oxygen, asking for on airplanes, 243
ozone
exposure and asthma, 126
dangers of, 66
vitamin E and, 193

Pal Dan Gum (eight silken movements), 88–97
pancreas, phlegm and, 54
pancreas meridian-related asthma, 15
pancreatic enzymes, 55
Panex ginseng (herb)
and the adrenal function, 120
and the lymphatic system, 52
pantothenic acid, 191
as antistress nutrient, 120
parasites, and candida albicans, 61
peanuts, life threatening reaction to, 136
Pepto-Bismol, 277
Percodan, 277–78

pessimism, as hinderance to health, 45–46

pest control, 209, 210

pesticides
exposure to, 203–4
reaction to, 138
in schools, 217

pets
cat-washing instructions, 263
as a common allergen, 131–32, 214

phlegm
and spleen/pancreas, 54
Dispel Phlegm Dish, 188

phlegm (what to eat and not eat)
cold, white stuck, 182
copious white, 181–82
hot, yellow or green stuck, 188
yellow or green (hot), 182–83

photocopy machines, 218, 225

Ping Chuan Wan (or Ping Chuan Pill) (Chinese patent herbal), 199

pituitary gland, natural light and, 121, 121–22

plants as air cleaners, 212

Po Chai Pills, 248

pollens as a common allergen, 127

poor treatment of asthma, 5–7

pork, giving up, 156

positive ions
as immune suppressor, 71
ion balance, 71–72

Postnatal Essence, 152

Prenatal Essence, 48, 54, 152

Pride, N. B., 12

problem solving
as step to coping with stress, 36
See also awareness

progesterone, 112–15

propranolol, 277

Proventil (bronchodilator inhaler), 10

pulmonologists (pulmonary specialists), 6

pulses, acupuncture and, 17

purpurea (Native American herb), 200

Qi (energy), 12–13
Kidney Qi, 152

Qi Gong, 13, 16

Quadrenol, 1

quinoa, 170

ragweed
as a common allergen, 128
foods that cross-react with, 140

rain barrel total load theory (Rea), 61–62

Rapp, Doris, 258

Rea, William J., 61–62, 66

reading aloud and breathing, 80

recipes, 165–88
See also under grains

recipes (desserts), 179–80
Fresh and Dried Pear Desert, 179
Sweet Congee with Raisins and Fresh Raspberries, 179–80
Sweet Kumquat Treat, 180

recipes (grains)
Cold Winter Energy Breakfast, 169–70
Millet with Carrots, Celery, and Fresh Herbs, 170–71
See also grains

recipes (for travel)
Rice Ball Recipe, 245–46

recipes (main dishes), 176–78
Astragalus, Codonopsis Stew, 177–78
Chicken Tomato Dish, 177
Watercress Fish Stew, 176–77

recipes (salads)
Carrot Seaweed Salad, 178

recipes (soups), 171–73
Aduki Bean, Water Chestnut, White Fungus Soup, 173
Astragalus Chicken Soup, 172
Basic Lentil Soup, 171–72
First Sign of Cold Soup, 186–87
Sweet Vegetable Soup, 171

recipes (stews and congees), 173–74
Astragalus, Codonopsis Stew, 177–78
Plain Rice Congee with White Fungus, 174
Recovery from Colds Stew, 188
Strengthening, Savory Congee, 173
Sweet Congee with Raisins and Fresh Raspberries, 179–80
Watercress Fish Stew, 176–77

recipes (teas), 161
Burdock, Lotus Root Tea, 168

steroids (*continued*)
  cortisol system, 118
  inhaled steroids, 274–75
  liberation from, 117–19
  nutrients and, 119–20
  oral steroids, 275
stomach, acu-point combination, 23
stress
  asthma as cause of, 32–33
  asthma as result of, 30–32
  and distress, 32
  other triggers, 32
stress (3 steps to coping with)
  awareness, 36
  awareness, acting on, 36
  a problem solving approach, 36
Stress of Life, The, (Selye), 117, 257
stretching, as exhalation practice, 77
sugar and sweets, 154–55
  on the plus side, 154–55
  why cut down, 154
sulfites, reaction to, 138, 139
Swedish massage
  and the lymphatic system, 52
synthetic material offgassing, 149
Szentivanyi, A., 115–16

Tae Kwon Do, 107–11
Tai Chi, 35
Tai Ji Chuan, 16
tamoxifen, 277
Taoism
  exercise for stopping asthma attack, 78–79
  herbalism, 14
  visualization, 44–45
teas, 161
  recipes, 165–68
Tedral, 271
Teeguarden, Iona Marsaa, 20, 36–37, 37, 88
terpenes, foods that cross-react with, 140
testing (for food allergies), 135
  cytotoxic testing, 143
  elisa/act test, 144
  provocative neutralization test, 143
  pulse testing, 142–43

sublingual food testing with
  kinesiology, 143
Theo-Dur, 10
theophylline, 146, 271–73
  side effects of, 273–74, 277
thirst
  what to eat and not eat, 183–84
Threshold Limit Value (TLV), 232
thymus gland, enhancing, 52
tiger energy, 107–9
  and emotion, 110
Tilade (nedocromil sodium), 276
Time Before Asthma Was Learned, A (sample visualization), 41
timolol maleate (timoptic), 277
timoptic, 277
Tintera, John, 116–17, 123
toiletries, 206
tongue, acupuncture and, 16–17
Townsend Letter for Doctors & Patients, 191
toxic substances, 65–72
  air, 66
  detoxification, 72–75
  food, 65
  heavy metals, 67–71
  water, 67
Traditional Acupuncture Institute, 17
traditional (allopathic) medicine, 7–9
  and alternative therapies, 8
trailers, 242
train, traveling by, 242
travel kit, 246–47
traveling (trigger free)
  air travel, 242–44
  on arrival, 247
  bed-and-breakfasts and apartment hotels, 247
  buses, 242
  cabin fever, 243
  city strategies, 250–51
  clean air, in pursuit of, 249–50
  dos and don'ts, 240–41
  eating carefully, 249
  food for travel, 245–46
  gas pump, at the, 242
  hiking the Gorge, 251
  hotel rooms, 244–45